Kingston Frontenac Public Library

W9-DGB-635

LYME
MADNESS

LORI DENNIS

Copyright© 2016 Lori Dennis

Cover and Book Design by *the*BookDesigners, 2016
Cover Self-Portrait by Matt Dennis, 2004

All rights reserved. No part of this publication may be reproduced, stored in a retrieval system, or transmitted, in any form or in any means—by electronic, mechanical, photocopying, recording, or otherwise—without prior written permission from the author.

Hardcover – ISBN 978-0-9951689-0-9
Paperback – ISBN 978-0-9951689-1-6
Audio Book – ISBN 978-0-9951689-8-5
eBook – ISBN 978-0-9951689-2-3

BISAC CODE: HEA039090
HEALTH & FITNESS / Diseases / Immune & Autoimmune

Manufactured in Canada
SoulWork Publishing™
http://www.soulworkpublishing.com

Legal Deposit – Library and Archives Canada, 2016

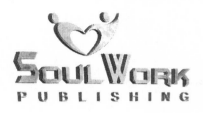

RESCUING MY SON DOWN THE RABBIT HOLE
OF CHRONIC LYME DISEASE

LYME
MADNESS

WHERE MILLIONS ARE SUFFERING
... AND FEW ARE LISTENING

*A Medical Odyssey
and Cautionary Tale*

LORI DENNIS

NOTE TO READERS

This publication contains the opinions and ideas of its author. I am not a medical doctor, nor am I endorsing, dispensing, or recommending any particular treatments, products, or health services as a form of diagnosis or treatment for any physical, emotional, or medical condition. I simply wish to share what has helped us and others in the search for answers. The content in this book is anecdotal and written for general, informational purposes only. This book is sold with the understanding that neither the author nor the publisher is engaged in rendering medical, health, or other professional advice or services. If the reader requires such advice or services, a competent and appropriate professional should be consulted. The content, ideas, theories, suggestions, and treatment protocols in this book may not be suitable for everyone. They are not guaranteed or warranted to produce any particular results. No warranty is made with respect to the accuracy or completeness of the information contained herein, and both the author and the publisher specifically disclaim any responsibility for any liability, loss, or risk, personal or otherwise, which is incurred as a consequence, directly or indirectly, of the use and application of any of the contents of this book. Neither the author nor the publisher shall be liable for any loss of profit or any other commercial damages, including but not limited to special, incidental, consequential, or other damages. Some names and details of some of the individuals mentioned in this book have been changed, including some Lyme sufferers who chose not to be identified. I have chosen to refer to certain doctors using an initial only in order to protect their identities and their practice. This protective practice is commonplace in the Lyme community as many doctors over the years have been met with punitive measures by their licensing boards due to their attempts to treat chronic Lyme outside of the prescribed guidelines. The doctors that I have chosen to name in full are those who have provided their consent and those who have been bold enough to talk about their practice in the public sphere.

CONTENTS

REVIEWS FOR LYME MADNESS

With Lyme Madness, Lori Dennis joins the Pantheon of alarmed mothers who have 'banged the teapots' to *force* dense and complacent governments *DO SOMETHING* to address the dangerous disease they perceived devastating their children, families and communities. Like the title of Polly Murray's book The Widening Circle, Lyme Madness is a triple *entendre*.

First is the irrational way the public health power structures have formulated their conceptualization of and response to the illness, the U.S.'s Centers for Disease Control, lost bellwether, leading its own as well as other nations off a cliff. Second, the patient population, abandoned and ridiculed by the medical establishment, government and private health insurers, is often left to fend for itself in an effort to find health and healing. This can sometimes lead down dangerous paths of uncharted territory as desperate patients cast about, like drowning rats, for something, anything, some 'life-line' to keep their sinking heads above water. Third, Lori Dennis and many other mothers of patients and the patients themselves (to borrow the classic line from the movie Network) are *mad* as *hell* and they're *not* going to *take* it anymore. Maddeningly too, increasing patient militancy is met with impunity. However, as more and more individuals at all levels of society are being impacted, power relationships are shifting and the Centers for Disease Control and the errant authors of the 2000 and 2006 Infectious Diseases Society of America Lyme Disease Guidelines are finding themselves increasingly on the defensive.

Lori Dennis, a psychotherapist, shares her and her son's experiences down what she calls the 'rabbit hole' of Lyme disease. Together, son and mother struggle to define diagnosis, traverse the vicissitudes of the illness and the challenges of discovering, of the available allopathic and alternative medical approaches, those which enable her son to recover. This eye-opener will be helpful to others who find themselves grappling with Lyme and other tick-borne diseases, navigating an arena full of contradictory advice and adversarial experts. It is also a clarion call to all to compel governments and their public health infrastructures to acknowledge the many problems with which these diseases confront us and to commit the financial, scientific and medical resources and the grit to solve them – to end the madness.

—KENNETH B. LIEGNER, M.D.

After reading Lyme Madness it raises the question—what is the more powerful force, a dysfunctional healthcare system or a motivated mother who wants the best for her son? The problems her son encountered accessing proper assessment and care is a story we have heard far too many times, in Canada, in the United States and in many other countries. It is frustrating to see clinical healthcare policy created by bureaucrats and researchers who lack true clinical expertise and are distant from the clinical realities and the full price of suffering and impairment caused by Lyme and associated diseases. Many will read this book and identify with her frustration, be motivated by her persistence and gain some insights on effective strategies. One thing is clear, when dealing with an illness that is controlled by dogma and special interests, it is necessary to do thorough research and to be a tenacious advocate. I am sure this book will help others who are searching for answers and solutions.

—ROBERT C BRANSFIELD, MD, DLFAPA

Lori Dennis' incredible commitment to helping her bright, competent, Lyme-infected adult son Matt is only seconded by the tremendous contribution she has made with this memoir. This is the book she and Matt and thousands of Lyme-impacted people needed four years ago ... 20 years ago. Don't be deterred by Dennis' periodic, though well-earned, polemics - if Lyme is somehow in your life, this one book can catapult you years ahead in your quest for understanding, and a path thru the Lyme labyrinth so vividly described herein.

This is a cogent, incisive, well-researched, well-developed contribution born of enormous frustration and disappointment with not just the allopathic (Western) medical system, its insurers, its pharmaceutical brethren and the endemic politics of power and profit that can so adversely affect any individual trying to overcome what Dennis presents here as this tremendously complicated illness, but all providers who are not Lyme Literate and "try" anyway, often, as evinced here, doing more harm than good. Epistemology is the study of how we know or make sense of things - Lyme Madness is a call to all providers to become Lyme literate and to make room for Lyme sufferers in their epistemologies and in their practices.

We can do much better! Ultimately, this memoir is yet another incredibly generous gift Lori Dennis offers her son, other Lyme sufferers, and those who love and care for them - and who just won't quit! A formidable read.

—DR. GREG O'DONOHUE, MBA (C.PSYCH)

"Lyme Madness is a compelling, heart-breaking story of a Canadian mother dedicating all of her time, energy, intelligence and love to get her son back to health. It reads like a travel journey. A journey into what the author rightly calls Alice's rabbit hole to Wonderland, set in the context of modern day health care. It is a well written and documented book.

This book clearly shows what the love of a mother can do and how many mothers are now standing up for their ill children. It will be a guide for other parents when their children suddenly fall ill, are misdiagnosed, mistreated and finally shunned or invalidated by the doctors you supposed would be knowledgeable and willing to help you. Or it may even be a clear warning to look into this subject, before they fall as ill as countless others have, all over the world.

Madness has two meanings. It is the experience of discovering the madness of a system invested by groupthink, vested interests, misinformation and corruption along with a system that punishes doctors who are willing to help parents like Lori Dennis. The second is the madness or anger that arises after years of frustration of seeing your own child and many like him suffer needlessly. This book deals with both.

The author's personal experience combined with her professional knowledge as a therapist will provide other parents with a guide through this rabbit hole and will save them much frustration, time and money. It provides them with insights into the many medical and psychological pitfalls in Lymeland, with practical approaches, with a brave investigation of reasons why the status quo has been like this for over forty years and with a range of stories by other people. These personal stories will validate other parents and Lyme patients' own sanity on an often lonely journey back to health——with the glimmers of light at the end of the tunnel that this book fortunately also provides.

May this book add to the mounting evolution of activities to end the Madness of negating and downplaying Lyme as the global epidemic that it is."

—HUIB KRAAIJEVELD, AUTHOR OF "SHIFTING THE LYME PARADIGM; THE CARETAKERS' GUIDE THROUGH THE LABYRINTH" AND FOUNDER OF THE ON LYME FOUNDATION, THE NETHERLANDS

I applaud Lori Dennis for her efforts in attempting to educate the public about this life-altering/life threatening infection misclassified as a simple nuisance disease.

Personal experiences described in her book "Lyme Madness" are not new however as stories like this have been hidden from the public for over three decades. The focus over this period has been to discredit the horribly sick and disabled as opposed to finding a cure for this antibiotic resistant/tolerant superbug; truly "Madness" for sure and a crime against humanity on a growing global scale. Those who have studied the wrongful handling of this disease believe that the rush to create a vaccine for Lyme led to its mishandling. In fact, the lead investigators of the two previous Lyme vaccines claim that Lyme is easily diagnosed and easily cured with 1-2 weeks of ABX. Prior to vaccine development, persistent infection (Chronic Lyme) was commonly reported in the literature. Shameful affair indeed as a congressional investigation is long overdue.

Kudos to Lori Dennis for writing "Lyme Madness", a must read for the ill-informed.

—CARL TUTTLE, LYME ACTIVIST
HUDSON, NH USA

This memoir is an act of empowerment.

Lori Dennis has transformed her personal experience of chronic Lyme and coinfections into a road map for navigating the complications of this medical and political disease. This memoir outlines the corporate capture of the CDC Lyme policy and shares the frustrations, sadness and anger of those denied access to treatment protocols that meet internationally recognized standards for evidence-based medicine.

Dennis validates the experiences of those living with Lyme and coinfections and presents a range of views regarding the nature of the illness. Her strong true emotions resonate with her observations of the CDC's and Canadian health establishment's deep discrimination against Lyme patients. Dennis also provides powerful examples of the resilience, innovation and growing power of those who reject these human rights abuses.

This is a memoir of a mother fighting for the survival of her son and she well understands how the madness embraced by the CDC Lyme policy is deadly for those living with chronic Lyme.

—JENNA LUCHE-THAYER, LYME ACTIVIST, FORMER SENIOR ADVISOR AT THE UNITED NATIONS AND OTHER ORGANIZATIONS

"In a mad world, only the mad are sane."
—*Akira Kurosawa*

"All truth passes through three stages. First, it is ridiculed. Second, it is violently opposed. Third, it is accepted as being self-evident."
—*Arthur Schopenhauer*

"Whenever a doctor cannot do good, he must be kept from doing harm."
—*Hippocrates*

"One doesn't have to operate with great malice to do great harm. The absence of empathy and understanding are sufficient."
—*Charles M. Blow, journalist*

"The world will not be destroyed by those who do evil, but by those who watch them without doing anything."
—*Albert Einstein*

"What strikes me is how desperately we all need to know that we are seen and heard."
—*Glennon Doyle Melton, author*

"Down, down, down. Would the fall *never* come to an end?"
—*Alice's Adventures in Wonderland*

"In the fullness of time, the mainstream handling of chronic Lyme disease will be viewed as one of the most shameful episodes in the history of medicine because elements of academic medicine, elements of government, and virtually the entire insurance industry have colluded to deny a disease. This has resulted in needless suffering of many individuals who deteriorate and sometimes die for lack of timely application of treatment or denial of treatment beyond some arbitrary duration."

—Kenneth B. Liegner, MD

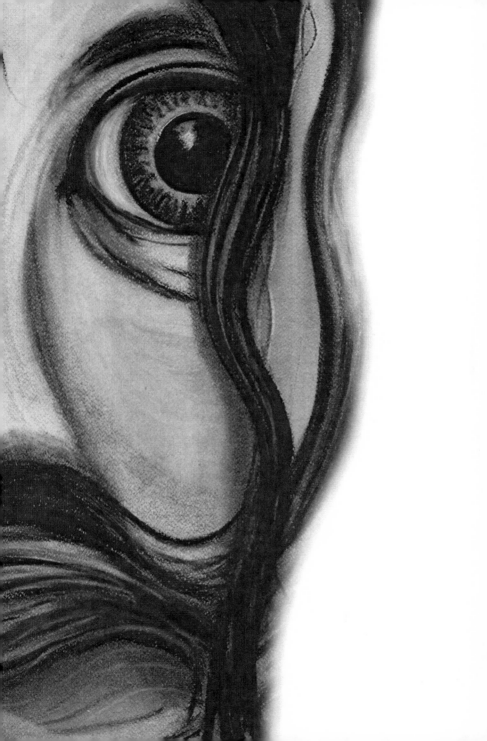

THE TICK THAT NEVER WAS

The legend goes like this,
If you know
you were bit
by a tick,
no bigger
than the head of pin
found it
on your person
somewhere
peeking its bum out in the air,
head burrowed deep inside
it's gourmet buffet
your blood,
or if you see a
dart board pattern reddening
of skin
they call it a bull's-eye rash
that appears around a
very tiny lump,

then it is very serious
and you must get treated
because a tick has been there
a clear sign
only lucky people get
but what happens
when you don't know
you were bit by a tick
no bigger than
the head of a pin
you didn't find it
anywhere
hiding on your skin,
they say it goes away
because you didn't know
but if you know
don't miss the treatments
this disease can kill you
only if you know

—Donna Y. Jacobs, illustrator, designer, Drawing Out Loud
Mother to Bronwyn, twenty-nine, Lyme sufferer

IMAGINE

Imagine waking up one day feeling shaky, dizzy, panicky, and light-headed.

Imagine standing next to your best friend and you cannot remember their name.

Imagine looking out the window and seeing two of everything.

Imagine having trouble sleeping, and sleeping pills do very little to help.

Imagine having an out-of-body experience like you are floating in space.

Imagine having shooting pains, electrical shocks going up and down your body.

Imagine getting so dizzy you can't get off the floor for hours.

Imagine feeling so tired and exhausted for no reason, like you just ran a marathon.

Imagine you can no longer work and you just lost your job, home, savings, marriage.

Now just imagine going to a medical doctor and hearing them tell you that all your tests are fine and what you are experiencing is all in your head and all you need to do is just get out more and things will be just fine.

You just entered the Chronic Lyme twilight zone.

Although we may look good on the outside, we are sick as hell on the inside as the Lyme bacteria wreaks havoc on our bodies.

—John Coughlin, Lyme sufferer, Syracuse, New York

DEDICATION

To Matt—my brave, inspiring, and tenacious Lyme warrior. You have shown Herculean strength and tremendous perseverance on this journey. I am in awe of your courage. I am in the trenches with you daily and I pray for you always—for your recovered health, resilience, vitality, and all that you wish for in your beautiful life. Thank you for letting me ride alongside you on this mad medical odyssey, every step of the way.

ACKNOWLEDGMENTS

To Jeff—for being a loving father to Matt and Allie, for always believing in me, for having great empathy, listening daily, understanding my hyperfocus, my worry, my angst, and my endless drive to get Matt well. You have been my rock, and I thank you from the bottom of my heart. I could not have created this life without you. Allie—I am so proud and in awe of the beautiful woman, the great human being, and the empathic doctor you've become. Shayna—I'm so grateful to have you in our lives. Thank you for your beautiful lightness of being and for standing so lovingly by Matt's side. Susan—for our lifelong promise to carry each other's hearts. Auntie Rosie—for always loving me like a daughter. Friends and family—for checking in, listening, and trying to understand the madness. Facebook "Lyme friends" who have made such valuable contributions and have helped me find sanity, humor, connection, companionship, support, understanding, encouragement, validation, quality research, shared passion, and endless drive in this battle we are waging together. Lyme doctors, Lyme activists, Lyme advocates, and Lyme warriors everywhere for your tenacity, support, voice, and courage. Dr. Kenneth Liegner, Dr. Robert Bransfield, Dr. Greg O'Donohue, author and Lyme activist Huib Kraaijeveld, Lyme activist Carl Tuttle, and Lyme activist and former Senior Advisor at the UN and other organizations Jenna Luche-Thayer, for your valuable content reviews, comments, and endorsements. Peter Economy for your brilliant editing. Gina Fusco and Michael Mandarano for your indispensable proofreading and fine attention to detail. Alan Dino Hebel and Ian Koviak of The Book Designers for your superb design work. Peter A. Downard, Sarah Goodwin, and Peter Jacobsen for your critical legal guidance. Kelly Drennan for your social media assistance and Joan Holman for your invaluable publishing and marketing guidance. The beautiful, light-filled souls at the Mastin Kipp Writing Retreat—all of whom helped me begin to heal. Finally, my deepest gratitude to the mothers who have been fighting this Lyme War for decades. As Dr. Kenneth B. Liegner so generously said, *"If it were not for mothers, we would be nowhere with Lyme disease. It is MOTHERS, concerned about their families, their children, that has sparked ALL progress in this field!"*

PREFACE

WRITING MY WAY THROUGH OUTRAGE AND SORROW

Sometimes the curiosity can kill the soul but leave the pain.
—ALICE'S ADVENTURES IN WONDERLAND

I begin writing in Ubud, Bali. How I arrived here in this spiritual wonderland is as mystifying to me as my crash landing in Lymeland so long ago.

I sit quietly now.

Listening. Thinking. Breathing.

Hoping. Wanting. Breathing.

Desperately needing to mend the broken pieces of my smashed-up heart.

My son is sick with chronic Lyme disease. I am reeling from a different kind of sickness. One that infects you when your son is ill and you can't find answers. One that you must bear when you spend every waking moment fighting for his life in a complex political war that has been waging since long before either of you were inducted. The kind of sickness that you carry when you realize you are on your own and it feels like *no one* can help you win this battle.

This illness of his—an illness that is terribly complex, unmistakably parasitic, and pervasively denied—has taken us both to the edge and back, many times.

I've come to understand that most of the things we worry about in life rarely happen. And the things we don't necessarily worry about often hit us so hard—from left field—that we buckle at the knees and fall down *flat*, truly believing we'll never get up again.

Well, I have gotten up and I have flourished. And, more importantly, so has my brave and tenacious son. I'm certain that our recoveries are closely intertwined.

Deciding to write this book has been my savior. It has given me a place to channel my angst. It has helped me manage this nightmare. It has forced me to expect less of those who cannot help, while allowing me to find a like-minded, supportive community—so many amazing Lyme warriors without whom I wouldn't be able to tell this story.

Writing *Lyme Madness* has been one long labor of love for my son—driven by fear, sorrow, confusion, overwhelm, the need for justice, the demand to find clear medical answers—and the relentless feeling of chronic outrage at a medical system that has failed him.

Our story is your story. It is *every* Lyme sufferer's story.

I hope *Lyme Madness* helps you cut through some of the confusion and allows you to feel less alone, more supported, and more deeply understood as you battle this highly complex, multisystem, politically charged, and perplexing disease.

I wish you continued strength in your chronic Lyme journey, my friends and fellow warriors, and please may we all find our way out of this crazy, mad, unending rabbit hole together—heard, understood and, above all, fully healed.

WHY "LYME MADNESS"?

Chronic Lyme disease is nothing if not complete and utter madness.

The illness itself, along with the political machinations of this disease, is complex, mind-bending, and entirely inhumane. The madness of chronic Lyme disease is multi-layered, never-ending, and head-spinning. The madness of chronic Lyme is precisely why I felt compelled to write this book—to try to make sense of it for myself and for others, as I continue to help my son recover.

When you're living with chronic Lyme, you are living in a parallel universe. Every day you are struggling to manage your illness while struggling to explain the madness of it all to colleagues, family, and friends—or anyone who will listen. Every day you see the confounded and wary looks on the faces of others. And at every doctor's visit, you are confronted with utter disdain, disbelief, and denial by those whose very duty it is to treat you.

For those who have been wholly invalidated in their suffering, as well as family, friends, medical professionals, and the like who don't "get it" but may want to understand the complexity of this disease, I hope this book sheds light.

Before you begin to read our story, here is just a taste of the madness that we collectively experience in the world of chronic Lyme disease:

Chronic Lyme disease is a pandemic, affecting tens of millions in eighty countries and on every continent except Antarctica. Yet in the popular media, the community at large, and the medical community in particular, we hear far more about the Zika virus than Lyme.

Chronic Lyme disease is a complex, multisystem, neurological, bacteria-driven, immunosuppressive post sepsis illness with relapsing fever and opportunistic infections, essentially destroying the immune system, infecting and affecting every organ, muscle, tissue, and cell in the body, including the brain and the nervous system, rendering the body a septic tank. Yet for decades now, the powers that be continue to narrowly define Lyme as a simple nuisance condition that can be treated with an aspirin or two at the very least—or twenty-eight days of antibiotics at most.

Chronic Lyme disease is medically ignored and universally negated, forcing sufferers—for the most part, save for a few heroic doctors—to diagnose, research, treat, and heal themselves. It's a *do-it-yourself* disease. A moment-by-moment guessing game where the guessing never ends. A road you are forced to travel for years and even decades, without a GPS.

Chronic Lyme disease forces sufferers to be amateur sleuths, medical researchers, and experts in so many medical disciplines, including microbiology, neurology, gastroenterology, immunology, rheumatology, endocrinology, pharmacology, nephrology, hepatology, and more.

Chronic Lyme disease is known as the new "Great Imitator" (some might say detonator), mimicking 350-plus medical conditions, including multiple sclerosis, Alzheimer's, Parkinson's, lupus, chronic fatigue syndrome, fibromyalgia, and more.

Chronic Lyme disease is "treated" more humanely on Facebook than in most doctors' offices worldwide.

Chronic Lyme disease is defined by the "powers that be" as an insignificant syndrome that is *"difficult to catch, easy to diagnose, and easy to treat."* This entrenched party line mimicked by the conventional medical community has not changed since the first large outbreak in Lyme, Connecticut, more than four decades ago, when Lyme was narrowly and incorrectly defined as a rheumatological condition known as Lyme arthritis.

Most maddening of all, chronic Lyme disease sufferers are victimized not once but multiple times. By the disease itself. By the majority of doctors who turn their backs. By loved ones who roll their eyes and walk away. By insurance companies who refuse to provide coverage. By the Centers for Disease Control and Prevention (CDC) and Infectious Diseases Society of America (IDSA) who claim that chronic Lyme does not exist.

It's been more than four decades since the first outbreak of Lyme. And it's been more than four decades that we've been fighting the widespread medical neglect, dismissal, and outright denial of this disease—while the number of cases continues to proliferate.

The madness needs to stop.

INTRODUCTION

LYME AWAKENING

Alice had not a moment to think about stopping herself before she found herself falling down what seemed to be a very deep well. —ALICE'S ADVENTURES IN WONDERLAND

I fell down the deep, dark rabbit hole of chronic Lyme disease sometime during the summer of 2014. My headlong descent was not by choice. *No awakening ever is.*

Without warning, I was forced into a painful and unending journey into the abyss of a disease I knew nothing about. Each day I awoke to once again find myself in a black void of confusion filled with chaos, disorientation, terror, helplessness, anger, loneliness, and frustration. I was completely overwhelmed.

Throughout the course of this nightmare, there were many days where I couldn't breathe, move, or get myself out of bed. My bed became my sole respite as I read every article I could find online about this new reality that had invaded our lives like a brutal, unsympathetic terrorist.

Two years prior, on October 30, 2012, my son, Matt—

twenty-five at the time—began to exhibit some very strange and unexplained physical symptoms. These symptoms started with what felt like a "bug"—a strange flu of sorts. But then his vision suddenly and briefly went "sketchy," and he felt dizzy with a dull, cloudy headache in the back of his head. Later that day, after a session on a rowing machine at the gym, Matt stood up, the room started spinning, and he fainted. The paramedics were called, and Matt was taken to the hospital where he was examined and told his episode was likely the result of low blood sugar and dehydration. Nothing to worry about, the doctors tried to assure him.

This was the beginning of a year and a half of a cascade of debilitating symptoms, with many missteps and misdiagnoses along the way.

Matt's predominant symptom was at first a severe generalized anxiety. We were concerned but assumed that Matt's transition from university to "real life" and his stressful job in New York City were the cause. Things gradually got worse. Other symptoms arose, including shortness of breath, a racing heart, sweating, and dizziness. Increasingly concerned about his physical state, Matt decided to see a psychiatrist to explore the possibility of taking antianxiety medication. This turned out to be a complete disaster. The medications he was prescribed made him feel dramatically worse. We didn't understand at the time the extent to which his nervous system was already impaired by the disease that was hiding deep within his body.

Enormously concerned about Matt's state of ill health, my husband and I made two separate emergency trips to New York. On the first visit, when Matt opened the door to his apartment, we were shocked by what we saw. He looked pale and wired, as if he had just stuck his finger into an electric socket. We immediately got him off the psychotropic meds and found a doctor who was an expert in integrative medicine. She ran an extensive panel of blood tests, which uncovered all kinds of systemic deficiencies, and put Matt on a whack-load of supplements. In retrospect, these supplements probably kept his immune system from failing completely while we continued to search for answers. For that I am grateful.

Matt's anxiety did not abate. He also began having odd head pain that he described not as classic headaches but rather as "something going on in my brain." His symptoms had settled into a steady routine of dizziness, chronic head pain and pressure, neck stiffness, nausea, and malaise. Matt made umpteen visits to his primary care provider, neurologists, an ENT, a gastroenterologist, a chiropractor, an acupuncturist, an orthopedist, a cranial-sacral therapist, and many others. He had several MRIs, X-rays, a beta-blocker for his chronic headaches, benzodiazepines for his anxiety, herbal supplements, made drastic gluten, dairy, and sugar-free changes in diet, and endured a series of trigger-point injections in his neck.

After eighteen months of running from doctor to doctor—diagnosis to diagnosis, treatment to treatment—there was no measurable improvement. In fact, Matt began to feel noticeably worse.

At a moment of crisis—when Matt reached a particularly desperate state, and we were making plans to take him to the Mayo Clinic—an idea flashed in my mind. What if this was Lyme disease? I thought about the daughter of a colleague who years before had become severely ill and was eventually diagnosed with chronic Lyme. However, my recollection was that her presentation of this condition seemed very different, so I wasn't convinced. Then a dear friend sent me an article about Lyme with a text message: "Just read this. Whew, it's a good thing this is not what Matt has!" I wanted to agree, but the article left me with a deeply nagging feeling.

It was not until Matt's symptoms began to physically migrate that it occurred to me this was a systemic problem and that it could be Lyme.

While it pains me to even begin to credit one of Matt's twenty-plus doctors—each of whom missed this diagnosis altogether—there was one specialist he had seen months earlier who actually thought to test him for Lyme. He ordered an ELISA test from a lab in New York City. The results came back negative, and the likelihood of Lyme was summarily dismissed. So we pushed the possibility aside

It was only when Matt's health declined further and he exhibited yet another seemingly odd and random, perhaps systemic, symptom—a rash on his elbows—that I Googled "Lyme disease" for the first time and instantly knew this was it. Matt's symptoms and experience matched up precisely. I felt it in my gut.

I quickly searched for a Lyme-literate medical doctor (LLMD) in New York City (who knew there was such a thing?), and managed to get an appointment within days, due to a cancellation. I later learned this was a "lucky" break, as some of the best LLMDs have waiting lists up to three years long. It took very little to convince Matt to see him—he would have done anything and gone anywhere at that point.

The LLMD conducted a thorough clinical assessment and knew that this was Lyme. For good measure, he did a blood culture test through Advanced Labs in Pennsylvania, and a Western blot from IGeneX, a lab in California. The results were positive.

We had finally found the answer to his suffering, but we had no understanding of the long and difficult road to recovery that still lay ahead.

Chronic Lyme disease (also known as persistent Lyme disease or late-stage Lyme disease) is complex, challenging, and confounding—on all fronts. From diagnosis, to treatment, to recovery, it is a journey that begs far more questions than answers. The disease itself is a constant moving target and presents with a wide array of ever-changing symptoms.

Chronic Lyme disease (caused by the *Borrelia burgdorferi* bacterium, named after its discoverer, Willy Burgdorfer) is the most common vector-borne disease worldwide. The disease is often accompanied by coinfections, such as babesiosis and bartonellosis; parasitic, viral, and fungal infections; immune issues caused by mycoplasma; inflammation; mitochondrial dysfunctions; heavy metal and detoxification problems; and more.[1] Dr. Richard Horowitz, a much sought-after Lyme specialist in Hudson, New York, has aptly named this disease Lyme-*MSIDS* (Multiple Systemic Infectious Disease Syndrome). Kathleen Dickson, an ex-Pfizer analytic chemist and LYMErix vaccine whistleblower, says that chronic Lyme disease is all about *OspA*—outer surface protein antigen—which unequivocally destroys the immune system.

While chronic Lyme disease has been detected and diagnosed for decades, medical awareness and scientific research into this devastating illness is still in its infancy. To make matters worse, the controversy surrounding the medicalization and politicization of chronic Lyme is highly complex, multilayered, and difficult to make sense of—preventing the majority of sufferers from getting the medical help they so desperately need.

For hundreds of thousands of sufferers, perhaps millions worldwide, chronic Lyme disease translates into a long, lonely, and terrifying journey of doctor visits, misdiagnoses, ineffective treatments—and precious few answers. When LLMDs are accessible to patients, it comes at a tremendous financial cost, and even then the treatment for chronic Lyme is long and arduous, and without a clear-cut resolution. Many say there is no cure.

For the most part, diagnosis and treatment is conducted by clinical presentation and guesswork, if you're lucky enough to find a doctor who is Lyme literate. When we asked my son's Lyme-literate doctor about his prognosis, he replied, "How many angels can dance on the head of a pin?" This from a seasoned medical doctor who has been treating Lyme for more than thirty years.

Lyme is recognized, diagnosed, and treated equally insufficiently in every one of the eighty countries where it currently resides.

In Canada, where I live, we are light-years behind. LLMDs do not exist here because our government won't sanction a longer, potentially more effective antibiotic treatment protocol than the conventionally prescribed twenty-eight days. Those in Canada's Lymeland can be treated by LLNDs (Lyme-literate naturopaths). However, other than in British Columbia, LLNDs are not licensed to prescribe antibiotics, thereby forcing Canadian Lyme sufferers to cross the border for long-term antibiotic care.

I want to be very clear at the outset that I am *not* a medical doctor or a medical researcher. Nor am I a scientist, a microbiologist, an investigative journalist, or a political pundit. *I am the mother of a Lyme sufferer,* and there is no greater impetus to get to the truth about Lyme disease than to be a mother who wants nothing more than to stop her child's suffering. Like all Lyme sufferers and their loved ones, I have been forced to be an armchair medical professional, scientist, and amateur sleuth, spending the majority of my time for years now trying with every breath I take to unravel the mystery that is chronic Lyme.

My unstoppable drive to get this message out has not only been fueled by my own outrage and heartbreak, but also by the stories of suffering, powerlessness, loneliness, and outright medical denial experienced by hundreds of people I've connected with in my research.

Since the day my son was formally diagnosed with Lyme disease, I have read anything and everything about this illness that I could get my hands on. I have been doggedly hyperfocused—reading, researching, and speaking with others who reside in this world of Lyme madness. Outside of my office hours, and sometimes within my practice as some of my clients are also sick with this disease, I live, breathe, overthink, analyze, and fret about Lyme daily. In my research I have read about, listened to, and witnessed hundreds of heartbreaking, excruciating stories of the terribly sick, sometimes broke and homeless, often isolated and lonely sufferers. The stories are tragic and compelling, and the inhumanity of it all is just so difficult to fathom. The question these stories leave you with is, "How can all of these people be so sick, and yet no one is helping them?" They're all alone, without medication, in severe pain and discomfort. Where is the humanity in the medical system? Why aren't we getting help? The answers to these questions—and more like them—remain elusive.

I wrote this book to put our experience and research to good use—to make it available to the world in hopes that

Lyme sufferers everywhere, as well as their family, friends, and colleagues, will better understand this terrible disease and stop doubting their illness and anguish. My hope is that with all of the research and investigative work that I've done, I may be able to expedite this journey for other Lyme sufferers and loved ones, hopefully saving you countless hours of research, confusion, and torment.

It's shocking to me that chronic Lyme remains an invisible disease, even though there are currently millions of cases worldwide. It's shocking to me that we in Lymeland know so much more about this disease than most medical doctors worldwide.

To give you a sense of the number of Lyme sufferers, Lyme activist Alison Childs of lymestats.org claims that there are eighty-three million cases in China, 1.5 million in Germany, several million predicted in Canada by the year 2020, and a highly underreported 300,000 cases per year in the US, up tenfold from the previous report by the Centers for Disease Control and Prevention (CDC) of 30,000 just last year.[2]

Governments and medical communities—in the US, UK, Australia, Canada, Germany, Netherlands, China, and elsewhere—are not listening, and are not doing nearly enough to deal with this pandemic. They are not even declaring it a pandemic, which it clearly is.

After all, what is a pandemic but a disease that spreads quickly over a wide geographic area and affects a high percentage of the population? It's essentially an epidemic of worldwide proportions. This seems to fit the experience of those with chronic Lyme disease. Although certain medical authorities would argue otherwise.

That said, according to US National Institutes of Health

statistics, Lyme disease receives less than 2 percent of the public funding devoted to the West Nile virus ($7,050 per patient), and just 0.2 percent of funding devoted to HIV/ AIDS ($57,960 per patient)—this despite the fact that the number of Lyme cases reported each year in the US far exceeds either of these diseases.[3]

Furthermore, there has recently been an alarming and aggressive response by the CDC in support of the Zika virus while Lyme disease remains in the shadows. We must ask why when the number of Lyme sufferers out- ranks Zika victims by a long shot.

On this long, circuitous voyage of ours, we must research daily to understand both the lack of medical and government response to chronic Lyme disease and how to become Lyme literate, with little medical guidance, as we search for effective treatment.

Matt and I, along with millions of others, have been required to learn an entirely new language—an unfamil- iar lexicon of scientific terms from microbiology, chem- istry, epidemiology, pharmacology, and the like. Terms that include (but are by no means limited to) antibodies, serology, titers, bands, spirochetes, neuroborreliosis, bor- reliosis, Lyme encephalopathy, *Borrelia burgdorferi*, Lyme- MSIDS, biofilms, OspA (outer surface protein antigens), Pam3Cys, blebs, b-lymphocytes, cytokines, lymphokines, macrophages, neurotoxins, quinolinic acid, zoonoses, enzyme-linked immune sera assay (ELISA), IgM Western blot, IgG Western blot, kilodalton (kDa), flagellin, agonists, adjuvants, toll-like receptors, autoimmune, immunoreac- tive, immunosuppressive, coinfections, Babesia, Bartonella, mold, parasites, cell walls, biofilm, mycoplasma, myco- toxins, leaky gut, brain fog, Hickman line, Doxycycline,

Rocephin, Flagyl, Azithromycin, pulse-dosing, GcMAF, Jarisch-Herxheimer reaction, rifing, bioresonance, dark field microscopy, PEMF, tDCS, current electromagnetic stimulation, and cannabidiol. The learning curve is steep and never ending. Every day there's a new term—or ten—to become familiar with as we continue our search for answers.

With any other illness, you expect your doctor to carry this knowledge for you. While you might want to play an active role in understanding your disease, you are never expected to take a crash course in every possible scientific discipline in order to understand your disease and medically treat yourself. With Lyme disease, the majority of doctors (save for a few open-minded and openhearted souls) have unfortunately rendered themselves useless at best, willfully ignorant, and even harmful at worst.

Never in modern medicine has there been a pandemic that has been so summarily dismissed by doctors and left for the sufferers to figure out and fix on their own.

This is why the Lyme community lives and breathes on Facebook. My "rabbit hole" on this long, long journey is located in the dark and uncertain—yet often comforting and supportive—netherworld of Google and Facebook. As much as doctors resent patients for "Googling" their own diagnoses and treatments, I shudder to think where my son would be without this vital resource.

So we're left to keep reading and researching and seeking and guessing as to what might work to relieve the suffering. It's a very desperate and terribly lonely road—with very few answers. It *is* the road less traveled. Those who don't "get it" look at us askance, with pity, judgment, and confusion. I don't blame them. The world of chronic Lyme disease, along with its political machinations, is simply too much for anyone's mind to comprehend. I can understand why their eyes glaze over.

People will ask, "Where did Matt get bitten?" or "Did he see the tick?" wondering how they can be more alert than we were to this life-altering disease. Of course, we don't know. As is true for the majority of Lyme sufferers. And I am always tempted to answer with, "Oh, how I miss the earlier and comparatively simpler days when I thought chronic Lyme disease was simply about ticks and woods and deer and bull's-eye rashes and spirochetes. If only."

This illness is complicated, to say the least. Equally complicated are the political and medical underpinnings that make chronic Lyme disease the most widely neglected pandemic in modern medicine.

The official party line of the US Centers for Disease Control and Prevention (CDC) and the Infectious Diseases Society of America (IDSA) is that chronic Lyme disease is *hard to catch, easy to diagnose, and easy to cure.*" For decades, this has detracted from the seriousness of this disease while deterring sufferers from getting the medical attention they so desperately need and deserve.

The CDC and the IDSA would have everyone believe that Lyme is a rare, self-limiting illness, a mere nuisance condition managed easily with an aspirin or two. The IDSA Lyme disease guideline authors claim that their stance is based on science when, in fact, there are seven hundred peer-reviewed journal articles that support the contrary—a plethora of scientific evidence demonstrating the persistence of Lyme and other tick-borne diseases.[4]

Herein lies the beginning of the madness that would become a decades-long story of chronic Lyme disease.

But there's much more to the Lyme story than just government lassitude and inaction.

The world over, conventional doctors ignore, negate, blame, shame, ridicule, and deny both the existence of chronic Lyme and the myriad of debilitating symptoms that accompany the disease—telling the sick and vulnerable every day that "it's all in their heads" and they should see a "shrink."

Lyme doctors in the US, Canada, and elsewhere have been threatened, harassed, bullied, and taken to court for prescribing antibiotics beyond the sanctioned yet ineffective IDSA twenty-eight-day period.

Insurance providers routinely refuse coverage for Lyme—denying the illness's very existence and creating so much red tape and paperwork that it is impossible for sufferers to get treatment coverage or disability payouts. As a result, Lyme patients are losing not just their health, but their homes, their savings—and their lives.

Essentially, chronic Lyme disease patients are victimized multiple times—by the disease that has invaded their bodies, by the medical system that has failed them, by loved ones who often roll their eyes and walk away, by insurers who refuse coverage, and by the CDC and IDSA who say that this disease we know as chronic Lyme does not exist.

Thankfully, change is in the air—a patient revolution is gaining momentum, and it promises to turn everything about Lyme right-side up. Chronic Lyme sufferers refuse to stay silent any longer. We're mad as hell and we're not going to take it anymore.

There is a term in clinical psychology known as *gaslighting*. Its origins are the 1938 play and 1944 film *Gas Light*. Gaslighting is "a form of mental abuse in which information is twisted or spun, selectively omitted to favor the abuser, or false information is presented with the intent of making victims doubt their own memory, perception, and sanity."[5]

This sounds outrageous. And it is. The years of lies, falsehoods, misinformation, greed, profit, ego, and arrogance enacted by the "higher-ups"—the very people that have prevented chronic Lyme disease from getting the medical attention it so deserves—have turned chronic Lyme disease into a case of gaslighting.

Gaslighting is a brilliantly orchestrated method of damaging your trust in yourself and in your own reality. When you've fallen prey to a chronic illness like Lyme, it's easy to be the victim of this tactic as you're already in a weakened position. Chronic Lyme disease is a perfect, yet tragic, example of this ploy—perpetrated by a global cast of characters against the most vulnerable among us.

I can assure you that chronic Lyme disease is very real, that the suffering Lyme patients are forced to endure is also very real, and that the number of people, organizations, and communities affected by the disease—both directly and indirectly—is growing exponentially while the medical establishment is doing little to address it.

For those of you who see your medical condition in our story—and in the others presented in these pages— and for those who know you have chronic Lyme disease and are struggling to get well, my deepest hope is that this book will allow you to take solace in our experience and the experiences of others. Know that you're not alone, and that many are working diligently to turn up the volume and advocacy for this disease.

Part of my mission in writing this book is to provide a platform for others to tell their stories. After all, "Stories are the creative conversion of life itself into a more powerful, clearer, more meaningful experience. They are the currency of human contact," says Robert McKee, a writer, teacher, and Fulbright scholar who also reminds us that, "In a world of lies and liars, an honest work of art is an act of social responsibility."

Lymeland is made up of so many stories—all frightfully compelling and filled with grief, heartache, suffering, perseverance, strength, and gut-wrenching honesty.

Apart from our story, I urge you to listen carefully to the stories of other chronic Lyme sufferers presented in this book. They deserve to be heard—by the public, the media, the medical establishment, the insurance companies, the universities, the pharmaceutical companies, and by family and friends. There is, after all, nothing more painful within the human condition than to be ignored and invalidated in one's suffering. Above all, in this life, we need someone to notice our pain, to witness our plight, to acknowledge what ails us.

The Institute of Medicine (IOM), a nonprofit organization established in 1970 as a component of the US National Academy of Sciences that works outside the framework of government to provide evidence-based research and recommendations for public health and science policy, seems to agree that patients should have a voice.

As stated on the National Academy's website: "In February 2013, the Institute of Medicine's Roundtable on Value & Science-Driven Health Care convened a workshop, gathering patients and experts in areas such as decision science, evidence generation, communication strategies, and health economics to consider the central roles for patients in bringing about progress in all aspects of the US health-care system. The discussions highlighted the critical role and capacity for patients and families to be leaders in informed care decisions, knowledge generation, and value improvement."[6]

Nice vision. But this is clearly not what Lyme sufferers are experiencing in the US or elsewhere.

It's time to give Lyme sufferers a voice. It's time to restore some semblance of humanity to the sick and the suffering. It's time to revolt against the greed, denial, ignorance, and willful harm that have brought chronic Lyme sufferers to this sadly abandoned and unconscionable place.

In my search for answers, I have spoken with a mycoplasma researcher in Japan, a mercury pathologist in Germany, interviewed a cannabidiol medical expert in British Columbia, and a PANS (pediatric acute-onset neuropsychiatric syndrome) expert in Massachusetts.

I have spoken with a range of medical doctors, including those who don't "believe in" Lyme, those who are currently treating Lyme, as well as those whose medical licenses have been threatened and stripped by the authorities simply for treating Lyme patients beyond the IDSA-sanctioned twenty-eight-day guideline. I have spoken with countless Lyme advocates, whistleblowers, lawyers, leaders, authors, and other experts on the subject. I have read about and spoken with hundreds of sufferers from all around the world—for almost two years now.

Here, I present you with my understanding of chronic Lyme disease as seen through my eyes, my son's eyes, and through the eyes of so many sufferers, supporters, advocates, and activists.

The only way I can tell this story is from my own sense of outrage. From our own personal experience. I do my very best to offer the most accurate sources of information and, in the Lyme world, this is no easy feat.

As author and spiritual guru Marianne Williamson said, "Only write from your own passion, your own truth. That's the only thing you really know about, and anything else leads you away from the pulse."

My "pulse" is that of a mother with a chronically unwell son and a medical system that has let us down—betrayed us, in fact. I will stay true to this framework as I take you on our journey through real-life medical trials and tribulations, anecdotal research, other Lyme sufferers' stories, interviews with experts, scientific journals, media reports, medical resources, and websites devoted to the disease.

Know that this journey will take you—as it has taken us—to places no one ever expected to go. Know that this struggle will reshape you, remake you, and remold you into a different being—hopefully for the better. Know that this journey is nothing if not humbling, echoing Thomas Edison's words, "We don't know a millionth of one percent about anything."

Please know that my voice is your voice. Our story is your story. If you multiply our story by tens of millions with countless heartbreaking details, you'll begin to get a clearer picture of the undeniable suffering—and reprehensible and shameful medical denial—faced by Lyme sufferers worldwide. While the mysteries surrounding chronic Lyme have yet to be unraveled, the untold suffering is unquestionable.

Above all, I trust that we *will* find answers to this madness we call Lyme.

Change of this sort—that is, moving an immovable mountain and facing some very dark and deeply entrenched forces—requires a critical mass rising up and taking action. Perhaps a whistleblower or two with enough power and authority to bring this to a head, so that change can finally take place. And in the meantime, resourcing treatment workarounds well outside of the conventional medical system, at a tremendous personal cost.

With millions of Lyme sufferers—and supporters—speaking out en masse, I am confident that together we will achieve a positive outcome. For the sake of so many, I hope we get to witness some form of resolution soon.

On this journey, I have been exposed daily to the vicissitudes of life—unbearable hardship and pain, loneliness and desperation, along with medical and political corruption—all of which I would give anything to unsee. There are far too many people in this Lyme world who are chronically ill, wasting away, sick and dying, alone, without financial resources and proper medical support due to a political landscape that is exceedingly more focused on lining their pockets than looking out for our health and welfare.

Surely we can and must do better.

1. CHASING A DIAGNOSIS

In another moment, down went Alice after it, never once considering how she was going to get out again.

—ALICE'S ADVENTURES IN WONDERLAND

My kids are my life.

When they're joyful, I'm joyful. When they're sad, I'm sad. When they're heartbroken, I'm heartbroken. And when they're sick, I'm sick at heart.

Call it codependence. Hypersensitivity. Or modern parenting. It's all the same. Especially when you're a mother and an empath.

I was never warned how hard parenting could be when our kids are struggling. I'm quite sure my own mother was far less affected when we were sad, heartbroken, or sick. For better or worse, she wasn't as keenly focused on us.

What I've come to know for certain in my twenty-nine years as a mother is that you really are only as happy as your unhappiest child—especially when you're deeply attached. This is true for many in my generation, whose style of parenting is primarily child-centric. Unlike my parents, and others of their time, we have strategically chosen, in stark contrast to how we were parented, to put the interests and well-being of our kids before our own. This, of course, comes with costs and benefits.

The cost is that we are always monitoring and self-sacrificing—leading some of us to micromanage our kids and, at the same time, forget to take care of ourselves.

The upside of child-centric parenting is that we meet the needs of our kids far more often than our parents met ours, rendering us more emotionally connected to them, with our lives being all the richer for it.

While I don't consider myself to be a helicopter parent, I know for certain there have been, and still are, times when I could have backed off more, let go more, and given my kids more space. It's a dance we learn as we go.

That said, there is nothing that can stop me from being right there when my kids are sick and suffering. I'm a mother bear protecting my cubs—even when they're adults. That's why I have written this book. I am compelled to get to the truth of this madness and help others do the same.

This crazy, mad journey that Matt and I have been on for the past several years began in October 2012. That's when Matt's unusual, seemingly undiagnosable, and quickly mounting physical symptoms first emerged.

It feels like forever ago when we started to worry and hyperfocus—or let's call it *obsess*—about Matt's health. And it was. The worrying began in earnest in the spring of 2008.

He had just graduated from Brown University in Providence, Rhode Island. The day after his convocation, Matt took a train from Providence to New York City where he was to begin his first full-time job, working for a hedge-fund company in the heart of Manhattan.

I worried terribly about Matt back then. In contrast to the three and a half wonderful years he had at Brown, in his final semester he had not been himself. His anxiety was at an all-time high. His hair began to fall out at the age of twenty-two. He looked pale, was unusually stressed, and his inner light seemed dim.

His job offer in Washington had been rescinded due to the economic crash. His apartment and roommate situation in New York City was not working out. Shortly after arriving in NYC, he found himself in an apartment without heat or electricity for two months until he finally decided to get a new place to live.

I chalked up Matt's "dis-ease" to his last minute scramble to find a full-time job and launch his adult life in a tough, fast-paced city. It may not have been apparent to most, but I knew he was not at his best—his spirit to me seemed somewhat dampened.

I worried plenty. Little did I know he was actually suffering from an illness that had already manifested itself in subtle, less pervasive ways.

Before long, everything changed.

One week after Matt received a flu shot in the fall of 2012, his symptoms became varied and acute, and he immediately questioned whether the vaccine he was given was the reason he felt so unwell. Maybe it was a bad batch, he wondered. At the time, I knew little about the potential harm of vaccines and flu shots—especially to those who are immunosuppressed, which we didn't know was the case. So I quickly dismissed this idea as a potential cause of his dis-ease.

The onslaught of Matt's symptoms began to present more dramatically.

At first, he felt a "bug" come on, including a mild sore throat and a cold that never fully materialized. The very next day, he had a moment at work where his vision suddenly but briefly went "sketchy," and he felt a bit dizzy the rest of the week. He was left with a dull, cloudy headache in the back of his head (which remains to this day and we're still working to eradicate).

The following month, Matt saw a neurologist who suggested an MRI. The results of the scan were unremarkable, which was a blessing, of course, but it meant we had to continue our search.

In January 2013, Matt went to the gym for the first time in a long time and exercised on the rowing machine. After he completed his set on the machine, he stood up and the room began to spin. He fainted and hit his head hard on the equipment. A gym employee called the paramedics and Matt was taken to the hospital, where he was told the fainting episode was likely caused by low blood sugar and dehydration—nothing really to worry about, as far as they were concerned.

As January rolled into February, headaches and dizziness were becoming a daily problem. By now, however, we were becoming very concerned about Matt's health. He became increasingly worried and anxious, developing severe anxiety. Matt returned to the neurologist, and he prescribed nadolol—a beta-blocker—believing Matt might be suffering from a migraine condition. When Matt took the nadolol, he had a panic attack. He also suffered from heightened light and noise sensitivity, and an increasingly cloudier head. At the same time, under the care of his general practitioner, Matt started taking meds for his anxiety and malaise, and the results were nothing short of disastrous for him. My husband made an emergency trip to NYC and consulted with a psychiatrist the following day. He prescribed other meds that were just as explosive to Matt's nervous system—causing us to have to make a second emergency trip to NYC.

When I arrived, I was shocked by what I saw. Matt looked as though he had stuck his finger in an electrical socket. His hair was standing on end. His expression was one of shock, as though his nervous system had gone into overdrive. It was terrifying. He broke down and sobbed in my arms. By now, I was really feeling afraid. I held it together for him.

The next morning, Matt gazed longingly out of his apartment window and asked me why it was that everyone else was able to go on with their day and he couldn't. He was scared—sad, confused, and unable to make sense of any of this. I felt helpless and desperately afraid as well.

I was convinced that Matt was suffering from an anxiety disorder—not a big leap as diagnoses go. After all, the physical symptoms of an anxiety disorder can include everything from dizziness to nausea to headaches to stomach upset— pretty much everything he was experiencing. And we figured he came by it honestly given our family history, on both sides.

Regardless, we clearly had to get Matt off these drugs. For reasons we didn't yet understand, they were pure poison for his nervous system. It was time to take a different medical path. At his follow-up session, when Matt told the psychiatrist we were going to try a more naturopathic route, he responded with a smarmy and sarcastic, "Huh, good luck." Unprofessional and disturbing, to say the least.

After being summarily dismissed by this doctor in such an unempathetic manner, I researched the possibility of seeing an integrative psychiatrist. I didn't know there was such a thing at the time, but I quickly learned there is a branch of medicine called *orthomolecular,* founded in Canada in the 1950s by biochemist, physician, and psychiatrist Dr. Abram Hoffer and Nobel Prize winner and molecular biologist Linus Pauling.

As defined on their site and coined by Pauling: "Orthomolecular is a term that comes from ortho, which is Greek for 'correct' or 'right,' and 'molecule,' which is the simplest structure that displays the characteristics of a compound. So, it literally means the 'right molecule.'"[7]

This approach to healing operates on the premise that anxiety, depression, and other psychological disorders can be treated far more effectively with natural supplements. Seeing how damaging the psychotropic meds were for Matt, I was excited about this discovery—hoping this would be the answer to what ailed him.

On the orthomolecular.org website, Dr. Hoffer is quoted as saying,

Orthomolecular treatment does not lend itself to rapid drug-like control of symptoms, but patients get well to a degree not seen by tranquilizer therapists who believe orthomolecular therapists are prone to exaggeration. Those who have seen the results are astonished.[8]

I found an integrative (that is, orthomolecularly trained) psychiatrist close to Matt's home and was able to secure an appointment for him that week. She ordered a ton of lab tests, put him on a whole host of supplements, determined that his adrenals were overtaxed and that his thyroid was sluggish, and his Krebs cycle was weak due to low levels of certain cofactors (explaining his low energy). In addition, the tests showed signs of a weak urea cycle, which the doctor thought might have caused Matt's cloudy headaches because of a possible buildup of ammonia. Further lab results showed high cortisol levels at night, as well as low melatonin at bedtime, explaining his poor sleep cycle. The doctor was surprised that Matt seemed to be absorbing little nutrition from the food he ate.

Clearly, there was work to do to get Matt feeling well, and we still had no official diagnosis or understanding of why all of these problems were occurring.

To this day, I do credit this integrative doctor's work for enabling Matt to get out of bed in the morning and function. At the same time, I have a hard time letting go of the fact that the diagnosis of chronic Lyme did not once cross her mind. Matt saw this doctor regularly for a year and it never occurred to her that an infectious disease could have caused all of these problems. How is that possible?

Even more disturbing to us is that several months after Matt's Lyme diagnosis—no thanks whatsoever to this medical doctor—she sent Matt an email sharing some instant cure for Lyme that she'd heard a celebrity had used, a six-hour remedy which everyone in the Lyme world knows is impossible. There simply is no quick fix.

A kitchen counter loaded with supplements for Matt's poor sleep cycle, his frazzled nervous system, his weak digestive system, and more, were now part of his daily protocol. Over time, his energy began to improve but his headaches and brain fog remained.

Matt next saw an ear, nose, and throat specialist who performed myofascial release and trigger-point therapy. This helped for a brief time, but the improvements were short-lived. He was, however, the first doctor to test for rare diseases, and Lyme was one of them. The results came back negative. (More on that in the chapters ahead.)

Over the course of the next several months, the list of doctors, tests, and protocols grew, as did our desperation for answers and relief.

A gastroenterologist tested Matt for food allergies on the premise that his symptoms could be caused by his digestive tract. (Years later, we learned that the gut is almost always affected by Lyme disease but is not likely the root cause.)

There was a second and then a third neurologist. Both assessed his headaches and ordered yet another MRI. Next came another ear, nose, and throat specialist who ruled out inner-ear issues. A nonsurgical orthopedist performed a series of Traumeel trigger-point injections on Matt, along with a cortisone nerve block in his neck. All to no avail.

Matt was prepared to try anything and everything, despite the fact that, at one time, he would have been fairly closed-minded about alternative therapies. Desperate times create desperate (or perhaps, medically unconventional and ultimately better) measures.

At my insistence, Matt tried a neurostimulation device for anxiety. Nothing. He tried acupuncture, biofeedback, meditation, massage therapy, and craniosacral therapy. No relief. At the suggestion of one of his physicians, Matt began a gluten-free diet, even though his tests came back negative to gluten intolerance. He tried amitriptyline—a tricyclic antidepressant that is often used for migraine prophylactic. He tried natural remedies for migraines and anxiety. And with the support of his integrative doctor, Matt continued to tweak his supplement regime in a desperate attempt to get some sustainable relief.

Still no change.

As time passed, he began to feel progressively worse. He would often get struck by debilitating and dizzying headaches, describing his condition as an unceasing, achy brain with neck cramps, dizziness, and nausea. In our desperation for answers, I would often revisit the idea of this being an acute anxiety disorder. But Matt would insist there was something physical going on in his brain—a feeling that was hard to describe.

Matt's daily symptoms continued to escalate unabated, in both their acuteness and frequency. Dizzying, debilitating headaches, wooziness, brain fog, nausea, anxiety, malaise, sore, stiff neck, sleep disturbances, faintness, blurry vision, optic neuritis, earaches, high sensitivity to light and sound were all part of his everyday experience.

Trips to CVS and Duane Reade were out of the question, as the fluorescent lighting would trigger an attack. The barbershop felt like a torture chamber as the razor's buzz sounded like a dentist drill and a jackhammer all at once, pounding in his ears.

Not a day went by when I wasn't Googling, researching, thinking, problem solving, listening, and looking for answers. As doctors continued to rule out disease after disease, we were left more and more alone—feeling afraid, desperate, and hopeless.

Where Are Marcus Welby and Dr. House When You Need Them?

The art of medical diagnosis was once the cornerstone of medicine. It has clearly become a lost art, with very serious consequences.

In the *Journal of the American Medical Association* (March 19, 1927), Francis. W. Peabody (1881–1927), a physician, teacher, and humanitarian who personified the Harvard Medical School's tradition of blending the medical scientist and the humane clinician, said, "The treatment of a disease may be entirely impersonal; the care of a patient must be completely personal."[9]

I grew up in an age when medicine seemed much simpler. We trusted our doctors. Revered them, actually. The popular television series *Marcus Welby, M.D.* epitomized our love of the general practitioner who cared deeply about his patients and went above and beyond the call of duty to solve medical problems.

Have times ever changed.

We now love TV shows like *House*, in reruns, because the protagonist—albeit an imperfect, narcotics-addicted misanthrope—is a medical genius and a diagnostician extraordinaire. The both adored and hated Dr. Gregory House is an iconic medical figure primarily because he is relentless in the pursuit of answers. He racks his brain, perseveres at all costs, and drives his team hard—not for the love of the patient, but because of his ego's need to find real answers to a serious problem. Whatever demons drive House to be such a gifted diagnostician are not certain or easily replicated. What *is* certain, however, is that he is able to navigate a host of seemingly obscure, unrelated symptoms, and then when things become most dire for his patient, he delivers a unifying, spot-on diagnosis that no other doctor would have thought of.

What is also certain is that doctors like House are impossible to find.

While chasing doctors and diagnoses for eighteen months, not one Ivy League—educated New York City doctor even considered Lyme to be a differential diagnosis, let alone the answer. To be fair, one of the twenty doctors Matt saw in this period of time did actually put on his thinking cap long enough to test for Lyme, but the test came back negative and it was never discussed or explored again. How can that be?

As medical students learn, there are two ways of approaching the diagnosis of a seemingly arbitrary set of symptoms: Occam's razor and Hickam's dictum. Occam's razor states that two complaints (i.e., headache and rash) are related symptoms of one unifying disease. Hickam's dictum says that the same two complaints are due to separate causes.

House seems able to correctly apply either or both when deciphering the most obscure disease. Where is Dr. House when you need him?

I am told there is a joke in medicine that goes something like this:

A family practitioner, an internist, a surgeon, and a pathologist go duck hunting. They decide to take turns shooting as the first flock of birds flies over. The family practitioner raises his gun, says, "It's a duck!" and misses the bird altogether. The next flock flies by. The internist raises his gun and says, "It's a duck...no, it's a goose...no, it's a swan..." while the birds fly away. The next flock flies by. The surgeon raises his gun, says nothing, and blasts away. A bird falls out of the sky. The surgeon turns to the pathologist and asks, "Okay, what is it?"

A good diagnostician is a doctor who has a depth of knowledge in his area of specialization and at the same time a breadth of knowledge allowing him to look outside of his own silo for connections and answers.

After all, "Sometimes a cough is hereditary angioedema caused by C1 esterase inhibitor deficiency. Other times, a cough is just a cough."[10]

Paging "A Real-Life Dr. House"

By May 2014, Matt was at his absolute worst. His health was quickly declining. I could hear the fear and desperation in his voice.

I was desperate, too. We were running out of ideas and doctors to consult with. No medical answers satisfied his condition, and he was feeling progressively worse. No one had figured it out.

In a moment of complete desperation, I Googled "real-life Dr. House." Lo and behold, my search revealed Dr. Bolte—right in NYC where Matt lived—a doctor who bills himself as "an unusual symptoms investigator." He claims to pick up the pieces where other doctors fail. Many of the patients Bolte sees are victims of iatrogenic, or doctor-caused, illness—people who have been misdiagnosed, overmedicated to the point of sickness, or given treatment inappropriate to their conditions.[11]

It was a Sunday morning. I immediately called Dr. Bolte. A gruff voice on the other end of the phone said, "Hello." I explained what I was looking for and he advised me to have Matt write him a letter describing his symptoms and medical history, as the instruction on his website indicated. Click. End of call. I did not get the reassuring or compassionate response of the rescuer I was hoping for.

Matt sent him a detailed letter that very day. The letter, several pages in length, provided a complete history and comprehensive description of his symptoms—from his very first bout of dizziness, all the way up to the terrible pit of suffering in which he was currently trapped. He talked about all the doctors, all the tests, all the drugs—in his calm and logical way.

We never did manage to connect with this "real-life Dr. House." So much for the promise of a savior. A notion I realize is fictional at best.

It was clear that no one was going to rescue us. We had only ourselves to rely on.

Deep in Crisis

It's excruciating for me to go back to the beginning—to relive and excavate the terror, the moment-by-moment haunting of this mysterious illness that was taking my son's health from him—and my son from me. While Matt was losing his health and vitality—day by day, week by week, month by month—I felt like I was losing *him*. It was my worst nightmare coming true.

My ability to help Matt was slowly waning. It felt like we were running out of options—and time.

As he became more and more ill, I began to panic. Matt continued to work which to me was a remarkable feat on his part. I kept asking him if he thought he should come home, quit his job, and take a long-term sick leave. Despite how bad he felt, he insisted that he'd rather be sick with a job than sick without one.

As months passed and we were no closer to figuring it out, I could barely operate. I don't know how he did it. I received daily texts from Matt, reaching out, leaning on me for reassurance, clarity, and direction. Or just to let me know how awful he felt.

He was afraid, and so was I. But I had to keep it together for him. We are very close and work well together—naturally synchronized in our thinking and our approach, although Matt is more logical while I'm more emotional. After work and on weekends, between texts and calls to each other, I cried every single day—to the very depths of my being. I didn't know that tears could flow so painfully and endlessly.

Matt did not cry much, and that worried me, too. What was he doing with all of his emotions? I wondered. I later understood why he seemed to be so numb.

I never stopped thinking, researching, analyzing, ruminating, suggesting, and advising while Matt continued to suffer. And we were physically miles apart.

The feeling that "no one gets it, no one is listening, there is no one to lean on, and no one understands" permeated my life. I'd never felt so alone and so helpless.

To be fair, my husband was always there to listen and support me. He was worried, too, of course. But as is always the case in our relationship, I overcompensate with worry and/or action, while he uses his preferred coping mechanism—burying his head in the sand. That is, until I pull his head out of the sand—again and again and again.

In May 2014, we decided our best course of action would be to take Matt to either the Mayo Clinic or Johns Hopkins—not that I had much faith in their diagnostic processes. We'd been let down by so many doctors, and I questioned why it would be any different at either of these places. But we were desperate and at the end of our rope. We didn't know what else to do.

In hindsight, I feel very lucky that my deeper intuition soon kicked in and we didn't go that route. Two separate, but meaningful, moments occurred that kept us from wasting even more time.

One day, in spring 2014, a dear friend read an article in the *Globe and Mail* on Lyme disease. She sent me the article with a personal message saying, "I just read this. Whew—good thing this isn't Matt!"

That message from my friend put Lyme top of mind for me. Something in my gut caused me to insist that Matt pull out his "negative" Lyme test results from months before to check them again. Were they really negative? If so, what did that mean?

Then came the clue we'd been waiting for. Matt casually mentioned to me that he had a brand-new symptom—*a rash on his elbows.* My mind immediately went to this line of thinking:

What!? Another unexplained symptom, a completely different, random manifestation…not in his neck or head…on a different part of his body…seemingly unrelated…but it must all be connected…migrating symptoms…this is systemic…I just read about Lyme…this is it… this is Lyme.

It's always amazing to me what we can pull from some deeper place within us when we get out of our own way.

I Googled Lyme. I read the long and detailed list of symptoms.

Then I wept all night—long, painful, grief-stricken cries mixed with trepidation and relief. I wept long and hard because I knew in my heart that *this was it.*

2. BECOMING LYME LITERATE

Either the well was very deep, or she fell very slowly, for she had plenty of time as she went down to look about her and to wonder what was going to happen next.

—ALICE'S ADVENTURES IN WONDERLAND

What a dizzying, mind-bending, frightening journey!

Eighteen months, twenty-plus doctors, twenty-plus misdiagnoses, twenty-plus different treatments. All a waste of time and money, while Matt continued to suffer.

The doctor visits and potential answers kept us moving, talking, connecting, thinking, and hoping. Matt and I are similar in that we're far more comfortable taking action than standing still—even if it's misdirected. Standing still is simply excruciating for both of us, and something we are just not willing or able to do.

That said, please tell me how it is possible that *it was left to me*—to us—to figure out what was wrong with my son. How is it possible that I—a nonmedical professional—could get to the answer when more than twenty-plus highly educated medical specialists could not? What does that say about our medical system, about the prevailing view of chronic Lyme disease, and the poor quality of diagnostic care? I quickly learned that our long and winding road to diagnosis is a common occurrence among chronic Lyme sufferers and sufferers of other chronic illnesses.

I've heard it said that the US doesn't have a health-care system—it has a disease-management system at best. At worst, it just sends people away to suffer when the patient's issues and complaints fall outside of the doctor's purview. Trust me when I tell you that Canada's medical system is not any better.

After eighteen months of agony, consultations with twenty top medical specialists, and just as many misdiagnoses, we were forced to solve this mystery completely on our own. Oh, how I wish that my intuition had kicked in earlier.

A knowing far deeper than we hold in our conscious brain is always available to us—especially a mother's knowing for her child. We just need to find ways to get quiet so we can access it. We certainly can't get to it in the midst of chronic worry.

Finding Some Relief

Once I knew in my heart that it was Lyme, I Googled the words "Lyme doctor NYC." Little did I know at the time that there was such a thing as a Lyme-literate doctor. I perused the first website which belonged to Dr. R MD.

The flood of information that poured out of his website was all so unfamiliar and so complex. I could see that Matt and I were about to enter a whole new world, one that felt strange, confusing, and completely foreign.

As stated on Dr. R's website, his philosophy of treatment views Lyme disease syndrome as a complex, infectious, neuroimmune phenomenon. A diagnosis is made based on the patient's comprehensive medical history, physical examination, symptom presentation, and advanced serological testing. Unfortunately, standard serological methods (ELISA, Western blot IgG and IgM) can be either false negative or false positive in up to 40 percent of cases.

Aha! That explained at a cursory level why Matt's initial Lyme test taken months prior came back negative. It had to have been a false negative. And the doctor he was seeing at the time was clearly not aware of this possibility. Something finally made sense.

Dr. R was a specialist in nutritional and integrative psychiatry/medicine. He became interested in tick-borne diseases, including Lyme disease, because of the chronic undiagnosed symptoms of his patients who lived in the endemic areas of New York's Westchester and Fairfield Counties.

I was impressed and comforted that he had successfully treated more than 3,500 cases of tick-borne disease (specializing in neuropsychiatric and neurocognitive complications). More than 90 percent of his practice was now devoted entirely to chronic Lyme disease and coinfections.

I was also comforted to know that he was a founding member and secretary of the board of governors of ILADS (the International Lyme and Associated Disease Society). He had been a featured speaker at more than forty workshops over the years on topics including psychiatry, drug abuse, psychoneuroimmunology, and tick-borne diseases, and he had appeared on national television (ABC, NBC, Fox) to discuss the medical concerns that pertain to tick-borne diseases.

According to Dr. R's website, "Most patients have seen a number of physicians before finding one who can make a correct diagnosis and initiate a successful treatment. The often variable nature of the patient's symptoms, combined with the negative serology, creates diagnostic uncertainty. This results in frustration for both the well-meaning specialist and the concerned patient."

I felt like I'd hit the jackpot—finding a medical doctor in NYC who seemed to mirror our own experience and might provide what we needed.

Someone who might finally get it!

I also found something that piqued my interest—disciplinary actions against Dr. R on the website casewatch. org. While this made me nervous, I have often found it is the doctors who have the courage to step outside of the medical rules and regulations—out of sheer necessity and human kindness—who are the heroes and true helpers in this profession.

So I took a chance and called his office. We got lucky— we were booked in on a cancellation just two days later.

Test Results Are Positive—It's Lyme!

Matt's first appointment with Dr. R was on June 14, 2014. Knowing he was going to see a Lyme expert, in short order, helped him to feel more hopeful.

At this point, I felt slight relief. I was also feeling like a hero—a supermom, donning a special cape. Unlike all of these useless doctors, I was able to finally figure out what I believed was making Matt so ill. But there are no heroes or glory in this terrible illness. There is only room for a momentary pause and a quick self-congratulatory pat on the back. To this day, the journey to recover Matt's health continues. There's still much work to be done.

While Dr. R undoubtedly had the expertise required to diagnose chronic Lyme disease clinically, in order to achieve diagnostic certainty, he sent Matt's blood sample to a lab in California called IGeneX, a name that would soon become part of our everyday vernacular (as is the case for every Lyme sufferer). I learned that the New York State Department of Health is one of the most highly regulated in the country and that IGeneX had been carefully vetted and fully approved.

Matt's IGeneX test results, which arrived a few weeks later, provided further evidence to Dr R's clinical assessment that it was chronic Lyme. His results included six double-starred bands on both the IgM and IgG Western blot which, says IGeneX, may indicate clinical significance. He had a positive result on bands twenty-eight and forty-one, which are "CDC-specific," and an indeterminate result on band thirty-nine which, as one of the most specific bands for Lyme disease, is considered to be a suspicious finding.

Understanding and interpreting IGeneX test results can be overwhelming. The bands reflect the reaction of your immune system to Lyme. It can be true but is not always the case that the longer you've been infected, the weaker your immune system and the less clear the results.

Most doctors, I've learned, do not know how to interpret diagnostic test results for chronic Lyme. This explains why Matt's first test was shelved—case closed. It's also important to note that a diagnosis should not be based on laboratory tests alone and should always be made in conjunction with clinical symptoms and patient history. A history which in Matt's case included many summers spent at an overnight camp and on canoe trips in northern Ontario, where ticks do reside. Followed by four years at university in Providence Rhode Island, where Lyme is endemic I've since come to know. [12]

While waiting for the IGeneX test results to arrive, we

sought out another diagnostic measure—a blood culture test conducted by Advanced Labs in Sharon Hill, Pennsylvania, which does not have the New York State Department of Health seal of approval and therefore required Matt to travel out of state.

According to some, the Advanced Labs culture test for Lyme disease can accurately and reliably determine whether the infection is currently present in your system, and is said to be more accurate than a serology (ELISA and Western blot), which can only measure your antibodies—indicating prior exposure. The sensitivity of most of these commercially available antibody tests has been so low that they may miss many cases—producing a lot of false negatives (as was the case with Matt) and sometimes—but far less often—false positives. In fact, the sickest people with Lyme symptoms are often the least likely to test positive using just antibody testing alone. This is because they may have a higher bacterial load that suppresses the immune response, or it can be due to species/strains not used in current antibody tests.

The sensitive high-quality blood culture test that Matt was to have was considered a tremendous breakthrough for the diagnosis of Lyme—finally giving Lyme patients a chance to be diagnosed with greater accuracy. It was deemed to be the gold standard in a disease world that is without reliable testing methods—an issue that has long been at the core of the Lyme controversy. At the same time, not surprisingly, this test has also been embroiled in an ongoing debate about its validity and effectiveness. We were grateful to have access to this additional diagnostic measure.

There are so many reasons why the ELISA and Western blot tests come back with false results. If you've recently been infected, antibodies may not yet be present in your blood. If you've been infected for weeks, months, or years, there may be too few antibodies in your blood for the ELISA test to register. Finally, antibiotics can suppress the level of antibodies in the bloodstream, also making it seem as though you aren't infected.

Advanced Labs is one of several labs in the US that has been denied permission to offer Lyme testing in New York State. For reasons that are unclear, Advanced Labs failed to provide independent validation studies of its test, and the US Centers for Disease Control and Prevention issued a warning for doctors and patients to avoid tests not recommended by the federal agency.

While this seems reasonable, there is so much more to this story than meets the eye. What I've come to learn is that just because a federal agency like the CDC issues a warning, this doesn't mean the warning or concerns are valid. I've come to understand there are always politics and a variety of competing stakeholder interests at play, which makes the task of deciding who to believe ever more difficult and complicated. Knowing what to believe and who to trust would be our daily quandary for years to come.

For now, however, we were grateful to have a doctor who we did trust and who was able to provide both a clinically sound and a laboratory test version of diagnostic certainty.

However, the fact that Matt, in his very ill state, could not get properly tested where he lived, the fact that he had to take a train from New York City to Stamford, Connecticut, where a Dr. S would take the blood sample and then send it to the lab in Pennsylvania, and the fact that in an eighteen-month period of time Matt couldn't get a proper diagnosis from any one of the twenty-plus specialists he saw, were among the first indications of the medical madness we were about to face.

It was just a matter of days before Matt received his blood culture test results. Results that we hoped would provide even greater assurance.

"Mom, it's Lyme," Matt told me on the phone. "My test came back positive."

I took a deep breath. Held back my tears for the moment. And said, "Okay, Matt, now we know. Now we can get you better."

We chatted for a bit and agreed to speak again later that day. We both needed to process the news and gather ourselves. Matt had to get back to work. It was a Friday, and I had the day off from my clinical practice. I called Jeff to tell him the news. I told my daughter and my sister. And then I crawled into bed, where I cried, and cried, and cried. And then cried some more. The tears were endless.

Who was going to look after Matt? I was so far away.

Given the unknown trajectory of this disease, I couldn't just assume that his beautiful partner, Shayna, would be his sturdiest and best support. She was and continues to be just that. She has handled these past few years with such ease and grace and so much love for Matt, and for that I am eternally grateful.

Facing a New, Frightening, and Unfamiliar Journey

Now that Matt was in good hands with Dr. R, I could finally let go, and let go I did—sinking into a deep, dark depression. Or perhaps the most broken of hearts.

Poet Hazrat Inayat Khan said, "God breaks the heart again and again until it stays open."

As Buddhist nun Pema Chödrön says in her book *The*

Places That Scare You, "Sometimes this broken heart gives birth to anxiety and panic, sometimes to anger, resentment and blame. But under the hardness of that armour there is the tenderness of genuine sadness. This continual ache of the heart is a blessing that when accepted fully can be shared with all."[13]

It feels like I have been here before. This place of grief, terror, anger, resentment, and brokenheartedness. I have experienced these feelings a few times too many in my life. Each time I've been in this dark place, my heart- and soul-crushing break was triggered by a huge emotional loss. This time I have chosen to share it—in the hopes of healing myself and others.

Loss is a tough thing to master. Especially when your only models are a grandmother who screamed during her husband's burial—in a voice so shrill, so loud, and so ear piercing that even the dead were scared stiff. And a mother who had a complete breakdown when her husband, my father, was sick and dying.

While life is always about loss and change, it seems as though we never really get good at it. Or, at least I never have.

My first heart-shattering experience was when my father died. I was twenty-five. He was my rock, or so I believed. Witnessing his three-year illness, and his untimely death at the age of fifty-seven (my age as I write these words) was a horrifying, life-changing experience.

The second time was when we lost our house due to a financial betrayal. The third was when my husband lost his business, thanks to some less than honorable partners. All very dark times.

But nothing, and I do mean nothing, could have prepared me for *this*. My heart has been so broken open, so completely shattered, there is no chance of it ever closing again.

When I wasn't at work, I was at home, falling into the dark abyss of Lyme research. The deeper I fell into the rabbit hole of Lyme literacy, the more anxious, sad, and helpless I felt. It was overwhelming to have to absorb so much information and have no one to bounce it off of. The task felt daunting. I understood I was entering a world that was unlike anything I had ever known before.

I read daily. Every evening after work. As I was falling asleep. Mornings before work. On weekends. I was overloaded with complex scientific data, I was immobilized by this daunting task, and I was flooded with tears and pain that I could not contain. My grief was ever present. Ever palpable. As was my burden of worry and fear.

There was so much to read. So much to understand. Everything was layered in scientific jargon, medical debate, political controversy, and endless confusion. It was so difficult to determine what was true and what was not. I couldn't help but get lost in the vortex of research while dealing with a daily onslaught of traumatic moments as my son continued to feel so unwell.

I studied some of the top Lyme sources—ILADS, Dr. Horowitz, Dr. Klinghardt, Dr. Burrascano, Dr. Cameron, The Better Health Guy, Lyme stats, CanLyme, and more.

I couldn't stop. I needed to know what we were up against.

Matt also has a persevering, tenacious character and is blessed with a logical mind. He began keeping a journal of his symptoms, which was a very sound way of coping. It was also useful in allowing Dr. R to help him more effectively.

June 11–17th—First week of treatment I started taking Cefdinir 300mg 2x per day. After one day I noticed a marked improvement in energy and mood. While *anxiety persisted it was more mild but depression and overall malaise was lifted rapidly. Also, I noticed a difference in gastrointestinal functioning as previously my stomach was loose, since starting antibiotics I feel a bit bloated and constipated at times but not to a concerning degree at this point. Unfortunately, the neck pains, muscle cramps/knots and headache symptoms saw little to no improvement. I should note that I continue to take Amitriptyline now at 30mg per day with Klonopin <1mg max per day but usually <0.5mg per day for symptom management. However, Klonopin was effective only for the first week or so in mitigating the headache symptoms. Further I continue to take supplements including fish oil, probiotics (Florastor and Culturelle), vit D3 10000IU, alpha lipoic acid, Genesa total amino solution, magnesium taurate, himalaya herbs stress care, migraine support formula, melatonin for sleep, megafood multivitamin, and body bio PC. I have ordered two supplements recommended by doctor R and will begin them when they arrive.*

June 18–19th—I just began taking Zithromax (250mg 2x per day) and oddly I am now feeling worse than just being on Cefdinir alone. I woke up this morning with that feeling like my sleep wasn't restful again. I also have seen a return of my headaches that rotate from being throbbing to just clouding and dizzying. I should note that I have been trying to reduce the amount of Klonopin having taken only 0.25mg the last two days whereas I was previously taking 0.5mg/day on average. I am looking to wean off Klonopin so that I can rely solely on the Amitriptyline, which is a better long-term migraine prophylactic. So, it is possible I feel worse only because of that and not the addition of Zithromax. One other change to note is that I just received my supply of Soothe & Relaxx (for mood and joints) and Transfer Factor LymPlus (for immune function) and started to take it last night. I have read that the Borrelia bacteria feeds off of glucosamine, which is an ingredient of Soothe & Relaxx so I wonder if that may have a negative effect while the bacteria is still present in my system.

__June 20th__—Last night I decided to increase my Amitriptyline dosage to 40mg given I don't believe it has been helpful with the headaches thus far and the neu-rologist noted the therapeutic dose tends to be at least "30mg or so." This morning I woke up a bit groggy but feeling a bit better than yesterday, although not as good as last week (my first week on Cefdinir). The headache today is less uncomfortable than yesterday, but the whole off-balance/dizzy sensation remains. Also the knot in the back right side of my neck seems to be back and is quite tender.

__June 21st–23rd__—Over the weekend I tried to com-pletely stop Klonopin having taken only 0.125mg 2x/day for a few days in a row; I felt OK, but on Sunday was feeling a bit cloudy headed and dizzy especially when up and walking; today I woke up at 5:30am and felt like I was only half asleep until my alarm and when finally having to get up felt a bit anxious and my back and neck were very stiff and sore; on my way to work I started to get dizzy and more anxious and finally relented once at the office and took 0.125mg of Klonopin at 9:20am and *felt some degree of relief within 20min; it is now 2pm and my neck and head are really bothering me and I feel a bit dizzy when I get up and walk; I don't believe that Elavil is having much of an effect other than making me more sleepy at night and sometimes in the daytime.*

June 24th–*Today I woke up feeling very anxious and shaky. I am now at work and feel anxious, nauseous and generally sick. I took 0.125mg of Klonopin again this morning, which may have helped slightly, but I still feel awful about 2 hours after the dose. I saw Dr. M today who offers vitamin IV capabilities, given this has been recommended to me by both several patients and practitioners who have experience treating Lyme. The IV contained mainly vitamin C but also had other vitamins/minerals such as B12, B6, magnesium, glutathione, etc. Immediately after treatment I felt worse with a heavy head and shaky/weak muscles especially in my neck. The malaise lifted within 30min and I felt a degree of improvement in my energy, although the headache remained. I believe the initial worsening of symptoms was likely due to a die off effect.*

June 25th–*Again this morning I woke up feeling anxious with my heart racing and feeling shaky. I took Klonopin (0.25mg), which took off the edge but feel an overall sense of malaise. It almost feels like hypoglycemia given the heart racing, shakiness, and almost woozy/foggy headache. This continued throughout the shakiness and woozy headache continued throughout the day. I also felt some cognitive symptoms like poor concentration and being somewhat forgetful/out* *of it. Symptoms did seem to improve as I consciously hydrated, however. From what I've read this was likely the height of my first 'herx' reaction.*

A Cursory Glance at Chronic Lyme Disease

By now, I had read a dozen books, hundreds of articles, and many websites devoted to the subject of chronic Lyme disease. I was becoming *Lyme literate.*

However, the more I read, and the more I studied, the less certain of anything I could be. While this is often the case in life, this is especially true of Lyme. There *is no certainty* about any aspect of this disease. Be it the testing methods, treatment methods, healing metrics, deciphering the cause—it's all an indeterminate mess.

While I have come to understand that chronic Lyme disease is one of the most controversial, complicated, politically corrupt disease entities in the history of medicine, at this earliest stage in my research, I tried to understand Lyme in its cursory form. Like the sound bites we get from the media. At the same time, as I found myself delving into the darker, more complex underbelly of this disease, I began to understand that I was being pulled into an alternate universe—one I had no choice but to enter. It felt so deep and unending, I often wondered how Matt and I would ever get out.

I have people constantly telling me that they read this about Lyme or heard that about Lyme and how great it is that the media is starting to cover it more often.

To this I say ignore all that you hear. The media thus far is just as uninformed, misinformed, backward-thinking, and decades behind on this subject, merely echoing a broken medical system. For all the awareness that the media is currently providing, it is often more damaging due to its inaccuracies and complete lack of investigative work and deeper analysis. We're clearly up against a propaganda machine that has been disseminating disinformation for decades.

Here I offer a cursory glance at this crazy, mad, confusing, directionless, unanswerable disease known as chronic Lyme.

But first, an important caveat. Be careful of the sources from which you glean information about chronic Lyme disease. This is the most controversial medical disease of modern times—even more so than HIV/AIDS in the early 1980s. The sources you think should be reliable are *not*. The sources that seem obscure and on the fringe may understand this disease best.

Everything is backward, sideways, and upside down in Lymeland. What you think makes sense gets turned on its head—over and over and over again, until nothing makes sense at all.

You've been warned.

The A to Z of Chronic Lyme
In the beginning...

Lyme disease was first publicly recognized in Lyme, Connecticut, more than forty years ago. However, much to their surprise, researchers have since discovered ticks fossilized in amber proving that the bacteria that causes it may have been lurking around for fifteen million years, long before any humans walked on Earth.[14]

Not only that. A research team from the University of Bath proved that Lyme disease, in fact, came from Europe—originating from before the Ice Age.[15] After DNA researchers probed bacteria inside one of the world's most famous mummies, they sequenced his genome. This revealed—among other findings—that Ötzi may have been a carrier of Lyme disease.[16]

In her book *Cure Unknown: Inside the Lyme Epidemic*, Pamela Weintraub tells us that the first American physician to document what would soon be called Lyme disease was a Milwaukee dermatologist named Rudolph Scrimenti who successfully treated a Lyme patient with intramuscular penicillin.

The next important player in this Lyme story was a woman named Polly Murray who in her book, *The Widening Circle: A Lyme Disease Pioneer Tells Her Story*, informs us of her family's struggle with this disease fifty-five years ago. Polly, an artist and mother of four who lived in Old Lyme, Connecticut, and members of her family were afflicted by a "mysterious illness." Her book—not unlike mine, and so many others—is an account of her struggle to convince doctors that her family's illness was real and that they were not malingerers or hypochondriacs.

Murray was accused of being a "doctor chaser," so she began to do her own research. (Sounds eerily familiar and simply outrageous that so little has changed decades later.)

In November 1975, Murray reported forty-three cases of children and adults around Lyme, Connecticut, who had mysterious, debilitating symptoms. Polly herself had been having severe health issues for almost two decades. By the time she finally got the attention of public health authorities, she and her family had been suffering alone, without proper medical attention, for a very long time.

Enter Dr. Allen Steere, a rheumatology resident at Yale who had spent some time at the CDC in Atlanta. He was asked to investigate and determine what this mysterious illness was all about.

Murray explained the myriad of symptoms she had been experiencing for years, including fevers, swollen glands, systemic pain, a debilitating stiff neck, numbness in her hands, skin rashes, nausea, diarrhea, constant fatigue, and more. Penicillin, she believed, seemed to be the only thing that improved some of her symptoms for a time.

After his initial investigations, Steere explained to the public on an NBC News report that Lyme was self-limiting, that aspirin was helpful, and that there was nothing to be overly concerned about.[17]

Before long, the "official" Lyme disease public relations campaign was launched and we were faced with what would become the CDC's decades-old party line:

"Lyme is hard to catch, easy to diagnose, and easy to cure."

From the start, the nation's leading Lyme disease experts would have everyone believe that Lyme was practically a nonissue.

Thomas Grier, a distinguished microbiologist and researcher in borreliosis diseases, notes in "A Short Historical Perspective of Lyme Disease" that it was from the time of the very first outbreak that many untrue facts were disseminated by the CDC.

Grier lists the many falsehoods we were told from the start as follows:

Lyme is only an Arthritic disease; it is easily cured with two weeks of tetracycline or doxycycline; it is only transmitted by infected Ixodes dammini ticks; it is only found regionally in the NE USA; the only host reservoir is the white-footed mouse; there is only one species of Borrelia causes Lyme disease; Borrelia burgdorferi is not related to Tick Borne Relapsing Fevers and is a separate disease;

unlike Syphilis it does not cross the placental barrier from infected mother to child; unlike Syphilis it does not enter the brain; all patients get a Bull's-eye Rash; Lyme bacteria do not enter nor inhabit human cells (intracellular disease); two-tiered testing is better than a single Lyme test and is 99 % accurate in Late Stage Neurological Lyme; adopting the Dressler Criteria for Western Blot Testing using five out of 10 selected bands is better than Western Blot interpretation based on known exclusive bands including bands 31 and 34 kda. (OSP-A and OSP-B); Lyme disease does not persist after two weeks of antibiotics but IgM antibodies can persist for months after treatment and are no longer significant; Lyme disease is not a Relapsing Illness; a Bull's-Eye rash is not diagnostic of Lyme disease; Lyme tests using the B-31 strain of Borrelia burgdorferi are adequate to diagnose all cases of Lyme disease even though six other species of Borrelia are now pathogenic in humans and cause Lyme disease.

Grier posits, "Imagine your self as a doctor who was completely new to understanding Lyme disease. Do you see how these completely untrue statements about Lyme-disease could lead to causing patient harm? Understand that most of these statements in the early days of Lyme disease were stated as absolute facts, and not something not to be debated or disputed!"[18]

Herein lies the foundation on which the story of chronic Lyme disease was falsely built.

In 1977, Steere published the first of many articles on his findings. He and several coauthors reported "An epidemic form of arthritis has been occurring in eastern Connecticut at least since 1972, with the peak incidence of new cases in the summer and early fall."[19]

It wasn't until the early 1980s that the spirochetal bacteria known as *B. burgdorferi* was recognized by namesake Dr. Willy Burgdorfer, a Swiss microbiologist, as the actual cause of the Lyme outbreak, and the name of the disease was changed from Lyme arthritis to Lyme. It's important to note that Burgdorfer noticed similarities to syphilis, which is also caused by a spirochete, presents with a similarly wide set of symptoms, and is treated with antibiotics.

During the forty-plus years since Polly Murray first brought this mysterious disease to the public's attention, Lyme has been the subject of outrageous controversy—and a great deal of untold suffering.

One of the best resources on the history of Lyme disease is a book called *Everything You Need to Know About Lyme Disease and Other Tick-Borne Disorders, Second Edition*, by Karen Vanderhoof-Forschner, with a foreword by the discoverer and namesake of the pathogen of this disease, Dr. Willy Burgdorfer.

Karen Forschner, who lost her son, Jamie, to Lyme disease in 1991—at the tender age of six—has been at the forefront of this war since the first known outbreak in Old Lyme, Connecticut. Karen and her husband, Tom, founded the first Lyme disease advocacy group in 1988, known as The Lyme Borreliosis Foundation, and later known as the Lyme Disease Foundation. Karen was also responsible for garnering a great deal of attention from the media and the scientific community in those early years. I don't know where she is today, but from one mother to another, I thank her for leading the charge for all these years.

It is a perversion of justice that little has changed or improved within the medical community and the political forces surrounding this disease in all these years. We're still trying to get the IDSA to change their guidelines. We're still trying to get infectious-disease doctors to diagnose and treat this disease with even a modicum of interest. We're still trying to get the CDC and the FDA to approve more reliable and accurate testing methods.

The political roadblocks to this disease have been large and immovable as you will come to see in the chapters ahead.

No Bigger than a Poppy Seed

I'd never had a reason to give a single thought to the eight-legged arachnid known as the *tick*. That is, until my son got sick. What I've since learned is that the tick, no bigger than a poppy seed, can *wreck you for life*.

We *all* need to be on high alert.

Ticks are bloodsucking external parasites of humans, pets, livestock, and wild animals. They are also vectors of a wide variety of disease-causing organisms. There are 889 species of ticks worldwide.[20]

The *Borrelia burgdorferi (Bb)* spirochete—the bacterial infection that manifests as Lyme disease—is a parasite that lives in deer, white-footed mice, and other rodents. The spirochete is transmitted from one animal to another through the bite of an infected tick. Tick species willingly suck blood from almost any animal they encounter.

In the United States, two members of the *Ixodes* family of ticks—the black-legged tick *(Ixodes scapularis)* and the Western black-legged tick *(Ixodes pacificus)*, more commonly known as deer ticks—are the most well-established carriers from animals to humans.

In Canada, we have approximately forty species of ticks, and only a few of them can transmit Lyme disease. Which is more than enough. Next to the deer tick, the Western black-legged tick is the second-most common Borrelia-carrying tick in Canada. As its Latin name suggests, this tick is found mainly on the Pacific coast.

Ticks have a life cycle of two years starting with the egg, and growing into larvae, nymph, and adult stages. It's the two later stages—nymph and adult—that appear to be primarily responsible for transmission of *Bb* to susceptible large animal hosts, including humans. It is said that larvae can transmit *Bb* to humans also. At this stage, ticks are the size of the head of a pin.

A tick feeds on blood by climbing onto vegetation and using its forelegs to feel and grab a host. When it attaches to its host—meaning *you*—the tick has a special way of anaesthetizing the spot they feed on so that you never even know that they've attached themselves, let alone potentially given you a dreadful disease. They are stealth from the moment they target you.

When *Bb* was first discovered in 1982, researchers believed there was just one strain of the infectious spirochetal bacterium. Since then, they have discovered there are about one hundred strains in the US alone and three hundred worldwide.

While commonly found in wooded areas, ticks can be found almost anywhere because they are carried by birds and other animals they feed on.

I've come to understand that ticks are only the beginning of this *Lyme Madness* story. The challenges extend so far beyond tick awareness and tick bite prevention. When people ask, "Where did your son get bitten?" I want to reply, "If you only understood that such a question is often impossible to answer, that the tick bite is so far back in our rearview mirror, and that ticks are only a fraction of the overwhelming obstacles that we face in this four-plus-year medical odyssey."

Lyme Is a Do-It-Yourself Disease

As Kris Newby, producer of the renowned, award-winning documentary *Under Our Skin*, told me, "Chronic Lyme is a do-it-yourself disease. You have to diagnose it yourself, understand it yourself, choose treatment protocols yourself, heal yourself." With chronic Lyme, there are very few experts in this world to rely on. Sufferers are forced to teach themselves and treat themselves.

We are all overwhelmed by the lack of knowledge about this disease. Even Lyme-literate doctors don't have many of the answers we need. And when we turn to them for help, they look puzzled and unsure about how to direct their patients. If you recall, Matt's first Lyme-literate doctor with decades of experience responded to our queries about recovery with a question of his own: "How many angels can dance on the head of a pin?"

Lyme is a complex disease, with a myriad of coinfections and varying states of immunity and symptomatology. The frontline treatment protocol among Lyme-literate doctors consists of a very long course of antibiotics that are efficacious for some, and not well tolerated by others.

So we're left to keep reading and researching and seeking and guessing what might work. It's a very desperate and lonely search with very few answers. Never in modern medicine has there been a pandemic that has been so summarily dismissed by doctors and left for the sufferers to figure out and fix on their own.

Faulty Testing

It is commonly known—at least among those medical practitioners who actually treat Lyme, and among those who suffer from it—that the diagnostic testing methods most commonly used for this disease are flawed, unstable, unreliable, and produce an inordinate number of false negatives.

Lab tests for Lyme disease include a CDC-mandated two-tier process:

1. **Enzyme-linked immunosorbent assay (ELISA) test.** Designed to detect antibodies to *B. burgdorferi*.

2. **Western blot test.** If the ELISA test is positive, this test is usually done to confirm the diagnosis. In this two-step approach, the Western blot detects antibodies to several proteins of *B. burgdorferi*.

According to CanLyme—the Canadian Lyme Disease Foundation—one of the most-trusted sources,

> *Lyme disease is a challenge to diagnose and can be even tougher to treat. Whether you have reason to suspect infection, or you've just been diagnosed, it's important to learn all you can about this complex illness.*

> *Lyme disease testing is not an exact science: patients often receive negative test results when the disease is actually present, and false positives are also possible, though less common. Experienced doctors recommend that Lyme disease be diagnosed clinically, meaning diagnosis is based on an evaluation of your risk and your symptoms.*

CanLyme wisely advises that people not get discouraged by a negative diagnosis, but rather seek out second and even third opinions if necessary.[21]

Lorraine Johnson, JD, MBA, and author of the Lyme Policy Wonk blog at Lymedisease.org, reported on April 18, 2014, that the CDC officially announced it recommends that only laboratory tests cleared or approved by the FDA be used to aid in the routine diagnosis of Lyme disease.

"This is a shame," says Johnson. "Waiting for FDA approval suppresses innovation in Lyme testing and furthers the interests of those who have vested interests in the current flawed lab tests, which miss as many cases as they detect. Neither of these is good for patients."

Johnson adds, "The CDC recently revised its case numbers from 30,000 to 300,000. These numbers tell us that there is a lot more Lyme around that is not captured by the surveillance system, which relies heavily on flawed FDA-approved tests. They also tell us that commercially vested interests and the researchers they consult with may have a stake in keeping the status quo in lab testing regardless of how bad the tests are."[22]

A doctor who shall remain nameless said, "There seems to be a lot of uncertainty about interpretation of Lyme testing, particularly Western blot interpretation. The criteria set by the CDC was chosen in 1994 and by design is purposely very restrictive, with specificity of 99.9 percent, which means that false-positive CDC results are virtually unheard of."

The bottom line is this: If you are presented with a negative finding and yet you are suffering with a spectrum of misdiagnosed or undiagnosed neurological and systemic symptoms that seem to mirror those of Lyme, search for a Lyme-literate doctor (MD or ND) to help you with a proper clinical diagnosis.

What Is Chronic Lyme Disease?

First, allow me to make a distinction between early Lyme disease and late-stage or chronic Lyme disease. (Not to mention post-treatment Lyme disease syndrome, which refers to those who experience prolonged, subjective symptoms following Lyme or, better still, a medical euphemism for, *"You may have had Lyme, you may not have had Lyme. Either way, we treated you for twenty-eight days, and oh dear you're still sick. Not our problem. Go home, see a psychiatrist, take an antidepressant. It's all in your head—we've done our job, too bad for you, nothing more we can do."*)

Early Lyme disease is this: if you are lucky enough, and I do mean lucky enough, to see the tick that bites you, or to see the infamous and often nonexistent red circular rash known as the bull's-eye—and if you get to a doctor immediately, and get treated with a twenty-eight-day regime of the appropriate antibiotics—then you may catch the illness in time, before it crosses the blood-brain barrier. If you don't catch the illness in time, and it has the opportunity to cross your blood-brain barrier, then it will almost certainly create all kinds of long-term, persistent neurological, cardio, and arthritic symptomatology. The majority of stakeholders in this mad and confusing Lyme story agree on this to some extent.

Where it gets complicated, muddled, and completely confusing is when we are referring to chronic Lyme disease (stages one, two, and three of this disease)—when it is *not* caught or treated in the early stages. This population is thought to make up at least 80 percent of all Lyme sufferers. Chronic or late-stage Lyme disease is the condition that the medical community is denying altogether, and the response is no better than it is for those deemed to have post-treatment Lyme disease syndrome: negation, mockery, misinformation, inane excuses, rationalizations, marginalization, and basically showing the patient the door.

The definition, treatment, and the very existence of chronic Lyme disease depends entirely on who you choose to believe. My obvious bias is toward the fringe of medicine, as the good majority of the allopathic medical system has all but abandoned its constituents. Their systemic denial, negation, abandonment, and invalidation of sufferers worldwide has given those of us in the Lyme world little choice but to find our answers elsewhere.

As Lyme sufferers gather together and share intelligences, resources, treatment protocols, and the like, certain members of the medical community have had the audacity to refer to sufferers as "Lyme loonies."[23]

Talk about adding insult to injury—*unconscionable*.

The powers that be deny the suffering and then bully the sufferer. Malignant, pathological narcissism and medical industry greed at its very worst.

Is it all to find ways to monetize chronic Lyme with a new vaccine perhaps? Or to monetize a wide spectrum of misdiagnosed chronic illnesses that may, in fact, all be interrelated and less profitable under one classification, where lesser priced antibiotics are the drug of choice?

While it's difficult to put all the puzzle pieces together, it is more than obvious to all of us in Lymeland that the powers that be simply don't want to acknowledge the existence of chronic Lyme. If they did admit to its existence, let alone its enormity, it would likely require billions of dollars to insure, possibly bankrupting the system. And then, of course, they'd have to admit to the many falsehoods and questionable misappropriation of funds that they may be responsible for over the past four decades.

Not a lot of upside for them it seems.

Forty years later, the denial and misrepresentations are far too big to admit. Therein lie the political underpinnings of the madness that is chronic Lyme.

About the Bacteria

Here is the "CliffsNotes" version of the detailed bacteriology behind Lyme.

Chronic Lyme disease is a systemic infection that causes tick-borne relapsing fever and immunosuppression. The infection is caused by a tick bite (among other means of transmission) that is not treated immediately—simply because the victim is not aware of the tick that bites him—thus poisoning our bodies with a bacterium known as *Borrelia burgdorferi*.

This bacterium is composed of spiral-shaped spirochetes and is unlike any bacteria ever studied before. It exists in three distinct forms:

- Cyst

- Spheroplast (or "L form," which doesn't have a cell wall—commonly called cell wall deficient [CWD])

- Typical spiral-shaped bacteria form that has a cell wall and flagella[24]

Lyme Borrelia has been proven to be pleomorphic—that is, it changes in shape or size in response to environmental conditions. Atypical cyst, granula forms, and colony-like aggregation of spirochetes into large masses have been observed when the organism is under stress. Once environmental bacteria return to normal, Borrelia bacteria revert back to their usual spiral shape.[25]

The Lyme spirochete can lay dormant in the system for years, in a nonmetabolic state. So just because a person is symptom free for a period of time, that doesn't mean they are not infected.

With the right conditions, the bacteria become activated. Once activated, they have high motility, meaning they can swim efficiently through the bloodstream and human tissue. In addition, Borrelia bacteria have a stealthy coat of armor—allowing the bacteria to hide from the immune system. It takes twice as long as most other bacteria to divide themselves, which means antibiotics take much longer to find and kill these bacteria.

The Lyme spirochete can show up in the brain, eyes, joints, skin, spleen, liver, gastrointestinal tract, bladder, and other organs, traveling through capillaries and cell membranes by attaching itself to the human cell's tip, and then working its way *into* the cell, evading the immune system and antibiotics. It can easily travel through the blood-brain barrier, creating neurological symptoms and relapsing fevers. The brain is designed to limit what can enter, as it has no immune system of its own. This stealthy Borrelia bacterium has found a way to override this protective system, causing neurological inflammation and a whole host of cognitive and physical symptoms.

Sunnybrook Health Sciences Centre in Toronto, Ontario (my hometown), has just announced a historic breakthrough. Dr. Todd Mainprize, in concert with other neuroscientists, has successfully broken the blood-brain barrier, opening the way for revolutionary new treatments for brain cancer, Alzheimer's, depression, stroke, Parkinson's, and more—including chronic Lyme disease, I presume.[26]

Three Diametrically Opposed Theories

As complicated as chronic Lyme disease is, what is even more complex are the political and medical underpinnings driving this disease.

There are essentially two factions at war.

On the one side there is the Centers for Disease Control and Prevention (CDC) who, together with the Infectious Diseases Society of America (IDSA), have firmly set the treatment, the medical definition, and guidelines for this disease. Most conventional medical doctors follow their lead, leaving chronic Lyme sufferers with little medical support.

On the other side is the International Lyme and Associated Diseases Society (ILADS) a nonprofit advocacy group and interdisciplinary medical society which advocates for greater acceptance of chronic Lyme disease and whose members are the only true medical support system for chronic Lyme sufferers. Some of the ILADS members have been met with punitive measures as a result of their medical treatment of Lyme.

The CDC and IDSA have worked closely together for decades—their theories and guidelines have gotten in the way of any real progress taking place in the treatment of chronic Lyme disease.

According to the CDC website, it is "the nation's health protection agency, working 24/7 to protect America from health and safety threats, both foreign and domestic." It says this yet offers so little information about Lyme disease that is helpful. What the CDC does offer on its site simply does not line up with the experience of most Lyme sufferers, especially when it says, "Most cases of Lyme disease can be treated successfully with a few weeks of antibiotics."[27]

The IDSA—a 9,000-plus member society including

practicing clinicians, scientists, and researchers, public health officials, hospital epidemiologists, and ID specialists around the world—tells us that "most cases of Lyme disease are successfully treated with a few weeks of antibiotics."[28]

More specifically, the IDSA tells us that "adult patients with late neurologic disease affecting the central or peripheral nervous system should be treated with intravenous ceftriaxone for 2 to 4 weeks."[29] These twenty-eight-day IDSA antibiotic treatment guidelines have been at the heart of the Lyme Wars controversy for decades.

According to the CDC and the IDSA—both of which we would imagine are the authorities on this subject—Lyme disease is a tick-borne infection that is "difficult to catch, easy to diagnose, and easy to cure." Together, these two powerful medical authorities have teamed up to dismiss the possibility of the persistence of symptoms over time, and unequivocally deny the real risk posed by this chronic Lyme pandemic, which exists in eighty countries worldwide and affects upward of tens of millions of sufferers—including between 300,000 and a million in the US alone.

To repeat, both the CDC and the IDSA insist that this easy-to-diagnose and easy-to-cure disease requires no more than twenty-eight days of antibiotic treatment and—*abracadabra*—you're *cured*.

To make matters even worse, some very large educational institutions, such as Yale University, have maintained a strong position on Lyme disease being easily detected and treated, with a high degree of success.

If only this were the case.

If chronic Lyme disease is so easy to diagnose, why did more than twenty medical doctors miss this diagnosis for my son? And why do the majority of chronic Lyme sufferers

consult with anywhere between ten and thirty specialists—
sometimes as many as eighty or more—before knowing that
their true diagnosis is chronic Lyme? Why have so many people succumbed to this disease—either by lack of treatment,
or by their own hand—due to years of suffering and years of
medical neglect?

In opposition to the CDC and IDSA, ILADS promotes
the idea that persistence of chronic Lyme does in fact exist,
and that it requires far more than twenty-eight days of antibiotic treatment to put patients into a state of remission.

According to ILADS members, Lyme disease is a multisystemic disease, which can affect virtually every tissue
and every organ of the human body. It is a disease that can
be mild for some and devastating for others. It can cripple
and disable and fog your mind. It can affect anyone and
everyone—including your family dog. (Ironically, by the way,
it's far easier to get diagnosed and treated if you are of the
canine versus human species.)

As in all wars, the two opposing sides could not be further apart in their thinking.

Now, to complicate matters further, there is a third
faction working hard to get the 'real truth' about chronic
Lyme disease heard and considered by the United States
Department of Justice (USDOJ). This group's fearless leader
is Kathleen Dickson, a former Pfizer analytical chemist
turned whistleblower of the shortlived LYMErix vaccine.
According to Dickson, chronic Lyme disease is a "Relapsing
fever borreliosis, post-sepsis syndrome that features chronically reactivated herpesviruses, which are well known to
lead to the 'New Great Imitator' outcomes."

Dr. Holly Ahern, an associate professor of microbiology at State University of New York Adirondack in

Queensbury, reports that "Lyme is the most misunderstood disease since AIDS."[30]

Writer and Lyme sufferer David Michael Conner offers a thought-provoking piece in the Huffington Post, "Is Lyme the new AIDS? Part Two: Life with Lyme and Controversies." In it, he tells us that while chronic Lyme disease and HIV/AIDS are very different diseases, they are similar in their severity and in their politics. Here, he also tells us that past ILADS president, Dr. Raphael Stricker, wrote him a note saying, "I often tell patients, Lyme Disease does not kill you the way AIDS does, but it often makes you wish it did."

It is not uncommon for those who are intensely ill with chronic Lyme to wish their lives were over. The pain, the suffering, the chronic fatigue, the anxiety and depression, the lack of understanding, the underrecognition, undertreatment, and next to no compassion from the majority of the medical profession would cause the strongest of sufferers want to give up the fight. For most, it's a wearying battle of slow and torturous decline.

Chronic Lyme disease tends to be so varied in its clinical presentation that, aside from the political and medical opposition to this disease, its highly variable symptom presentation also makes it difficult to diagnose for those who are ill-trained in this infectious disease, which happens to be the majority of doctors. But most strikingly, it's nearly impossible to recognize a disease when the disease itself is believed among the majority of the medical community to be nonexistent.

Take a poll here in Canada—most doctors will tell you that ticks don't cross the border.

Yet chronic Lyme disease could not be more real. Apart

from my own son, I've witnessed the suffering of so many.

And while I would never want to minimize Matt's suffering, and he has suffered terribly over the duration of these past few years, he is one of the "lucky" ones who has been able to continue to function. In this time, he has managed to not only keep his job, but also get promoted. I know plenty of people who have been bedridden, wheelchair bound, with feeding tubes, experiencing unyielding seizures, and excruciating, unrelenting pain due to Lyme. This is not Matt. And for that I am profoundly grateful.

But I am also terribly saddened by the suffering and deaths—yes, deaths—of Lyme friends that I have made along the way.

Matt's illness has been primarily neurological. At his worst, Matt has been dizzy, woozy, faint, systemically weak, sleepless, nauseous, anxious, and fatigued for months on end. None of which he would wish on his worst enemy. He likens it to having a chronic flu layered with a wired nervous system, an internal storm that gets more intense at various times. At his best, he has a never-ending brain fog and wooziness that is almost impossible to describe, and very difficult to manage 24/7. But manage he does. Throughout this nightmare, he has shown greater strength, tenacity, and perseverance than I could have ever imagined.

Like us, most sufferers simply want answers. Now.

As long as the medical community continues to be so deeply schismatic and so polar opposite in their approach to this disease, little progress can be made.

Apart from Ticks, How Is Lyme Transmitted?

Lyme disease is a vector-borne illness—from the bite of an infected tick. Some claim that Lyme can also be transmitted from the bites of mosquitoes, fleas, flies, mites, and spiders.

According to Dr. Charles Ray Jones, the world's leading pediatric Lyme disease expert, there are "at least nine species of ticks, 13 species of mites, 15 species of flies, two species of fleas, and numerous wild and domestic animals (including rabbits, rodents, and birds) [that] have been found to carry the spirochete that cause Lyme disease. Lyme Disease symptoms may appear days, weeks, months, or even years after initial infection."[31]

Further evidence suggests that "although Ixodes dammini is the chief vector of B.burgdorferi in the northeastern United States, Wisconsin, and Minnesota, other arthropods, such as mosquitoes, horse flies, and deer flies, have also been found harboring this bacterium."[32]

While the research is not conclusive, some studies and anecdotal evidence tell us that Lyme disease can also be passed from mother to child in utero and through breast milk, blood transfusions, and through sexual intercourse.[33]

"There is always some risk of getting Lyme disease from a tick bite in the woods," internist Dr. Raphael Stricker, one of the researchers involved in the study, said in a press release. "But there may be a bigger risk of getting Lyme disease in the bedroom."[34]

As Dr. Jones warns, "Absence of proof is not proof of absence. And it's better to be safe than sorry."[35]

According to this article,

Not only can Lyme be passed among sexual partners— it might also be passed from mother to child before birth. It's unclear the extent to which this happens.

There's some evidence to suggest that the worst harm to a fetus occurs when the mother is infected during pregnancy rather than prior to conceiving. For this reason, one study suggested that the harm to the fetus is really due to a maternal response to infection rather than fetal infection itself.[36]

The real kicker, I learn, is that there were people who claimed that they were sickened by the LYMErix vaccine itself—the very vaccine that was meant to prevent Lyme back in the early 1990s. I'm told I might lose readers if I talk about vaccines. But vaccines are part of the madness and, therefore, a part of this story.

Many theories abound on how this infectious disease has become a pandemic in eighty countries across the globe, infecting and affecting millions.

On July 18, 1989, *The New York Times* ran an article that asked the question, "Can Lyme disease be spread through blood transfusions as well as by ticks?" The article's author, Dr. Lawrence K. Altman, went on to say, "The answer is not clear and the matter is the subject of increasing concern, despite assurances from health officials that such transmission is highly unlikely. The officials admit that it is theoretically possible, but they note that there have been no documented cases of Lyme disease associated with transfusions."[37]

Lyme Coinfections

To make matters more complicated, chronic Lyme disease is also known as Lyme-MSIDS—Multiple Systemic Infectious Disease Syndrome. This term was coined by Lyme expert Dr. Richard Horowitz—a board-certified internist in Hyde Park, New York, who has treated more than

12,000 chronically ill patients with Lyme disease.

If you suspect that you may have Lyme and any of its coinfections, do a Google search for the *Horowitz Lyme-MSIDS Questionnaire* and complete it. This questionnaire will give you a very clear indication of whether you're in the ballpark.

Chronic Lyme sufferers may have more than one infection—and for many, Lyme is not always the most predominant. So if you thought that Lyme in its *Borrelia burgdorferi* form was all we had to be concerned about, think again. Many Lyme sufferers must also contend with Babesia, Bartonella, and Ehrlichia. Depending on the geographic area, ticks can carry pathogens responsible for mycoplasma, Rocky Mountain spotted fever (also known as rickettsia), tick paralysis, Tick-Borne Relapsing Fever, and more.[38]

There is also a disease called Morgellons that is often associated with chronic Lyme as a coinfection or an opportunistic infection. Naysayers in the scientific community call it a condition of sheer delusion and tactile hallucinations, where sufferers, they claim, falsely believe that they are infested with parasites, bugs, insects, or other pathogens. I encourage you to research Morgellons, view the many photos showing people with open, oozing skin lesions from stem to stern, and tell me how this painful and debilitating condition which can cause fibre like growths on the skin can be anything but real, regardless of the genesis.

In the world of infectious diseases, it seems that there are always new findings. In a study recently published in *The Lancet Infectious Diseases*, Mayo Clinic pathologist Dr. Bobbi Pritt and her colleagues tested more than 100,500 clinical specimens. These specimens—which included such things as blood, cerebrospinal fluid, and tissue—were collected from US patients with suspected Lyme disease between 2003 and 2014. The research confirmed the existence of a new microbe that has, in fact, never been documented before. The researchers propose to name the new species *Borrelia mayonii*.[39]

Lyme Cofactors

The common belief at the surface level of the scientific community and the population at large is that Lyme disease is caused by a tick bite. When you peel back the layers, however, it is important to note that research now suggests that certain vaccine viruses actually enable Lyme disease. The tick bite is only a cofactor.

When I first understood this to be the case, and then watched a video presentation by Dr. Thomas Rau of the Paracelsus Clinic in Switzerland, everything began to make slightly more sense.

In his research, Dr. Rau discovered that not everyone with a tick bite manifests symptoms. He also found that the difference between those who were able to heal themselves and those who could not had viruses and underlying toxicity from heavy metals and mercury. In addition, his research showed that specific vaccine viruses acted as cofactors, including the tick-borne meningoencephalitis vaccine, hepatitis B vaccine, flu vaccine, Coxsackie vaccine, and Epstein-Barr virus (EBV) vaccine.[40]

In fall 2012, Matt had his annual flu shot. While he was not at the peak of health for a few years prior, it was one week *after* he had his flu shot that he began to show a variety of unexplained symptoms.

Matt's intuition kicked in right away. His very first thought as to why he wasn't feeling well was because of the flu shot he had just had. I quickly dismissed this theory at the time, thinking there was no basis to it. Now the picture became clearer for us. Matt's flu shot might very well have been the catalyst for his chronic illness, as was his original guess.

You can read more about vaccines in Chapter 5. But here I need to say that while vaccines, including flu shots, may be safe for the majority of the population, I have come to know with certainty that they are not safe for some. Do doctors ever think to check the health of their patient's immune system before administering vaccines? If not, why not? Why are there no checks and balances in place to determine this? Isn't it a doctor's duty to know whether the patient they are about to immunize is immunosuppressed and possibly susceptible to further immune system damage?

Why Lyme Disease Is Called "The New Great Imitator"

This is what typically happens to an undiagnosed Lyme patient. Please put yourself in their shoes for a moment.

You go to your physician and you complain about a number of vague, seemingly unrelated symptoms. Your physician will then send you to a neurologist, a rheumatologist, an endocrinologist, and so on. Depending on which specialists you consult with, you will likely be diagnosed with any one of the following maladies: depression, generalized anxiety, chronic fatigue syndrome, fibromyalgia, rheumatoid arthritis, multiple sclerosis, ALS, or Parkinson's disease.

You'll be given all kinds of meds, and months later you will not feel any better.

When the treatments don't work, your doctor will insist that you need to see a psychiatrist to deal with your apparent stress or psychosomatic issues.

The irony is that Lyme actually *is* primarily all in your head, as it is a neurological disease that directly affects your brain and nervous system. The psychiatrist will insist that you start psychotropic meds and therapy for your anxiety, depression, and "phantom pain." But it might be much more than stress and childhood issues that are causing you to feel so bad. And I work as a therapist helping people heal childhood wounds every day.

The consequence of this journey comprising one misdiagnosis after another will sentence you to a life of prescription drugs and supplements for a disease you don't have. Sadly, you'll probably never find complete relief from the real cause of your pain and suffering.

For reasons that are complex and multifaceted, chronic Lyme disease is the last thing that the majority of doctors—including infectious-disease specialists—consider.

What makes Lyme even more complicated to diagnose is that it can imitate more than 350 *other* diseases, including multiple sclerosis, Parkinson's, lupus, fibromyalgia, Lou Gehrig's disease (ALS), rheumatoid arthritis, and heart disease (Lyme carditis).

As syphilis in the nineteenth century was known as the Great Imitator, Lyme disease has come to be known as the new "Great Imitator."

In a 1988 PubMed abstract titled "Borrelia burgdorferi in the nervous system: the new 'great imitator,'" author A.R. Pachner draws several parallels between Lyme and syphilis, including "their spirochetal etiology, the ability of the spirochetes to stay alive in human tissue for years, occurrence of clinical manifestations in stages, early disease in the skin and later disease in the brain, and susceptibility to antibiotic treatment. Thus, one can assume that many of the same lessons learned from the centuries of experience with syphilis will apply to Lyme disease."

Here, Pachner also states, "One of these lessons that should be constantly borne in mind is that spirochetal disease of the brain can mimic many other neurological diseases. Thus, the 'effective clinician' must take special care to consider Lyme disease primarily because of the excellent response to antibiotics early in its course in relationship to some of the diseases it mimics."[41]

A researcher from Yamaguchi, Japan, that I spoke with insists that mycoplasma infectious diseases (MID) are *the* missing link for many medical problems, including chronic Lyme disease. Could mycoplasma—a genus of bacteria lacking a cell wall and impervious to common antibiotics—be the underpinning of so many diseases, explaining why Lyme is The Great Imitator?

According to Dr. Dietrich Klinghardt in the documentary *Under Our Skin*, it is now well established that chronic *infection* is an underlying factor in most chronic illnesses. Diseases such as Parkinson's, multiple sclerosis, and chronic fatigue syndrome are all turning out to be expressions of chronic infections. Says Dr. Klinghardt, "Right at the center of that is the ongoing discovery of Lyme disease."

Dr. Klinghardt goes on to say, "We never had, in the last five years, a single Alzheimer's disease, Lou Gehrig's disease/ALS, Parkinson's disease, multiple sclerosis/MS patient who did not test positive for *Borrelia burgdorferi* (Lyme disease bacteria), not a single one!"

Just ask Dr. David Martz about his experience. He was diagnosed with ALS, only to discover as his health spiraled downward—by happenstance, as he connected with a Lyme disease specialist and began taking hard-hitting antibiotics—that his deep fatigue, systemic pain, and inability to get out of bed could be reversed because he was actually suffering from Lyme disease masquerading as ALS.[42]

Dr. Neil Spector—a top Duke oncologist—describes his own painful near-death experience with Lyme disease in his recently published memoir *Gone in a Heartbeat: A Physician's Search for True Healing*. Years of living with undiagnosed Lyme disease left this doctor's heart so badly damaged that he needed a heart transplant. What makes his story so compelling is that even as a prestigious medical professional, he struggled to be heard by his own doctors. His health issues, including arrhythmia and arthritis pain, began in the early 1990s. And even though he lived in an area highly endemic for Lyme, it took years to receive a positive diagnosis for Lyme disease. The way in which he was pushed around, misdiagnosed, and ultimately ignored by the medical establishment mirrors the experience of every Lyme sufferer.

In a Huffington Post piece by singer/songwriter/Lyme sufferer Dana Parish, Spector tells us that Lyme is *"The infectious disease equivalent of cancer"*.

Spector continues,

Throughout the years, there've been a lot of links made between infectious agents and cancer. For anyone who says it's impossible, I'd ask, who would have ever thought thirty years ago that H. Pylori was the causative agent for stomach cancer? Or that HPV virus can cause cervical and head and neck cancers? Or that Epstein Barr can cause lymphoma? So it is not far-fetched to say that a bacteria that causes inflammation can cause the perfect storm for developing a tumor.[43]

Dr. Alan B. MacDonald, a hospital pathologist and diagnostician of microscopic images who was featured in award winning documentary *Under Our Skin*, was the first to discover a link with Borrelia and Alzheimer's. In the documentary, MacDonald tells us,

> *I extracted DNA from 10 Alzheimer brains that came from the Harvard University brain bank. Using molecular methods, I was able to find the DNA of the Spirochete which causes Lyme disease in 7 out of 10 of the Alzheimer brain specimens that I received from Harvard.*[44]

From 1999 to 2001, Dr. Martin Atkinson-Barr tested 150 ALS patients for Lyme disease. According to Dr. Atkinson-Barr, "Effective treatment of late stage ALS is possible with aggressive antibiotic therapy that must include metronidazole. Other researchers have recently reported success in treating early stage ALS with antibiotic therapy."[45]

In a 2015 feature article for *Maclean's* magazine, writer Anne Kingston reports on the new branding by the Multiple Sclerosis Society of Canada—a campaign which leaves us all wondering why it is that Canada ranks first in the world for this chronic degenerative disease.

Kingstone reports that one MS Society billboard reads: "Welcome to MS nation."

The EndMS.ca website says that Canada is the "world leader in hockey, maple syrup and multiple sclerosis. In Canada, you have a greater risk of developing MS than in any other country. Is it our climate? Our diet? A lack of vitamin D?" the site queries.[46]

Dr. Ernie Murakami of Hope, British Columbia, thinks

he knows exactly why the numbers are so high. He believes that many patients who have MS symptoms can, in fact, be suffering from chronic Lyme.

"We have the highest number of MS (patients) in the world and the lowest number of Lyme," says Murakami.[47]

In a PubMed article titled, "Chronic Lyme borreliosis at the root of multiple sclerosis—is a cure with antibiotics attainable?" author, M. Fritszche claims that "Worldwide, MS prevalence parallels the distribution of the Lyme disease pathogen Borrelia (B.) burgdorferi, and in America and Europe, the birth excesses of those individuals who later in life develop MS exactly mirror the seasonal distributions of Borrelia transmitting Ixodes ticks."[48]

According to the National MS Society,

"Lyme disease can cause delayed neurologic symptoms similar to those seen in multiple sclerosis (MS) such as weakness, blurred vision caused by optic neuritis, dysesthesias (sensations of itching, burning, stabbing pain, or 'pins and needles'), confusion and cognitive dysfunction, and fatigue. Lyme disease symptoms may also have a relapsing-remitting course. In addition, Lyme disease occasionally produces other abnormalities that are similar to those seen in MS, including positive findings on magnetic resonance imaging (MRI) scans of the brain and analysis of cerebrospinal fluid (CSF).

These similarities in symptoms and test results have led some people with MS to seek testing for the presence of antibodies to Borrelia, to determine if their neurologic symptoms are the result of Lyme disease or truly MS. The distinction is important because Lyme disease, especially when treated early, often responds to antibiotic therapy, whereas MS does not.[49]

According to an informal study conducted by the Lyme Disease Alliance (LDA), most patients diagnosed with chronic fatigue syndrome (CFS) are actually suffering from Lyme disease. In a study of thirty-one patients diagnosed with CFS, twenty-eight patients, or 90.3 percent, were found to be ill as a result of Lyme.[50]

And those who are Lyme literate would agree that Lyme disease can contribute to every psychiatric disorder in the Diagnostic Symptoms Manual IV (DSM-IV)—including major depressive disorder, generalized anxiety, attention deficit disorder (ADD), obsessive-compulsive disorder (OCD), antisocial personality, panic attacks, anorexia nervosa, autism, and Asperger's syndrome (a form of autism), among others.

Top Lyme disease expert Dr. Richard Horowitz says, "When you include the actual known cases of Lyme, and then you add to it all of these other diseases that are mimicking Lyme disease without good testing, you realize that you may be dealing with millions of people per year who are getting it.

"When you're looking at the future generations of America—playing on the lawn, the mothers transmitting it, the blood supply—the numbers that the CDC are seeing, which we know are underestimates because the tests are not picking it up, you're really dealing with a very major healthcare crisis at this point that has not been properly dealt with."[51]

In a Facebook post, Elsie Gordon says,

"I thought it was hard to get a doctor to believe me when I had fibromyalgia. When I was diagnosed with Lyme, I thought, "Oh, thank god, I have a real disease. They'll

take me seriously now. What's even more nuts ... my doctor is Lyme-averse so I have to pretend I have fibro to get the meds I need to survive. I'm sure glad I got diagnosed with a disease that isn't a disease before I got diagnosed with a disease that doesn't exist."

Even Dogs Get Treated Better

It seems evident to us humans trying to navigate the world of Lyme that, by comparison, dogs have it easy. Dogs don't have to fight for testing like their human counterparts do. They don't have to bump up against medical nonbelievers in the veterinarian world. Dogs even have access to a vaccine known as LymeVax—a two-strain, multiantigen vaccine that induces an antibody response to bacterial proteins OspA and OspC.[52]

Over the course of my research, I've uncovered anecdotal evidence that some people have scored antibiotic medication for Lyme from their dog's veterinarians who, despite the risk to their own professional licenses, were more than willing to help those in dire straits. I've also heard people ask if the diagnostic test for dogs with Lyme works on humans as well. Desperate times, desperate measures.

For obvious reasons, seeking diagnosis and treatment for Lyme disease from your dog's veterinary doctor is not a viable option. No harm in asking, I suppose. But having to even think about getting medical care from your local veterinarian certainly adds one more layer to the madness that is chronic Lyme.

Wake Up, World!

Lyme disease is a pandemic.

My understanding is that a pandemic is an epidemic that occurs over a wide geographic area and affects an exceptionally high proportion of the population. This sounds like chronic Lyme disease to me.

Do we need to shout it from the rooftops? Why isn't anyone protecting us?

With chronic Lyme disease victims likely numbering in the tens of millions worldwide, why isn't the CDC responding? Where are their pandemic preparedness efforts? Why isn't the World Health Organization, along with the CDC, the IDSA, and other stakeholders in the medical-industrial complex, working to control and manage this disease?

Is it because the mortality rate from chronic Lyme disease is not yet high enough for them to bother with it? Is it because lifelong suffering from a vector-borne bacterium is not enough of a crisis to take some real action? Is it because doctors see chronic Lyme victims merely as whiners and malingerers whose suffering is "all in their head"?

Oh yes. It's because *"chronic Lyme disease does not exist."*

3. LOST IN LYMELAND

Have I gone mad? I'm afraid so…You're entirely bonkers but I'll tell you a secret—all of the best people are.

—ALICE'S ADVENTURES IN WONDERLAND

I'm lost in Lymeland.

As Dante once said, "In the middle of the journey of our life, I came to myself within a dark wood where the straight way was lost."

The picture keeps unfolding. I travel deeper and deeper. Into a dark and unfamiliar place.

Before long, I fall fast into an overwhelming abyss—a bottomless pit of research where it feels impossible to keep track of who said what. So hard to decipher what's real, what's made up, who to believe, what to believe, who are the good guys, and who are the bad. So little direction in my quest to discover what is sound or safe or true.

I read about Lyme daily—every chance I get. I can't look away or shut it off. And I feel terribly alone on this journey. There is no navigational system to rely on. Only our own hard work, research, and intuition.

I feel like I'm drowning. Drowning in research. Drowning in confusion. Drowning in decision making. Without a map or a GPS.

Matt and I are partners on this medical odyssey. Trying to stay afloat while living in an alternate universe. Speaking a foreign language that no one in our circle knows. Having been plunged into a strange and perplexing land, we're doing our best to immerse ourselves and feverishly catch up on all that we need to understand. It's beginning to look like we're stuck here for an indefinite period of time. And it looks like we're pretty much on our own.

The recovery picture feels a great deal bleaker than Dr. R is letting on. Do we follow him blindly? We can't. We need to keep reading, learning, understanding.

I hyperfocus. I am unable to concentrate on little else. I make it a full-time job. The more I read, the less I know or understand. The research is endless. The answers hard to find. So many conflicting reports. Who are the true experts? Who can I trust? The mountains of evidence based on double-blind studies are being trashed—called fraudulent, unreliable. The only thing that matters to me is that I solve this and solve it soon.

I continue my professional practice while feeling pretty broken. Work serves to keep me grounded and functioning. I try to practice what I preach about coping under stress. I move from mastery to helplessness to mastery to helplessness again and again, depending on what action I take or whether I'm inadvertently rendered frozen for the moment.

We all have our own private logic or mistaken beliefs about ourselves, others, and the world in which we live. From the time I was little, my own private logic went something like this: "No one can help, no one gets it, I'm on my own. Either make yourself useful or get out of my way." During the course of my fifty-seven years—and now in this crisis of all crises—it's all I know to survive.

It just so happens that, in the world of chronic Lyme where few can or will help you, my conditioned worldview has been further solidified.

In Lymeland, there is very little support. Very few can help. Most doctors negate your experience and suffering. And while many in the Lyme world are lovely and helpful, some are territorial and hypersensitive about their own findings, thereby treating you like a threat. To top it all off, friends and family look at you with a cocked head—not getting anything you're saying, or just plain skeptical about it all.

They say things like, "You can't talk about subjects like vaccines or conspiracies. People will think you're crazy and you'll lose all credibility." Perhaps, but I'll take my chances. Or when they ask about Matt they might say, "Well at least it's not cancer," or "Matt said he was feeling better today; that's good." As if one moment or one hour or day of feeling somewhat decent is the measure of healing in this crazy Lyme world.

I assure you, it's not.

When Matt is put on a whole host of rotating oral antibiotics, his symptoms do seem to improve somewhat. However, he is not the same—he is flat, distant, lethargic.

Nothing is the same. I'm not the same. I'm fixated on this maddeningly complex and destructive disease, disinterested in anything else, and disconnected from family and friends—feeling alone in this battle to save my son. I try to come to terms with the fact that I'm on my own and no one can be of any help.

I read about Lyme deaths and put myself into a complete

and utter panic. Despite what some misinformed authorities would have us believe, these deaths are real—just ask Rossana Magnotta, president and CEO of Magnotta Winery, whose husband, Gabe, succumbed to Lyme carditis several years ago. And he is only one of so many whose lives have been destroyed and ultimately cut short by this disease.

Yet no one is paying attention to this pandemic. No one in my world gets it or is taking this as seriously as I need them to.

I'm feeling alone, overwhelmed, in a twilight zone. An alternate universe. So afraid to lose my son. I'm losing him every day as his personality becomes flatter, as he becomes increasingly disconnected, and as we look for answers that don't seem to exist.

I read about chronic Lyme's similarities to AIDS. I read about how it is similar to syphilis, in both bacteria and politics, as I research the Tuskegee Syphilis Experiment—a US-government-sponsored human experiment that withheld potentially lifesaving antibiotic treatment to hundreds of African-American test subjects.

I read about how the Lyme vaccine, which was introduced in 1998, was pulled off the market by 2002, as patients said they were literally sickened by it. Some filed lawsuits against the maker, GlaxoSmithKline. Was the introduction of this vaccine a human experiment—similar in many ways to the syphilis experiment in Tuskegee? Some believe it was.

I read about the immune system and how AIDS and Lyme are similar in that they are both immunosuppressive diseases, damaging the immune system and making sufferers prime targets for opportunistic infections.

I read that, like AIDS, there is no cure or treatment that works. Some would beg to differ, so it depends on whom you choose to believe. Some people do recover, but their immune system is forever compromised and vulnerable to other infections for life.

I read that Lyme is the infectious-disease equivalent of cancer. Dr. Neil Spector, a top Duke oncologist—and long-time undiagnosed Lyme sufferer whose own illness resulted in irreversible heart failure and a heart transplant—says, "With cancer, we know that administering one algorithmic form of treatment doesn't work. I think we need to start thinking this way about Lyme."[53]

Matt is my heart. And my heart is breaking into smaller and smaller shards, each and every day, with every new source of Lyme research I consume. Chronic Lyme is a multilayered abyss of information that is extremely difficult to sort through. And the loss of Matt's health feels simply unbearable.

Loss meets us in all forms. And in a myriad of ways. The loss of a home, career, finances, marriage, health, a loved one. Anything that makes our lives feel upended—any unexpected severing of a close bond, any major change that affects our core identity—can render us grief-stricken.

In our grief, we often retreat. We are trapped in a different reality—a parallel universe—and we often find the "real" world terribly hard to relate to. We look for ways to escape because the pain is so intolerable. We lose the ability to think straight. We lose interest in social connection, although we are desperately in need of it to heal. We lose the ability to function.

"Grief does not change you, it reveals you," says author John Green.

Poet and writer Anne Lamott says: "It's like having a broken leg that never heals perfectly—that still hurts when the weather gets cold, but you learn to dance with the limp."

Author José N. Harris says, "Tears shed for another person are not a sign of weakness. They are a sign of a pure heart."

My heart must be fully pure by now, as I cry buckets of tears each day.

This earlier stage of grief is all about brokenness. In the loss of my vibrant, brilliant, beautiful son, I had begun to lose hope in a promising future for him. I was stuck in a searing state of pain—one that my husband assured me would find its way to the light again.

What I needed most was to feel that those closest to me could and would comfort me and accept the pain I was experiencing, so that I could continue to find the strength I needed to support my son.

Jeff was that person. Every day, he held me. He allowed my tears. He didn't judge me. He worried with me. He, too, became depleted by my grief. His conditioned defense is to bury his head in the sand. With this crisis, I wouldn't let him. I needed him. I needed someone to listen—someone to hear what I was learning. To understand all that frightened me.

I am compelled to learn more every day—to make sense of this, to heal my son—even if it kills me. I am pursuing this learning at the expense of my other relationships, downtime, fun safety, health, and life.

This is not how my life was supposed to go. I never intended to live out my story with my son being chronically ill. Who does? But here we are, and I will fight to the death to solve this.

The Statistics Are Astounding, Overwhelming—and Horrifying

How does the world not know what is happening with chronic Lyme? The true number of people suffering? That the numbers are growing exponentially?

It might be of interest to note that Alison Childs, the creator of lymestats.org—a site that those of us in Lymeland rely heavily on as a trusted source—received an officious letter from the executive director of the American Lyme Disease Foundation (ALDF). The ALDF, not to be confused with Karen Forschner's Lyme Disease Foundation (LDF), is a public service that refers patients to the IDSA treatment guidelines. In this letter, the executive director accused her of posting false information on her site and asked her to remove it. Is Child's site posing a threat to the powers that be?

Here are just a handful of stats that are important to know. None of us in the Lyme world can know exactly what the numbers are with full certainty. What we do know, however, is that the numbers tend to be highly underreported. What we do know, with certainty, is that the official statistics represent a small fraction of reality.

- **The US now claims there are 300,000 to one million new cases** each year, the majority of which are unreported.[54] According to the CDC's rough estimate of 300,000 new cases per year, by the end of this year, close to one million new cases would have been diagnosed in the US since the initial estimate. However, several states have reported surges in Lyme cases in the past two years due to climate change and vector expansion. The CDC figure does not include undiagnosed, misdiagnosed, chronic cases, nor does it include vector-borne coinfections.[55] "When the CDC says the number is 300,000, you always have to multiply that by ten—which makes the number of Lyme cases in the US closer to three million."[56]

- In **Canada,** our number is always **10 percent of the US** for any disease, infection, colds, or virus.[57] According to recent vector expansion models, by 2020, 80 percent of the Canadian population will be exposed to the deer tick, a main vector transmitting Lyme Borrelia.[58] (Yet Canadian doctors still insist that ticks don't cross the border! And across the country, doctors refuse to and are forbidden from acknowledging or treating any cases of chronic Lyme beyond the twenty-eight-day guideline. More on this in Chapter 8.)

- Lyme disease can be found in more than **eighty countries worldwide.**[59]

- Lyme disease has been diagnosed in **every US state** and on **every continent except Antarctica.**[60]

- Only 3 to 26 percent of people see the tick that bites them.[61]

- **Lyme is six times more prevalent than HIV/AIDS.**[62] HIV funding eclipses that of Lyme disease by nearly 135 times.[63]

- **Lyme is persistent.** A total of 230 peer-reviewed studies show evidence of persistent—that is, chronic—Lyme disease. The CDC claims that Lyme doesn't exist in a chronic state, and that an early, short-term course of antibiotics cures the disease. In a recent study of more than 6,000 Lyme patients, half were sick with the disease for more than ten years.[64]

Physical and Psychological Symptoms of Chronic Lyme

As the New Great Imitator of 350-plus conditions, Lyme disease presents with an astounding range of symptoms—many of which mimic and can be easily mistaken for other diseases, including ALS, Parkinson's, Alzheimer's, chronic fatigue, fibromyalgia, and multiple sclerosis, among others.

Polly Murray, one the of earlier pioneers of this disease, observed, "I am struck by how Lyme disease never seems to act exactly the way it is supposed to, how each individual seems to respond differently to the spirochete."[65]

Murray's prophetic words come back to haunt us all these years later:

I'd been "in the field" for awhile, and I knew it wasn't going to be easy to figure everything out so fast. Whatever this illness was, it was complicated, in that it involved so many systems of the body, and my instincts told me it was going to elude definition for some time to come.[66]

To help us understand what chronic Lyme disease can feel like, Canadian Lyme sufferer Ryus St. Pierre says,

"Do you think it would be painful to drill a corkscrew through your hand? Lyme disease is literally millions of microscopic corkscrew bacteria that drill their way through skin, muscle, joints, bones, nerves, organs, and brain tissue causing out of control inflammation and a myriad of disabling complicated symptoms."

Observing and listening to my son and so many other Lyme sufferers, it is clear that Lyme feels like you are living in a daily torture chamber. The symptomatology can differ from one hour to the next. Most commonly, it feels like you have a chronic flu every single day for years on end, with symptoms that include but are by no means limited to: indescribable fatigue while simultaneously feeling wired; dizziness; wooziness; migraines; a deep ache from head to toe and sometimes pain that is simply intolerable; nerves that fire without notice, resulting in electric shocks; an internal storm; sleeplessness; anxiety; malaise; depression; nausea; visual and auditory sensitivities and disturbances; brain fog; grogginess; a loss of mental sharpness; memory loss; a leaky gut; stabbing and burning sensations; muscle tremors; and more.

These sensations can all be felt in the course of one hour, one day, one week. The body is constantly crying out for help, telling the sufferer that something here is terribly wrong and you need to pay close attention. So sufferers learn to tune in to their bodies, trying to determine what is causing or exacerbating the latest symptom and how best to respond. And there are a myriad of ways to respond, which, for the most part, amount to a moment-by-moment guessing game. And sometimes, there is absolutely nothing you can do but simply bear with and try to breathe through the latest symptom that is shouting out the loudest at that moment.

I'm sure I haven't described it perfectly. And I know that many sufferers can offer even more gruesome details of what it feels like to have Lyme.

Lyme-literate MD Joseph G. Jemsek says, "Most of my HIV patients used to die ... now most don't ... Some still do, of course. My Lyme patients, the sickest ones, want to die but they can't. That's right, they want to die but they can't."

What matters most here is that the world needs to understand that chronic Lyme is real. That it is affecting millions worldwide. That the conventional medical community continues to turn its back on sufferers. That the number of cases is growing exponentially around the globe. And that we need to understand this disease and find helpful medical solutions...now.

Thanks to the CDC and the IDSA, Lyme sufferers, with all of their daily struggles, are forced to be warriors on this medical odyssey—navigating this disease primarily on their own, with very little guidance. It's time that the medical community stop negating and debating the existence of this chronic illness and start listening to the sufferers and their suffering. Before long, they, too, will be affected. Maybe then they will get off their high horses and pay attention to this undeniable level of anguish and affliction.

Here is a list of symptoms—by no means exhaustive—that Lyme sufferers face. This list is gleaned from CanLyme, Lyme Research Alliance, and other trustworthy sources, as well as what I've personally witnessed with Matt and so many others suffering from this disease. It's important to note that not everyone suffers in the same way, with the exact same set of symptoms or from all of the symptoms listed here.

Unexplained hair loss, headaches, migraines, seizures, pressure in the brain, white matter lesions in brain, brain fog, twitching of facial or other muscles, facial paralysis, stiff or painful neck and jaw, tingling of nose and tip of tongue, cheek or facial flushing, dental problems, sore throat, clearing throat a lot, phlegm, hoarseness, runny nose, double or blurry vision, increased floating spots, pain in eyes, swelling around eyes, oversensitivity to light, flashing lights, peripheral waves or phantom images in corners of eyes, decreased hearing in one or both ears, plugged ears, buzzing in ears, pain in ears, oversensitivity to sounds, ringing in one or both ears, diarrhea, constipation, irritable bladder (trouble starting, stopping), interstitial cystitis, upset stomach (nausea or pain), leaky gut, GERD (gastro-esophageal reflux disease), bone pain, joint pain or swelling, carpal tunnel syndrome, stiffness of joints, back, neck, tennis elbow, muscle pain or cramps, fibro-myalgia, shortness of breath, can't get full/satisfying breath, cough, chest pain or rib soreness, night sweats or unexplained chills, heart palpitations or extra beats, endocarditis, tremors or unexplained shaking, burn-ing or stabbing sensations in the body, fatigue, chronic fatigue syndrome, weakness, peripheral neuropathy or partial paralysis, pressure in the head, numbness in body, tingling, pinpricks, poor balance, dizziness, dif-ficulty walking, increased motion sickness, light-head-edness, wooziness, psychological dysregulations including obsessive-compulsive behaviors, attention deficit issues, restrictive eating, personality changes, sensory sensitivities, mood swings, numbness, anxi-ety, panic attacks, irritability, rage, bipolar disorder, intractable depression, disorientation (getting or feel-ing lost), derealization (out-of-body experience), feel-ing as if you are losing your mind, heightened emo-tional reactions, crying easily, sleep disturbances such as too much sleep, insomnia, difficulty falling or stay-ing asleep, narcolepsy, and sleep apnea, memory loss, confusion, difficulty thinking, difficulty with concen-tration or reading, speech difficulty (slurred or slow), difficulty finding commonly used words, stammering speech, forgetting how to perform simple tasks, loss of sex drive, sexual dysfunction, unexplained menstrual pain, irregularity, unexplained breast pain, discharge, testicular or pelvic pain, phantom smells, unexplained weight gain or loss, extreme fatigue, swollen glands or lymph nodes, unexplained fevers (high or low grade), continual infections (sinus, kidney, eye, etc.), symptoms seem to change, symptoms come and go, pain migrates (moves) to different body parts, a "flu-like" illness, low body temperature, allergies or chemical sensitivities, increased effect from alcohol and possible worsened hangover.[67]

Lyme Is Numbing

I've noticed that those with neurological Lyme disease often post about their inability to feel much. In fact, they wonder if they'll ever feel *anything* deeply again. Their effect tends to be flat, which can wreak havoc on their own self-esteem and on their relationships with others. One woman posted online, "My husband wonders if I'll ever be able to feel anything for him again." Lyme survivors assured her that as the symptoms abate, her range of emotions will return and her ability to express love for her husband will be reborn.

I know there were times when—as close as I am and have remained to my son, perhaps closer than ever as we battle this disease of his together—I have felt an emotional chasm, a sense that he's not quite there. I have not witnessed him cry very often—not in a very long time. I have often wondered where he puts his emotions—where he bottles them up. I am all too aware that when his affect is flat, it is just another way that neurological Lyme presents itself and impacts its sufferers.

It's awful for them, and painful for those of us who just want to love them. We can easily misinterpret their emotional disconnect as a lack of interest or caring, when in fact it's simply the unfortunate result of their nervous system operating in so many dysfunctional and unfamiliar ways.

Herxing—Another Lyme Symptom

Herxing is part of our daily lexicon and new Lyme language. Short for the Jarisch-Herxheimer reaction—and first identified with syphilis—a *herx*, as I understand it, is an exacerbation of symptoms caused by toxins released within the body during some form of antibacterial or detoxification treatment.

When you take an antibiotic, ingest an herbal remedy, or do any one of the hundreds of available and possible treatments for Lyme, you will likely experience a herx. It is a heightened inflammatory response caused by spirochetal die-off. It's a feeling that Lyme sufferers know all too well and often have a tough time describing.

It can manifest in so many ways, including fever, chills, headache, sweating, dizziness, hyperventilation, muscle pain, exacerbation of skin lesions, sleeplessness, irritability and anxiety, just to name a few. The intensity of the reaction can vary from person to person and from day to day. It generally reflects the severity of inflammation.

Herxing is yet one more very difficult, sometimes daily or weekly challenge in a series of health challenges for chronic Lyme sufferers. To begin with, herxing is very hard to control. Some say it is self-limiting. But it can be so intense as to be intolerable.

Herxing is unavoidable. In order to heal from Lyme, the systemic bacteria *has* to be killed and released—making its way out of your system.

As every chronic Lyme sufferer will respond to treatment

differently, so will they respond to herxing in their own way. Lyme sufferers need to become highly attuned to their bodies and monitor how they're feeling—noticing and managing their own range of discomfort.

Anything can bring on a herx—antibiotics, herbal tinctures, a change in supplements, infrared saunas, detoxification baths, and more. Anything that is good for a Lyme sufferer can also cause further suffering—all in the name of healing.

Herxing can start anywhere from an hour to days after you begin a new treatment. It's also possible to have a delayed herx reaction to a treatment you recently took.

So when you feel sick, you never really know for sure if it's the Lyme illness presenting itself, a herx detoxing response, a new infection that has taken hold—or all three. This makes for a never-ending and frightening guessing game, rendering it extremely difficult to know how to manage it or what to do next.

In short, Lyme sufferers become excellent sleuths, always having to monitor their symptoms in order to make their best guess as to what to do next.

Brain Fog

Brain fog is the most common and lingering symptom of chronic Lyme disease, and it is one of the first symptoms that Matt complained about. I remember doing a Google search for it and finding all kinds of sources more than three years ago. While many of Matt's symptoms have improved over time and with treatment, brain fog still persists. I believe it's one of the toughest Lyme symptoms to eradicate.

In trying to make sense of Matt's brain fog, I visited the website of Dr. Lawrence Wilson who provides a clear explanation of what it is:

*Brain fog may be described as **feelings of mental confusion or lack of mental clarity**. It is called brain fog because it can feel like a cloud that reduces your ability to think clearly. It can cause a person to become forgetful, detached and often discouraged and depressed.*

Brain fog is not recognized as a clinical diagnosis because it is not easy to test for it. [...] I hope that medical doctors will soon expand their diagnostic ability to assess brain fog, but for now it is a subjective condition, though it is very real.[68]

Brain fog has been described to me in a myriad of ways including...

having a slow and achy brain...feeling chronically lost in a familiar place like your own home...not being able to find the correct word to describe *something such as 'table' when you mean 'chair'...the inability to retrieve names and simple facts...the inability to focus on anything for more than a minute or two at a time...constantly losing your place in a TV show or a book that you're reading...at a loss for short term memories including what you had for lunch that day... finding it impossible to multi-task...feeling mildly high or drunk...feeling spacey and hung over...having difficulty processing information...losing the context or meaning of things...nothing that runs through your mind makes sense...no ability to retain information... listening intently without hearing the words or processing what is being said...getting easily distracted...*

unable to stay focused in a conversation... *your train of thought is like a runaway freight car...everything in your brain seems misfiled...swimming against the tide in a sea of sludge.*

I see brain fog in my practice daily, with clients who are experiencing emotional distress, trauma, and grief. With Lyme, the fog is not an emotionally driven response but rather a physiological response to toxic overload, hidden viruses, and bacterial infection. And it makes life hard because you never feel "normal" and your brain never feels quite right. What's even harder is not knowing or understanding why this is happening to you, and having doctors who aren't equipped to acknowledge, explain, or help you with this condition.

We've also come to learn that Lyme—which can wreak havoc on every organ, including your liver, kidneys, heart, and so on—can also create a leaky gut, causing your intestinal walls to be weakened and food particles to be released into your cellular environment. This is yet another cause of brain fog for Matt and so many others, requiring a very restrictive diet for healing to take place.

David's Lyme Story

We were first introduced to David Feldman several months into Matt's Lyme treatment. David was more than willing to share his story in all its gruesome detail. His suffering and bravery further compelled me to write *Lyme Madness*. Apart from finding it frightening to hear the depth of David's agony so early on in Matt's journey, his story also provided us with hope. We had to believe that if he could heal, then so could Matt.

Here is David's story.

*In August of 2012, my family went on a canoe trip in
northern Ontario. I don't remember any tick bite, nor
did I notice a bulls-eye rash. Three weeks later I was
driving in my car and felt my heart rate pounding out
of my chest, dizziness and like I was about to pass out. I
was rushed to the hospital thinking I was having a heart
attack. I was released after five hours. It took that long
for my heart rate to normalize. I was released with a cardiac referral.*

*Over the next few days, I felt like I was buzzing with
many extra beats in my heart. Three days later, I was
lying in bed and had another attack of increased heart
rate, dizziness and numbness all over. I kept saying to
my wife, "I feel like I'm going to die." It continued for
24 hours with an indescribably terrible feeling in my
chest and upper abdomen. I was feeling weak over the
next few days and then had many heart tests with a cardiac specialist. ECG, echo, stress test, holter...everything.
All was normal. Over the next three weeks, everything
worsened. I had severe attacks of increased HR, dizziness, nausea, pre-syncope, neck pressure, 10/10 headaches, severe fatigue, etc. I felt like I was "on fire" or lit
up and it went in waves. We had three 911 calls over
the next week as I felt like I was going to die. The chest/
abdominal discomfort I had was so terrible, I had no
peace in my body for a second.*

*Over the next few days I had many more ECGs,
bloods, ultrasound of my aorta, abdominal ultrasound. Everything normal. My symptoms only continued to worsen with many "attacks." Finally, I was*

admitted to hospital in late September 2012 for a few days of tests…nothing…except on the way out they told me to meet with the psychiatrist who told me that I should stop doing tests and accept that I had a panic and anxiety disorder and that I should be on medication. I couldn't accept this and I was glad I didn't. I knew something was definitely wrong with me. I was not an anxious person before.

I kept getting worse. I started seeing an internist who checked my thyroid and adrenals, I was referred to another cardiologist and gastroenterologist. I had an endoscopy and colonoscopy. I had an MRI of my brain looking for a brain tumor…NOTHING! Throughout the month of October 2012 the attacks were less but the symptoms were becoming chronic—including the "terrible" chest feeling (it wasn't chest pain but worse if that makes any sense), severe fatigue and yawning beginning at 45pm daily, periodic episodes of shortness of breath, air hunger, weakness in my legs, dizziness, lightheadedness, and lots of nausea. The medical system at this time had nothing left for me. I began seeing a homeopath, chiropractor, osteopath, cranio-sacral therapist, and many different energy workers (you wouldn't believe). I went gluten free, started taking many vitamins, remedies, etc.

In late Oct. I was tested for Epstein-Barr and had Ontario Lyme testing (ELISA). All normal. I was then told to do a sleep study. I was diagnosed with sleep apnea and put on a CPAP machine. In late November I could barely move with fatigue, weakness or some kind of discomfort. My stool began to be bloody all the time.

Throughout November/December/January—all symptoms were more and more chronic, some days would have some symptoms, some days others, it would always switch around, one day it would be shortness of breath and dizziness and fatigue—another day would be weakness, headaches, weird chest feeling, leg numbness, jaw pain.

Starting in January 2013 and into February, I began having severe pain for the first time. Most of all of the symptoms previous to that were not pain. I started having moderate to severe chest and rib pain most of the time. This would often occur with bad shortness of breath. My neck was constantly stiff with decreased ROM. I would often have a feeling that I was going to drop to the ground, or a feeling that I missed a step. There would often be a wave of extreme nausea and dizziness that would then follow with chest pain, numbness, weakness, etc.

In late Jan, I had an appt. with another internist who ordered a Chest and Abdominal CT and more blood tests including ESR, thyroid panel, Amylase, Urinalysis—all normal—he said I should be on an SSRI (yet again). Month of February—started using the CPAP machine regularly—was not sleeping well at all on this—was given Tryptophan by my psychiatrist to help me sleep. Used it for two days—then started getting horrible burning in my chest bilaterally in the upper chest as well as 10/10 upper to mid thoracic back pain. I could not move without severe pain. Stopped the Tryptophan thinking that it may be the cause. Finally, was convinced to try an SSRI for one day but had vomiting and severe nausea so stopped it after one day. But the burning and pain continued. Now I had the burning and pain on top of all my other symptoms.

I started to get extremely depressed. I contemplated suicide.

I had never felt that before. Everything continued to get worse and worse. I had to stop work (I'm a chiropractor). Late Feb—Had IGeneX testing for LYME on the advice of someone I met randomly (thank-god). In mid-March my results came back definitively showing that I had Lyme and likely Babesia as well. Since March 1/13— everything continuing to pile on and worsen. At least I had a diagnosis.

Every day from waking—started with burning chest pain, shortness of breath, pressure in the chest, the burning moved down into my upper arms, was having severe left jaw pain (which began after dental work in early March for a cracked tooth) and constant tingling on my left face, fasciculations in my right triceps, left eye, chin, and other random areas.

Days of mostly lightheadedness and brain fog. No memory, couldn't concentrate. Waves of dizziness and nausea that come and go, severe back pain all the time, feeling like I'm on fire inside, being lit up. Sleep disturbances are more severe—intense terrible dreams, waking dreams—stopped using the CPAP to try and get more sleep. I was getting extreme headaches and migraines, heart palpitations or missed beats were increasing, electrical shock feelings in my head especially left side, indescribable acute head/facial "shock," loss of equilibrium right ear started ringing, neck pain and stiffness, the fatigue was so severe that even rest, when I did get it, did not help, occasional issues with balance, anxiety when watching a TV show that had emotional content, bouts of crying, memory loss.

Beginning of April, I saw Dr. P, a LYME specialist in Buffalo. She reconfirmed the LYME and started me on all the antibiotics (six of them at first including Doxy, Rifampin, Hydroxychloroquin, Mepron...and others I can't remember off hand. I was on the drugs for three months, April, May, and June 2013.

The herxes obviously were awful. In beginning of July 2013, I didn't think it could get any worse. Dr. P. said the drugs weren't working and I needed to be on IV antibiotics.

As of April, I had also begun taking many different other supplements too. I went home from that appointment and cried for two days. I had had enough. I decided to go off of the drugs fully, not get the IV antibiotics and just stay on all the natural stuff. I just couldn't do it anymore (the drugs, herxes, etc.). In August '13 I felt 2% better.

September I started to see a doctor in Toronto who did IV cocktails. I started doing those weekly and rotated between a Hi C cocktail and an IV of Hydrogen Peroxide. September/October '13 I felt another 10% better. November and December another 1020% better. I never really knew why. To this day I question it. Maybe the three months of drugs worked, maybe it was the IVs, maybe it was the supplements. I still don't know. I went back to work in January '14 and felt slightly better every month. I would have the odd attack or my symptoms *would return but it didn't last. I slowly felt like I was getting my life back. Even so, I had developed a post-traumatic stress type anxiety disorder, which was mostly based around fear that when I didn't feel so good that the disease was all coming back.*

Today, I would say I'm 98% improved. I have very rare occurrences of symptoms and when I do, I have become better equipped at handling it all through mindfulness and mindfulness meditation.

I see a therapist every two weeks, I still go for monthly IVs and have continued taking all the supplements that I started in April '13 to this day. These include an herbal formula called tick-attack, other herbs including a lymph, liver and kidney drainage, and glutathione. D and A drops, garlic, alpha lipoic acid, Magnesium Bisglycinate, three compounds that help methylation in the body (ATP, transfer factor and something else I forget), digestive enzymes (called Nattozyme). I'm sure a few more that I could get the names of for you if you'd like.

I have not gone for any more testing. My wife, kids, and I are still in a healing phase but every day life gets a little bit more back to normal.

I pray, Matt, that your last 20% of healing will come quickly and that you can one day put this behind you. I am a changed person from who I was before, and I have to say, mostly good changes. It's too bad I had to go through all of the above to figure certain things out about myself, but I have to say that the little problems in life definitely don't seem so tragic anymore and I get great joy with just being able to lie down with my body feeling some peace. I never thought I was going to be able to do that again. As I said, I still live in fear that this will come back again one day as so little is still known about how all this works. I now have tools that can help me deal with this fear. I am becoming a complete person again.

Neurocognitive Lyme Disease

Yes, it's true. Chronic Lyme disease is, in fact, in your head. But not in the way that doctors intend it to mean.

Contrary to medical consensus, chronic Lyme disease is not a made-up illness. Nor is it ever a case of malingering, Munchausen, hypochondria, laziness, or "craziness."

Chronic Lyme disease is, however, *all in your head* because it is primarily a neurological disease, wreaking havoc in your brain and your nervous system—as well as your heart, your liver, your kidneys, and so many other organs.

Lyme disease patients can—and most often do—experience anxiety, depression, panic attacks, rage, attention problems, short-term memory loss, depression, personality changes, mood swings, and learning disabilities. They also often experience detachment, dissociation, depersonalization, isolation, suicidal ideation, and suicide.

As with any cognitive impairment, chronic Lyme sufferers may have trouble keeping track of their daily tasks, they may lose things easily, including words and objects, they may have trouble retrieving information, forget appointments, and struggle with holding a conversation.

Sufferers are desperate for mental health professionals (along with all other medical specialists) to understand Lyme so that they will use Lyme as a differential diagnosis before plying them with psychotropic meds that may make matters worse. There have been so many Lyme sufferers misdiagnosed as bipolar and institutionalized when, in actual fact, the patient who has been committed to a psych ward has Lyme encephalitis.

Consider the story of John Caudwell—the UK's multibillionaire founder of Phones4U—and his twenty-year-old son Rufus. Rufus had been struggling with Lyme for nine years of his life before the disease was diagnosed in February 2015. His illness began at age eleven with acute psychiatric symptoms, including panic attacks, agoraphobia, and a health anxiety.

In an interview with *The Telegraph*, Mr. Caudwell, sixty-two, described the disease as "a kind of alien microbe in Rufus's body, slowly but surely destroying his life.[69]

"It is a public health scandal, a travesty, a tragedy that people are being left to suffer," he said.[70]

Lyme and Suicide

Suicidal ideation and completed suicides are certainly not uncommon among Lyme sufferers.

I clearly understand why this is the case. I have personally witnessed the intolerable suffering of those who have wanted to end their lives. I have also read plenty of stories about those who have taken their own lives as a result of Lyme—stories that are heartbreaking and tragic, and perhaps could have been prevented.

There are a number of reasons why people commit suicide. Chronic Lyme is the perfect storm. It's a disease that matches up with so many reasons for not being able to see a way out of the darkness. It is so clear to me how and why chronic Lyme sufferers, in particular, so often succumb to this disease by their own hand.

Lyme sufferers are often anxious and depressed. Anxiety and depression are commonly experienced neurological symptoms of Lyme. After all, with Lyme, the brain is inflamed and therefore subject to all sorts of neurological imbalances. This, compounded by the lack of and often outright negation of medical attention, leads to discouragement, fear, helplessness, frustration, loss, grief, loneliness, and, at times, little hope for recovery. When an illness is chronic, and there is often unrelenting suffering and inadequate relief from the myriad of debilitating symptoms, anxiety and depression can become even more pronounced. Lyme depression is often intractable—that is, resistant to treatment. Lyme can also affect the endocrine system, potentially creating mood disorders. Among other symptoms, Lyme sufferers can experience psychotic episodes, attention deficit, panic attacks, obsessive-compulsive disorder, dissociation, and depersonalization.

Lyme sufferers are sick for years and even decades and get worn down over time. The collection of symptoms— including brain fog, headaches, fevers, joint pain, nerve pain, anxiety, depression, shakiness, instability, dizziness, vision and auditory disturbances, hallucinations, seizures, paralysis, and more—experienced day in and day out, can wear you down, making even the most resilient warriors eventually want out.

Lyme sufferers are socially isolated, medically denied, crying out for help, and no one is listening. Family and friends don't know how to help. Some loved ones all but abandon the Lyme sufferer because they get fed up with the constant complaining and limitations. As doctors are showing

Lyme sufferers the door—dismissing, mocking, and negating their disease and suffering, and offering no answers for finding relief—it becomes more and more difficult for loved ones to understand and support those with Lyme.

Lyme sufferers feel like a burden. They lose their independence, their livelihoods, and their ability to function. They feel like they're losing their minds at times. They live with constant brain fog and cognitive limitations, making every task far more difficult. They get worn down by the chronic pain and illness, by the fear, the inactivity, and the inability to plan or have anything to look forward to.

Lyme sufferers have to face loss every day. Loss of health, loss of the person they once were, loss of independence, loss of dreams and goals, loss of missed opportunities, loss of the life they once had, loss of an identity, loss of self-esteem, loss of loved ones who abandon them, loss of hope, loss of finances, loss of employment, and loss of a future.

Lyme sufferers are victimized many times over—by the disease itself, by doctors who turn their backs, by family and friends who roll their eyes and walk away, by insurers who refuse coverage, and by a medical system that negates the very existence of this disease.

In short, Lyme causes a multitude of neurological problems, and when our brain isn't working well, *we* are not working well. Depression and anxiety can cast a very dark shadow over our thoughts. This, along with the pain and exhaustion of chronic daily suffering, a lack of support, medical negation, gaslighting, and abandonment—it's no wonder that suicide can sometimes feel like it may be the only way to stop the madness.

Jenn's Lyme Story

Twenty-nine-year-old Jenn has been suffering with Lyme and several coinfections since infancy, but was officially diagnosed only a year ago when her illness became acute. Here is her description of what it feels like to have this disease.

Today I can finally type and my arms don't feel like I either lifted hundreds of pounds of weights or like needles are going into them, so I will take advantage of that and try and write. This is one of the hardest things I have ever gone through. I often can't believe what's happening. A part of me knows that I have to be strong, believe that this will all work out some how, find solace in the fact that others have gone through this and made it. I am fortunate to have someone pushing me along and supporting me so much through this. I know I should appreciate what I have and stop looking around for what I am still missing.

No matter how many times I break down there is still a part of me that says, I am not done yet and I need to get back up. So far I have made it through 100% of my worst days, so I'm sure I will get through this one, as much as in certain moments I wish I wouldn't.

This changed my whole life so quickly. I was never asked for permission, no one ever gave me an option, I just woke up one day and my life was never the same. I'm afraid I will never know anything different. I am afraid I will never get back all the things that I lost. To get my physical health back is one thing, but to repair my spirit and soul that has been broken—I don't know if you can come back from that. Regardless of what my future holds, regardless of what treatment looks like, I will never be the same person. That doesn't mean it'll be for the worst, but I just won't be the same. I guess being challenged in life is inevitable, being defeated is optional. It's scary when you wish, hope and pray for defeat. That's when you know the pain, and the hurt is very real. No one should ever know what it is like to wish for the end. Some days it doesn't matter how you keep going, how you move forward, what that looks like, you just keep moving because it's what you do. Graceful or not, you just keep moving. Most days I keep moving and I don't know why, but I hope that along the way I will find the reason why.

I am grateful that I am not totally alone in this; there is at least one person that believes me, and has faith I can get through this. Today that has to be enough. Despite it being difficult to walk, despite that plane taking off on Monday for Bali without me, this has not beaten me yet.

Being sick has taught me a lot about the people around me. I never ask anyone to understand, I just ask that they don't doubt. For those that doubted, they made their choice and that was their right. Now I have to make mine. I will never demand support from someone, I will never tell them how they can help, it's not who I am. Sometimes it's not just about having someone want to help you it's knowing how to accept that help that can be even harder. Believing in others when it's near impossible to believe in yourself.

This journey has just started, and I've already threatened to quit more times than I can count. This has been and will be the hardest thing I have ever gone through. I will never be able to prepare myself fully for tomorrow, I will never be able to know what will happen, but

tomorrow will come and I just have to take it one minute at a time, remember the moments that inspired me
in the moments that threaten to break me. Sometimes
you have to hold your own hand through life, be your
own witness to your pain, and some days that just needs
to be enough, and that has to be ok. I'm sure there will
be plenty more days when I give up, cry, and scream that
I am done. You know that when the first thing you do
when you wake up in the morning is cry, this will be a
tough moment, a tough morning but I try to believe that
doesn't mean it has to be a tough day. I'm sure that there
will be more days where I wonder why I am doing this.
I hope on those days if I can't find the strength, someone
can help me find it.

I don't want pity; I don't need to be talked down to.
I need to be believed, and have someone care. I know I
can't do this alone every single day and I hope I won't
have to. Just have to remember the kind and comforting
words from the days when I wasn't alone, and let those
carry me through the days when I feel I am. This is my
journey, one I don't understand yet; don't know where
it will lead me or how bumpy the ride will be. I am terrified, but I am here. Today that just has to be enough.
Today I wrote something, and that matters. I may not
know or understand why but something tells me it
matters. As my arms start to hurt and typing becomes
harder, I am reminded how far I still have to go, but then
I can scroll up the page and see how far I have come.
One day I will live not just survive. For now, I will try
and make surviving look good. Sometimes strong is the
only choice you have left."

Years to Diagnosis and Treatment

In an informal survey conducted by the author of the blog whatislyme.com, chronic Lyme sufferers were asked how long it took them to get diagnosed. The answers ranged from months to years. People reported being misdiagnosed with everything from multiple sclerosis, to Alzheimer's, to Parkinson's, to ALS. Some reported being sick for as long as forty years or more without knowing why.

If the number of doctors one is forced to see is a reasonable measure of this madness, one story that trumps them all is that of Lisa Gumieniuk, an Australian woman and "high-flying corporate IT manager" who fell ill in 2013 and had no idea what was causing her strange symptoms. The *Daily Telegraph* reported that "the 34-year-old from Drummoyne suffered facial paralysis, blurry vision, stiff joints, insomnia, fevers, memory loss, speech difficulty and ended up losing her career. She went through *88* doctor appointments before she found a visiting US doctor in July, who correctly diagnosed her debilitating condition: Lyme disease, an infectious disease transmitted to humans by tick bites."[71]

The Treatment Protocols Are Innumerable, Unproven, and Primarily Hit and Miss

Can you imagine having cancer, not having it confirmed by your doctor because he refuses to do so and—having been forced to self-diagnose—you have to figure out how to treat it, all by yourself? This would never happen with any other disease known to modern man. Only with chronic Lyme.

When it comes to treatment, it's critical to know that it requires a three-pronged approach, and not always in this order:

- Part 1: Antibacterial agents to kill the spirochetes and other infections

- Part 2: Detoxification to release the bacteria from organs and tissues

- Part 3: Immune and gut-strengthening support

All three steps are typically repeated many times, and all three steps are necessary to get well—all without knowing how or when, in what combination, or in what sequence. Hit and miss. Trial and error. Figure it out. Do it yourself.

Bewildering to say the least.

For jaw-dropping impact, which I imagine this will have, I have compiled a list of the treatment protocols that Lyme sufferers are using to reclaim their health. This list is by no means exhaustive. There are many, many more protocols than those I've listed here that are being used to treat Lyme.

I do not offer details about each of these treatment protocols, as there is plenty of information readily available. I offer this list only for the purpose of helping you understand what Lyme sufferers are up against in deciding how to treat their illness.

Many of the following protocols—listed in no particular order, other than antibiotics, which are typically the first line of defense—are summarily dismissed and even mocked by members of the medical profession. We are accused by the "old Lyme guard" of living in a pseudoscientific echo chamber, of being delusional and succumbing to quackery and snake-oil promises of renewed health and magical healing.

Lyme sufferers are desperately sick people willing to use desperate measures—measures that can, at times, be more efficacious than anything conventional medicine has to offer thus far.

Perhaps if the medical profession were doing its job and working on solutions rather than mocking us and forcing us to find our own protocols, we wouldn't have to go on such a desperate search for things that may or may not help. Perhaps if we had more so-called evidence-based research on some of these protocols, they wouldn't seem so ridiculous after all.

Here are just some of the treatments that Lyme sufferers use in their desperate search to escape this nightmare:

Extended antibiotics. Oral, intravenous (IV), and intramuscular (IM). Typically, a rotation of tetracyclines, penicillins, macrolides, cephalosporins, and amino-quinolines. Antibiotics are the go-to, first-line treatment for chronic Lyme. The best approach seems to be pulse-dosing. Antibiotics can only be prescribed and administered by a licensed medical doctor, with the exception of naturopaths in British Columbia and perhaps elsewhere. In the case of chronic Lyme, long-term antibiotic treatment is administered—usually quietly and under the radar—by Lyme-literate doctors. Most doctors refuse to acknowledge the disease and will not prescribe at all, some may prescribe antibiotics for twenty-eight days if they "believe in" Lyme, or they may be part of a small subset of doctors who have been brave enough to prescribe outside of the limited IDSA guidelines but at a cost to their personal and professional life, including having their practices shut down. In Canada, with a few rare exceptions (as revealed in Chapter 8), you cannot find a doctor who will give you antibiotics beyond the

IDSA twenty-eight-day sanctioned antibiotic protocol. Most Canadians have to travel to the US for antibiotic treatment. In order to function at all, the majority of chronic Lyme sufferers are on antibiotics for months and even years, and most do so with the help of just a small handful of US LLMDs.

Probiotics. Taken daily to avoid intestinal yeast overgrowth from long-term antibiotic use.

Gluten-free/sugar-free/dairy-free diet. To keep yeast at bay, regulate blood sugar, inhibit spirochetal growth, strengthen the immune system and the gut.

The Gerson diet. A natural treatment that activates the body's extraordinary ability to heal itself through an organic, plant-based diet, raw juices, coffee enemas, and natural supplements.

Herbal protocols. Developed by a number of practitioners, including Lee Cowden, Stephen Buhner, Byron White, Dietrich Klinghardt, and others. Some Lyme sufferers use these antimicrobial protocols instead of, or as an adjunct to, antibiotics.

Wellness protocols. Check out the protocols developed by Drs. Dietrich Klinghardt, Joseph Burrascano, Richard Horowitz, Marty Ross, Joseph G. Jemsek, and David Jernigan.

Cannabidiol. Also known as CBD, from hemp seed with minimal THC (psychoactive properties). Read about

Dr. Ernie Murakami and check out Dr. Sanjay Gupta for more details.

Bee venom (apitherapy). Google Ellie Lobel for her remarkable story and how bee stinging became a popular Lyme protocol. Many people are stinging themselves with live bees in the hopes of healing, and swear by their success.

Rifing. The Rife machine, developed by Royal Raymond Rife in the early 1930s and replicated by modern manufacturers. With his machine, Rife claimed he could cure cancer and other diseases by weakening or destroying pathogens using specific frequencies of electromagnetic fields that vibrate at the same frequency as the bacteria cells.

Low-level laser. Cold laser and low-level laser therapy using LED (light-emitting diode) light. The energy in the light waves is absorbed by the ATP in the mitochondria in our cells. When a cell isn't getting enough oxygen and blood sugar to make energy, this additional energy will help the mitochondria work better, and the cell returns to health. Wounds can heal more quickly, muscle spasms may relax, and inflammation can be reduced.

Genetic testing. 23andMe or Younique, for example, determine pathways and genetic sequencing that can help you with personalized molecular medicine.

Infrared saunas. Detoxifies, relaxes, relieves pain, and improves circulation and immune function.

Detox baths. Detoxifies the body and relieves pain, but it also seems to stop many infections quickly and helps the body regain balance.

Air and water purifier. Removes contaminants in your water and air, lessening the body's toxic load.

BioMat. A state-of-the-art medical device that delivers therapeutic, far-infrared rays and negative ions, relieving pain and improving immune function.

Acupuncture. Regulates immunity and manages pain.

Lymphatic massage. Stimulates the lymph flow within the lymphatic system, as it can become sluggish while battling Lyme disease.

Chiropractic medicine. Can help with aches, pains, and improve immune system.

Craniosacral therapy. Improves and balances the flow of the fluids (cerebrospinal fluid)—bathing the brain and spinal cord, which in turn helps calm and relax the entire nervous system.

UVLrx—ultraviolet light. A form of intravenous therapy where low light energy is introduced directly into the circulatory system to support red blood cell oxygenation and a healthy immune system.

Diamond Shield Zapper or Hulda Clark Zapper. A groundbreaking, multifrequency zapper that offers six important improvements, including sweeping, micro-currents, and constant voltage.

Hyperbaric oxygen therapy. Breathing pure oxygen in a pressurized room or tube.

IV ozone therapy. Ozone is injected into the bloodstream to kill pathogens and boost the immune system.

Bio-oxidative medicine. Introduces small amounts of medical ozone (O_3) or hydrogen peroxide (H_2O_2) into the body for the prevention and treatment of disease.

Cryotherapy. Noninvasive cold therapy focused on athletic recovery, pain management, and overall health.

Low-dose immunotherapy (LDI). Helps restore immune tolerance to the environment outside and inside the body.

Advanced cell training (ACT—formerly immune response training). Uses the same premise as muscle memory.

Bicom/MORA/bioresonance. Electromagnetic waves used to diagnose and treat human illness.

Vega machine testing. A type of electro-acupuncture device used to diagnose allergies and other illnesses as well as sensitivities to supplements.

Ondamed. A pulsed electromagnetic frequency device designed with principles based on biophysics.

Claritin. This antihistamine may starve Lyme bacteria by preventing them from gathering manganese, which they need to harm the body.

Whole stevia leaf extract. Shown to possess antibiotic activity against the Lyme pathogen.

Colloidal silver. Antifungal, antibacterial, and antiviral.

Vitamins, minerals, lipids, enzymes, and amino acids. To support immune system and organs.

Yoga, qigong, tai chi, Reiki, and other energy work. For balancing your system.
Oil pulling Lyme in mouth and teeth. An ancient Ayurvedic remedy mentioned in *Charaka Samhita*.

Dr. Dakin's solution. Twenty parts water to one part bleach in Waterpik for teeth and gums where spirochetes hide.

Ritchie Shoemaker mold protocol. Cutting-edge research and treatment for mold.

Colonics/enemas. Eliminates waste buildup, detoxifies, and reduces fatigue.

Lyme bomb. Cocktail of Young Living Essential Oils (YLEO)–Thieves, frankincense, and oregano.
Heavy metal detox. Cilantro and Sun Chlorella.

IVIG. A plasma protein replacement therapy used to treat disorders of the immune system or to boost immunity.

GcMAF. Gc protein-derived macrophage activating factor is a vitamin D–binding protein naturally found in the human body, whose function is to repair tissue and stimulate immune cells to attack foreign substances and infectious microbes.

Marshall protocol. A medical treatment used by physicians worldwide to treat a variety of chronic inflammatory and autoimmune diseases, including (but not limited to) sarcoidosis, chronic fatigue syndrome, fibromyalgia, Crohn's disease, and rheumatoid arthritis.

Zhang formula. A combination modern Chinese medicine treatment protocol designed to kill Lyme and its coinfections, as well as support various organ systems in healing.

A Lyme sufferer who writes the Will There Be Cake blog ran an informal survey for five weeks to determine who does what for Lyme treatment. When asked the question, "Which treatment options have you personally tried upon receiving a diagnosis of Lyme disease?" the results ranged from 66.7 percent who tried conventional antibiotics and herbal protocols to 21 percent who tried the Rife machines or similar, to 1.5 percent who tried Zhang.[72]

As to which protocol(s) work best and in what combination, your guess is as good as any.

Do People Ever Recover?

Yes, but it all depends on what you mean by *recover*.

With chronic Lyme, you will never be the same. Like any illness, it forces you to slow down, practice better self-care, and pay more attention to your stress levels, health, and well-being.

Recovery means *remission*; it does not mean *cured*. It's always possible—perhaps even probable—that you will have a relapse. The most important thing I've learned on this journey is that Lyme sufferers have to pace themselves, listen to their bodies carefully, slow down, and give themselves what they need at all times. Using your energy wisely is important—not pushing yourself too much, even when you feel better.

Recovery is all about pacing yourself, getting adequate rest, great nutrition, gentle exercise, and continuing with herbal and nutritional supplements.

Above all, recovery is about strengthening the host (your immune system) while killing the bugs (spirochetes and company), and eliminating the toxins from your body. Healing requires an unspecific, hit-and-miss, idiosyncratic dance between the use of antibiotics, herbals, probiotics, and enzymes to strengthen your gut, kill off the bacteria and the biofilm, and release the toxic load.

No matter what, recovery is a long, hard-won battle. And no matter how defeated you feel, it's all about keeping a balance between strengthening your immune system and killing off the bad stuff.

There is no silver bullet for treating tick-borne diseases. There are so many variables, including how long you've been infected, what type and how many types of infections you have, how your illness has manifested, the severity of your symptoms, the strength of your immune system, how well you detox, genetic mutations, and how you manage the other stressors in your life.

The key to recovery is to spend time fine-tuning your self-care and gaining acceptance of your state of health. The longer you remain angry and feel victimized (understandably so), the harder it will be to get well.

To receive this overwhelming burden of information and misinformation about Lyme and Lymeland—all at once—is just too much for the human psyche to withstand.

I fully understand what poet Anaïs Nin meant when she said, "There are very few human beings who receive the truth, complete and staggering, by instant illumination. Most of them acquire it fragment by fragment, on a small scale, by successive developments, cellularly, like a laborious mosaic."

Perhaps this is why so few in our life can tolerate hearing about all that we're learning. Perhaps this is why so few are neither willing nor able to join us in this dark abyss.

It's simply too much for most to bear.

4. NO ONE IS LISTENING

There is a place, like no place on earth. A land full of wonder, mystery and danger! Some say to survive it, you need to be as mad as a hatter. Which, luckily, I am.

—ALICE'S ADVENTURES IN WONDERLAND

I am outraged.

I am outraged that it took eighteen months to figure out why Matt was so sick. I am outraged that not one doctor was able to detect Lyme. I'm outraged that the mainstream medical community is not only *not* listening, but some are getting on their soapbox and brazenly bullying the victims of this disease.

To medical doctors who are so willing to label chronic Lyme as a nondisease, I challenge you to spend a day with a group of chronic Lyme sufferers, understand how sick they are—and the damage this disease has done—and then tell me there is no such thing.

How do you know there is no such thing as chronic Lyme disease? Is that what you learned in medical school or from medical journals? The articles we have come to understand are sometimes misleading and skewed? Have you taken the time to speak to a group of sufferers, listen to their experiences, witness their pain? Do you, by the way, have any other suggestions as to why millions are suffering without answers? Perhaps you should spend more time trying to figure out that conundrum and less time patronizing and bullying the sufferers.

No One Gets It—No One Is Listening

Every day, in every city, in most medical offices worldwide, doctors are showing Lyme patients the door, making them feel as if they have no right to investigate this disease, treating them like they are modern-day lepers, and refusing to discuss the possibilities of their illness.

Across the continent and across the pond—in eighty countries, and on every continent except Antarctica—doctors are saying the stupidest, most uninformed, most damaging things to patients, and as a result are doing harm.

Doctors refuse to take you seriously, as they pronounce with uncorroborated certainty, *"There's no Lyme here."*

They believe the party line, they don't bother to do their own reading or research, and they just repeat what they've been told. Like sheep in a herd, they follow. If you bring them a positive test, they'll tell you it's a "false positive." If your test is negative, there's nothing further to discuss.

This is a closed loop—sealed tight. And millions of people are paying with their health and their lives.

Amber Robinson, who knows all too well that when it comes to chronic Lyme disease there is no one listening, shared this:

"I saw a man in my local community the other day at the grocery store. Known him since 1983. I didn't have

time to stop & chat. But I envied the man, knowing his reckless past. He has doctor appointments paid, meds paid & support & disability. He's positive HIV. I thought "You lucky fucker."

US Lyme sufferer Erica Maurin bravely videotaped a few minutes of herself in pain to show the world how excruciating Lyme can be. It's difficult to watch and is not for the faint of heart.

In the video she pleads:

I want the world to see the pain and suffering of thousands of Lymies across the globe with hopes that the CDC, Insurance companies, doctors, friends, and family WAKE UP and HELP instead of saying we are crazy or turning the other way. Lyme disease is BIGGER than AIDS has ever been and much more prevalent than ANY OTHER disease in the world. We need the CDC to buck up and face the fact that Lyme is a pandemic and needs new research, new more effective test, and better treatment and we need insurance to freaking pay for Lyme treatments also. If this were cancer, then people would be getting treated so fast their heads would spin. It's just sickening to me how our government, CDC, Big Pharma and greedy money-hungry doctors ignore patients like me. I have been misdiagnosed for 16 years!!!!!! Now I'll be lucky to ever be Lyme free. It's all about awareness. Episodes like this last anywhere between 15 min to 1 hr. I'm a prisoner in this body...This IS NOT ME! I MISS ME SO MUCH.

As Canadian rock start Avril Lavigne—who has been suffering with Lyme for quite some time now—told reporters in tears:

> *I was in Los Angeles, literally, like the worst time in my life and I was seeing, like, every specialist and literally, the top doctors, and they were so stupid, and they would pull up their computer and be like, "chronic fatigue syndrome," or "Why don't you try to get out of bed Avril, and just play the piano? Are you depressed?" This is what they do to a lot of people who have Lyme disease. They don't have an answer for them so they tell them, like, "You're crazy."[73]*

Here is a grueling description of how it feels to be the mom of a kid with Lyme as described by Thaiadora Katsos-Dorow, author of *What's the Big Deal About Lyme?* Thaiadora posted this on Facebook. It immediately caught my attention and she happily agreed to share:

> *This is what sucks to be a mom of a kid who is invisibly sick. She has a western blot that still lights up like a Christmas Tree even after being on treatment since 18 mos. Yes, Lyme CAN persist. She has Autoimmune Neurologic Encephalopathy. She has Inflammatory Response System. She could have just one, or more than those. It doesn't matter. Your child's primary doc won't treat because the infection is too complex. The docs who will treat are thousands of dollars every two months; they treat beyond CDC stringent guidelines therefore can't/won't be covered by insurance. So, when your child is sick, you can't just pick up the*

phone and get help. You must travel. You must come up with the money for the appointment, the lab work, your lodging. And all the while during the wait, more things happen to your child. Neurologic symptoms start increasing after she has had an infection, they are numerous and start to scare you. Some people might think you over react and see more than is there. Others might think that you UNDER REACT because if a kid is slurring and dropping things and having pain, why aren't you freaking out and making noise??? You've been there, you understand the symptoms too well. You know how the system works, and you watch in despair as your child suffers, fearful of what may come if you don't get help fast. You manage to get your kid to school, to keep her involved in social events even if truly she needs to be in bed by 4pm, because you desperately want to keep her kid life as normal as possible. You don't want Disease to define her or be in her vocabulary, but as much as you try to protect her, you know you can't trick her 6-year-old brain anymore when she is wailing, "What is WRONG with me lately, Mommy?" So after you finally manage to drop her off at school, with her fatigued, pale brother who you are also trying to create a very normal world for, you pull into your driveway and sit in your car and cry.

I hear so many of these stories, every single day.

Lyme sufferers are visiting doctors' offices and emergency room departments in local hospitals daily, only to be turned away. They are suffering from seizures, indescribable pain, shortness of breath, immobility, and black-outs, only to be told to go home, there is nothing they can do, that there's no such thing as Lyme here, that it's all in their heads.

The medical denial of this disease is all so painful and outrageous, and we're left with little recourse other than to find a Lyme-literate doctor—one of a small subset of medical professionals who are not easy to locate and can be cost-prohibitive for some.

What would happen, I wonder, if each and every Lyme sufferer who gets mocked, bullied, misdiagnosed, or invalidated by their doctor reported their doctor to their licensing and regulatory body. What if we inundated the authorities with complaints in unprecedented numbers? Would it eventually force them to take action against this madness?

I'm afraid that the answer is "no." Those who have led the charge in decades past have written books, alerted the media, rallied, protested, and marched on Washington, met with all kinds of officials, including congressmen and MPs, and served the Department of Justice with criminal charge sheets. Yet here we are—still clamoring to be heard, considered, and understood.

Although there are plenty of "rules" in Alice's Wonderland, true justice is nothing more than a parody where anybody can be executed for reasons known only to the sovereign Queen.

In Lymeland, the powers that be have made all kinds of inane rules, and as in Wonderland, true justice is no more than a mockery, a travesty—causing suffering and pain for so many.

Under Wonderland rule, the monarchy is above the law. Under the medical establishment's rule, it, too, seems to be beyond reproach.

Here's a shocking story about a film interview with Dr. Willy Burgdorfer, and the National Institute of Health (NIH), which tried to stop it:

On February 28, 2007, the UNDER OUR SKIN film crew interviewed Willy Burgdorfer, Ph.D., M.D., and Scientist Emeritus at the National Institutes of Health (NIH), for three hours at his home in Hamilton, Montana. Dr. Burgdorfer is the discoverer and namesake of the spirochete (a type of bacterium) that causes Lyme disease, called Borrelia burgdorferi.

Just as we began filming, there was a pounding on the door, and we found ourselves facing someone who turned out to be a top researcher at the nearby Rocky Mountain Laboratories, a biolevel-4 NIH research facility. Standing on the porch, our uninvited guest said, "I've been told that I need to supervise this interview. This comes from the highest levels. There are things that Willy can't talk about."[74]

What was the NIH trying to keep under wraps? What were they afraid would be revealed in this interview? What secrets are they keeping that caused them to send a representative to muzzle this doctor—a private citizen who was instrumental in the understanding of Lyme disease, had been retired for years, and was a candidate for the Nobel Prize?

Our hope lies in the truth about Lyme disease being told. And here the "truth" was silenced. The Lyme community is grateful that Dr. Burgdorfer was willing to talk—under obvious stress and strain—before he passed away in November 2014.

At a Lyme rally, lawyer Michael Schopmann pointed out this equally chilling fact: "If a doctor begins to treat Lyme disease in any significant percentage of their total practice, they are guaranteed to face investigation—either private or public or both—by managed care, insurance companies, and state licensing agencies."[75]

Just ask Lyme-literate doctors Jemsek, Jones, Burrascano, Murakami, and others—each of whom has faced years of investigation, who collectively have spent millions of dollars fighting the medical establishment, who were forced either directly or indirectly to close their practices, and some who suffered ill health as a result. All because they tried to help chronic Lyme sufferers.

What Doctors Are Being Taught

Medical students are taught about tropical infections such as malaria, yet bacteria in their own backyard are primarily ignored. I'm told that Lyme disease occupies no more than a paragraph in most medical textbooks. I'm told it is barely covered in courses on pathology and infectious diseases, and that it is hardly given mention in the preparatory materials for the American board exams.

Not surprisingly, up-and-coming doctors are being taught little about Lyme, and even less about compassion and empathy. In fact, medical school applicants worldwide are selected more for their biochemistry intelligence than for their emotional and social intelligence—including their natural empathy and humanistic values. They should matter equally. However, in my experience, it's rare to find doctors who are balanced and adept at both. It's no wonder they aren't listening. So many don't know how.

Doctors Who'd Rather Patronize and Bully

I don't know who the author of the Relative Risk Blogspot is. From both the content and tone, I gather it's a disgruntled doctor or a scientific researcher.

In an October 21, 2015, post titled "I Believe, So I Don't Have to Know," the author says,

Belief is an amazing force among Lyme activists, (not to mention among fundamentalists and American Republicans). They won't believe anything CDC says or the data from any journal article that is in conflict with their ideology of chronic Lyme disease. On the other hand, they eagerly swallow any improbable nonsense offered by anyone who takes them seriously.[76]

In reference to a Lyme sufferer's pleas, the same author posted this:

Yes, it's a fiendish conspiracy to reduce the population of white, middle-aged women with nonspecific, subjective complaints of pain, discomfort and depression. Of course, this same nut insisted in 2011 that she was infected with 13 different bacteria, viruses, and parasites. Not even the mangiest mutt in India or Egypt or South Africa would be so burdened. But then it's hard to tell crazy people that they're crazy.[77]

To the author of this blog, I have to wonder: Why don't you spend your valuable time and higher education trying to understand why so many people are so terribly sick? They are not "Lyme nuts" or "mangy mutts," as you call them. They are not crazy, but rather desperate with nowhere to turn. Your tactics—bullying, patronizing, dehumanizing—don't help the cause. Your blogs may be entertaining for you; they're nothing but destructive for the sick and infirm.

The SkepDoc is a retired family physician who writes about pseudoscience and questionable medical practices. In an online post, she admonishes a US pharmacist for her Huffington Post article "Feel Bad? It Could Be Lyme Unless Proven Otherwise" where the pharmacist says,

> *Lyme is a multi-systemic illness, and may affect every part of the body causing fatigue, stiff neck, headaches, light and sound sensitivity, tinnitus (ringing in the ears), anemia, dizziness, joint and muscle pain, brain fog, tingling, numbness and burning sensations of the extremities, memory and concentration problems, difficulties with sleep (both falling asleep and frequent awakening), chest pain and palpitations and/or psychiatric symptoms like depression and anxiety.*

So what exactly drew the ire of the SkepDoc? Here she tells us,

> *That pretty much covers everyone. Who hasn't experienced one or more of those symptoms? I've personally had 10 of them just in the course of the past week, none significant and none requiring a hypothesis like CLD for explanation. If I wanted to identify myself as "sick" and to believe these symptoms were due to a single underlying cause, it wouldn't be hard to fit them into the CLD framework.*[78]

To the SkepDoc I say:

Stand face-to-face with the hundreds of thousands, if not millions, of chronic Lyme sufferers so you can tell them that their symptoms are something we *all* have. I promise you these sufferers will respond with anger and outrage, and justifiably so, because they have spent years listening to medical opinions just like yours—none of which have helped them get well.

What we need are answers. And we welcome those anytime.

Then there's the MD who wrote an opinion piece in the *Montreal Gazette* titled, "Lyme disease is very real, but it's no epidemic."

In the article he claims, "In the end, many of the symptoms will disappear over time (usually about six months)."

Healed in six months. Really? How do you explain why millions are sick for years and even decades?

He continues,

Advocates of post Lyme disease syndrome generally try to scare the public by saying that Lyme disease is a quickly growing epidemic. It is true the number of cases has been rising, partly because global warming is allowing the Ixodes tick to move north and survive the now milder Canadian winter. There were 682 cases (not deaths, mind you) of Lyme disease in Canada in 2013, and remember, we're a country of 35 million people. To put that in perspective, we had 889 non-hockey related ice-skating injuries in 2011. There were also 2,158 fatal car accidents and 3,728 suicides. Finally, in 2013 we had 1,640 new cases of tuberculosis.[79]

First, let's make it abundantly clear that the author's numbers, research, and understanding of chronic Lyme disease do not reflect the reality of Canadian Lyme sufferers.

Lyme is the fastest-growing vector-borne disease in the United States—300,000 cases per year and counting—up to a million by the end of 2015. And contrary to what Canadian doctors have to say, ticks do, in fact, cross the border, and as with most diseases, I am told our case numbers are typically 10 percent of that of the US.

As the author correctly points out, due to climate change and vector expansion, Lyme disease is growing. In fact, one expert predicts that 80 percent of the Canadian population will be exposed to deer ticks by 2020.[80]

I recognize that doctors are human, flawed, and not miracle workers. I recognize that doctors who behave badly may do so because of long hours, excessive stress, and the demands of a high-pressure field. They may do so because of outsized egos, arrogance, and a lost sense of care and humanity. And they may feel entitled to offer opinions without being fully informed.

If this is the case, then let's fix the system. Change the demands. Reduce clinical hours. Choose candidates for medical school based upon their emotional intelligence and their sense of humanity, as much as their scientific intelligence. Demand that doctors do their homework rather than spread misinformation and confuse the public at large.

But doctors, please do not take out your own frustrations on the very people you are charged with helping. Cockiness, disinterest, mocking, patronizing, manipulative, and disrespectful behavior will not be tolerated. Too many people are sick, without answers. They need your attention, not your disdain.

There Is Medical Muzzling Going On

There's something strange going on in Lymeland.

Doctors won't commit. They won't confirm what you've got. They are secretive, cryptic, uncommunicative, patronizing, defensive, and unwilling to validate a chronic Lyme patient's suffering as anything tangible or real.

Lyme sufferers need answers. Something to hang their hope on.

So whether you call it chronic Lyme disease, post-treatment Lyme disease syndrome, late-stage Lyme, or post sepsis non-HIV/AIDS, Lyme patients don't really care. Call it what you will. Call it whatever your legislative body requires. Just hurry up, make up your mind, remain consistent, and acknowledge that Lyme sufferers are ill and need answers.

Stop changing the terminology to confuse us. Tossing mixed jargon around as if it makes any difference to those who are infirm. This is a perfect example of the "crazy-making" that doctors create for patients.

They don't know what it is. So how can they help? And if they do know, they're not helping. They're just creating confusion with their topsy-turvy language that means nothing in the end—especially if it's merely a smoke screen to hide behind.

Can doctors be trusted?

UK Lyme patient Paul Gill thinks not:

Today I went to see my Infectious Disease Consultant at Aberdeen, who last year diagnosed me as having a "chronic infectious disease." This year, he is telling me that he did not tell me that, and in fact, he had diagnosed me as having "post infection syndrome" which was never mentioned last year.

I said if this was what he had diagnosed me as having, why was it that while he was flicking through the letters he had sent to my GP, it quite clearly said he had diagnosed me as having "chronic fatigue syndrome."

Gill asks us to witness the illogical medical trail:

1. *I get bitten by a tick, I remove tick, I get EM rash.*

2. *Get diagnosed with "chronic infectious disease" possible "Lyme" and get treatment for Lyme, but, he informs my GP I have chronic fatigue syndrome.*

3. *Today doc tells me that I can't possibly have Lyme or a co-infection, since I had three weeks of Doxy, also denies that I had herx while on Doxy.*

4. *I asked about Doxy killing all the infections and he said I no longer have Lyme or co-infection. Mention biofilms and he said "show me one medical paper on biofilms" my answer was "give me your email address, I'll send you fifty."*

5. *According to him I have in fact got "post-infection syndrome" and my own immune system is attacking my body, and that I no longer have any bacterial infection.*

What a f-cking joke!!!

I'm not one for using profanities but I am frustrated not just for me but for everyone who has been lied to and ignored by doctors who ignore the facts. Before I became ill, my chosen area of interest was Quantum Mechanics, String Theory, Quantum Chromodynamics, Quantum Field Theory, Quantum Electro Dynamics. I have an Upper Quantile IQ. I don't appreciate doctors treating me like an idiot.

Kris Newby, the award-winning screenwriter, science writer, and producer of the medical documentary *Under Our Skin*, is one highly educated, intelligent person who is certainly listening. She understands that when it comes to chronic Lyme disease, doctors are, without a doubt, being muzzled.

It was her own case of chronic Lyme disease that drove her to produce this important work, which has validated the medical madness that so many of us have experienced.

Says Newby,

I had Lyme during the filming of Under Our Skin. *I'm a relentless researcher and yet it still took me a full year to get diagnosed. It was not a matter of just having a bad set of doctors in California. This is a systemic problem and a complicated set of circumstances. As we know, testing is inadequate and unreliable. The alliance between the government and their funded researchers was unified in denying this.*

The biggest thing this film did was give a voice to patients.

Validation is what they need—so that they can look their doctor or family members in the eye and say with confidence that they aren't whiners, hypochondriacs, or malingerers. It helped patients and their families know that this was a real disease. It helped them to understand the political landscape.

There was a good reason why we didn't interview a balanced number of mainstream doctors and Lyme doctors for the film. At the very beginning, I didn't understand the political landmine I was about to enter.

Newby described how difficult it was for her to get any of the significant IDSA spokespeople or representatives to speak with her at the time of filming, making it next to impossible to get their viewpoint firsthand.

As Newby explained,

...one of the lead authors of the IDSA guidelines, refused to be filmed at the society's annual conference in San Francisco, so we had to fly a film crew out to his office instead. It was an expensive way to get the IDSA official position on the disease.

During the interview, [this particular IDSA spokesperson] had a PR person with him in the room and didn't say much—he called Lyme sufferers hypochondriacs. He reiterated the party line. He had such arrogance in his eyes.

Then we arranged a private interview with [another IDSA official] at Yale-New Haven Hospital. Uninvited, the head of communications of the IDSA showed up as his minder. It was all very carefully controlled.

After these interviews, it was difficult to gain access to IDSA members. We were stonewalled.

Newby then phoned a significant IDSA member to interview him, a certain renowned professor of medicine and microbiology who in 1980 worked with Willy Burgdorfer to help identify the cause of Lyme disease. She asked if he'd explain how the Lyme bacteria cause disease. Instead, he hung up on her.

She concluded,

The IDSA-affiliated doctors didn't want to talk with us. But the LLMDs, the community-based Lyme clinicians, were more than happy to discuss the disease. In comparison, they seemed to have nothing to hide.

Doctors Are in Utter Denial

Every Lyme story has the underlying theme of the sufferer not being heard, not being acknowledged, and not being attended to by the medical system. The very medical system that we once thought was on our side, and was designed to take care of us, has failed us miserably. With Lyme, the expectation that doctors will listen is turned on its head.

Here is **Donna Y Jacob's Lyme story** about her twenty-nine-year-old daughter Bronwyn, their uphill battle with a medical system that is wholly ineffective, and what was required to get her doctors to "listen":

Imagine you are in a room with a raging fire surrounding you. The firefighters come into the room and tell you that the fire is all in your head. You can feel the heat, you are choking on the smoke, you feel the very real danger you are facing, yet no one wants to acknowledge the reality you know is very present and extremely dangerous.

This is how Bronwyn feels all too frequently. This is how she felt laying on a hospital bed not able to keep anything down, even water. Severe vomiting and diarrhea had been plaguing her for years only now it was a real problem. Her weight for her 5'7" frame was 98 lbs. Her gallbladder was removed two months earlier, and sent off to a lab because the surgeons said they have never seen a gallbladder in such decay in such a young woman.

The doctors kept insisting that pills would solve her problems. A neurologist also visited her room to tell her that if she went for psychiatric therapy her problems would disappear. It was after this encounter that she called me, unable to fight for herself any longer. She needed my help and nothing could keep me from her side. I flew from Montreal to Kansas, and settled into a routine at the hospital.

I would drive in with her husband and stay all day. A much-needed relief for Max, he could work without worrying about the medical care they are so used to fighting for. Mom was present to take up the gauntlet.

Each day I would sketch while Bronwyn slept. Too weak to do anything else, I would put the sketches up on the wall next to her "medical white board" to keep her attention away from the "facts and measurements." We soon realized that the sketches broke down the medical barriers of formality into a real person. Nurses and doctors would comment on the sketches and how alone, or in pain, or sad the drawings were.

"Good," Bronwyn would say. "They are starting to see this is a real problem." The medical staff would talk to Bronwyn as a person and began to see when she was

being brave and not admitting to how badly she felt. The nurses would intercede for her making sure that painkillers were not forgotten along with all the supplements she needed to take.

Lyme disease is not mentioned when you are in the hospital for fear that that word would alert insurance companies not to pay for the expensive care required. After much reluctance and observation, they finally ran some definitive tests that told them that her problems were not in her head but very real.

What was finally discovered was severe gastroparesis— her stomach would not empty. Everything just sat there and rotted. They also found damage to the vagus nerve. That is a nerve that regulates digestion. A tube was then inserted into her intestines, bypassing the stomach to deliver nutrition. It was a very long road of recovery from severe malnutrition and uncontrolled seizures and heart problems that surfaced as well.

Several methods of nutrition were tried in the next two years. TPN (direct to blood nutrition) was the most successful but could not be maintained as she suffered from two bouts of sepsis—a life-threatening, whole-body inflammatory response to an infection.

We spent the next two years on this merry-go-round of ups and downs. This is when we decided that the sketches needed to scream out the realities of Lyme disease and "Drawing Lyme Out Loud" was created.

There are no apologies about how dark and sad the art is. This disease takes more than just one life; it affects everyone. Bronwyn now typically hears from all her doctors and specialists that she is beyond the medical boundaries of their experience. They do not know what to do anymore to help her. This is the reality of Lyme Disease, treatments for the disease when antibiotics do not work are expensive and alternative.

The real-life threatening dangers are always present and everyone lives on edge. Along with the anger that no one diagnosed her until 20 years into this battle because doctors in Canada are ignorant to Lyme and the country lacks proper testing. Therefore, together, Bron and I are fighting for recognition and education of the impacts of this disease, and pushing for Lyme to be screened in an annual blood test, since exposure is not always known.[81]

The following are comments that chronic Lyme sufferers all around the world hear from doctors in response to their pleas for help.

Every single day, Lyme sufferers are told by their doctors that they can't have chronic Lyme because...

I don't believe in Lyme...You were nowhere near a tick-infested region, were you?...I would have tested you for it if I thought it was Lyme...Something would have shown up in your blood test...Your blood tests were indeterminate, so you can't have Lyme...Your blood tests were negative so you don't have Lyme...It's a false positive, you don't have Lyme...You got better after a round of antibiotics so it's cured...This disease is very rare...There is no Lyme in this country, city, town, region...If you didn't see the tick, then you can't have Lyme...Did you have a rash?... If you didn't see the bull's-eye rash, then you don't have Lyme...It's Post-treatment Lyme disease syndrome--don't worry, it will resolve itself...It's Post-treatment Lyme disease syndrome and there's nothing more we can do...Go home and find some distractions...Everyone with Lyme has made it up...It's a figment of your imagination...There is no such thing...The Internet is wrong...Stop Googling... When did you get your medical degree?...With all due respect, Google is not medical school...Remember, I'm the one with the credentials...I can assure you that ticks don't cross the border...You didn't go hunting in the highlands of Scotland, did you?...You don't have an elevated white blood cell count so you can't have Lyme...You don't have arthritis so you can't have Lyme—your joints are fine, aren't they?...No one gets headaches with Lyme disease...Lyme doesn't cause your symptoms...I don't know anything about Lyme disease but I can tell you, you don't have it...No one can have that many symptoms...No one can be that sick...You look too good...You're a beautiful girl and you don't need this illness to get attention...It's just menopause...These are just normal signs of aging... Everyone feels tired...You're just lazy...Get some fresh air and exercise...You just need to get out and get busy...You're depressed...You're stressed...You're just feeling anxious... It's likely an inherent weakness...You just need to think positively...It's all in your head...Stop dwelling on your problems...Try praying...If you just stop thinking about it, you'll feel better...Are you familiar with Freud?...Here, I'll refer you to a psychiatrist...An antidepressant and some therapy should do the trick.

Arghhhhhhh! I wonder if doctors know how maddening they sound to those suffering. Do they even think twice before they offer such empty platitudes and mindlessly mimic what the IDSA and the CDC have so boldly pronounced—that Lyme is "hard to catch, easy to diagnose, and easy to treat," and/or that "Lyme doesn't exist at all"?

Doctors around the world have sick people coming in and out of their offices every day, begging for answers, being stonewalled, and being blamed for making it up, being ridiculed for Googling their own symptoms, and for thinking that Lyme could be the answer—when it quite likely is.

How are doctors rationalizing all of this? How are they sleeping at night? Do they even care? It doesn't seem so.

Doctors, please remember your duty and your oath to "do no harm." Such statements are thoughtless at best, and damaging at worst. And they are uttered by you and your colleagues every single day. And by the way, Lyme is not a religion, a philosophy, or a cult that you "choose" to believe in. It's science—take a good, hard look at the existing research. Seven hundred peer-reviewed, evidence-based studies that are accessible to you.[82]

I know my son. And I know what my son has been through and what he continues to experience. No one can negate our experience ...or that of millions.

Matt went to twenty-plus doctors in New York City before *we* figured it out, no thanks to any of them. The average number of doctors that Lyme sufferers see before they are even diagnosed lies somewhere in the range of ten to thirty. Some see upward of eighty. This journey—before you even get to treatment—is a long and painful one for all chronic Lyme sufferers.

Why are you doctors not acknowledging this disease? When you listen to countless sufferers describe their personal experiences, when you really listen to the stories in all their horrid detail, how can you believe that chronic Lyme disease does not exist? How can loved ones believe Lyme sufferers if their doctors don't recognize their illness? How can insurance companies support disability claims if the medical community deems chronic Lyme to be nonexistent? How can Lyme sufferers ever get better when they are told it's all in their head?

Over time—months, years, and even decades for some—the suffering, the pain, the discouragement, and the sheer helplessness that chronic Lyme patients are forced to endure becomes simply intolerable.

To feel sick every day from a systemic, neurological, immunosuppressive chronic illness that shows up in all kinds of horrific ways—from dizziness, nausea, joint and muscle pain, and sharp, electric jolts, to brain fog, memory loss, tinnitus, light sensitivity, numbness, fainting, seizures, and sleeplessness—is, in itself, hard enough. Then to be told by your doctor that "you're making it up," or made to feel as if you're just plain crazy, is a torture beyond description.

Every single day, I read post after post on Lyme Facebook groups by people—just like you and me—who were perfectly healthy one day, and then they were not. A sudden onslaught of weird and mysterious symptoms then sets them on a path of seeing one doctor after another, being referred from one specialist to the next, being given one misdiagnosis and then another, receiving false negative test results, and being confronted by doctors who throw up their hands at best, and bully and shame these sufferers at worst.

When it comes to chronic Lyme disease, the level of medical disregard is unconscionable.

Debra Hovagimian, who was positively diagnosed, then mistreated and neglected by the medical system, wanted to share her horrors:

> *After a surgery last year, I found out that on my patient profile there was a comment that "the patient thought she had Lyme despite two negative tests." This explains why I never got follow-up care and my health is a mess. The tests, in fact, were positive and I had encephalopathy diagnosed by a real neurologist in Massachusetts. I had lesions on my brain. Can someone tell me why this comment was going around the whole HMO. I did not talk about it, but thanks to electronic medical filing, it will always be there. They had no right to make that remark and once again I am fighting for my life because they did not take any of my health concerns seriously. This is discrimination plain and simple. It has to be brought to the courts. If I were well enough, I would fight to my last breath so that no one has to lose their health or feel ashamed for having a disease. I pray for this because too many take their own life in despair. I knew a young man last year who hanged himself because he could not fight anymore!*

I often hear Lyme sufferers say they are ready to give up the fight. Who can blame them? They shouldn't have to fight so hard to have somebody hear them and help them. Isn't it a doctor's duty to believe the patient when they're reporting their experiences, and to work with them to understand it and find a solution together? Isn't it their professional, ethical, and moral obligation? If they can't do this, then why bother? Then, it seems to me, it's time for them to take down their shingle and look for another profession altogether.

Family and Friends Disappear

To make matters even worse, Lyme sufferers are not only suffering from the disease itself and the medical neglect they are forced to bear, but also by the actions or inactions of family and friends who simply disregard their suffering or abandon them altogether.

Here are the words of Michelle Root, a chronic Lyme sufferer, who agreed to share her Facebook post:

Yesterday my brain was on fire and I was feeling pretty freaked out because I "felt" like I couldn't get a deep breath. So I called my mom because I didn't want to be alone. She came over and attacked me for what I eat, the supplements that I am taking and suggested I see another medical doctor because there was something "wrong" with me but it wasn't Lyme. All I want is support and not to be berated by her. I think I have to cut ties because I can't listen to that or be treated like that. I am sick. I am not mentally ill—just physically ill. I want to be believed. Makes me sad that she is so clouded by a medical system that doesn't help people.

Marriages are disintegrating. Friends and loved ones are looking for the nearest exit. Savings are being depleted. Homes are being refinanced and, ultimately, taken by the bank. Children are losing out on their ill parent's ability to parent. Children are being taken from their parents by the courts. Adults are moving back into their elderly parents' homes—if they'll have them.

One Canadian Lyme sufferer had no choice but to live in her car because she had nowhere else to go. "I didn't fit into an acute care patient, necessarily, but there was nowhere else for me," said the forty-six-year-old from Canmore, Alberta.[83]

If *Lyme Madness* can accomplish just one thing, my hope is that more people—doctors, politicians, family, friends, and the public at large—will begin to take this health crisis far more seriously. For all of the friends and family members out there who are doubting their loved ones, remember the words of J.K. Rowling's character Dumbledore when he says to Harry Potter:

...of course it is happening inside your head, Harry Potter, but why on earth should that mean that it is not real?

The suffering that people feel with Lyme couldn't be more real.

Of course Lyme is happening *inside* your head—that's where it resides. Inside your brain, your mind, and your nervous system—as well as your tissues, your joints, your other organs, your cells, your bones, and your bloodstream. That's what is meant by the terms "multisystemic" and "neurological." That's the reality of chronic Lyme.

Faking Good

Instead of receiving love and support, Lyme sufferers have to fake good while enduring naive, ill-informed, and unhelpful comments from friends and family daily.

Utterances and platitudes that negate, dismiss, and shame sufferers such as,

You look good; you must be feeling better...You went out today, so I guess you're okay...Go for a walk; I'm sure that will help...You're so thin—I'd like to be on the Lyme diet so I can look like you...Have you asked your doctor what to do?...Have you thought of this?... Have you tried that?...You try too hard...You worry too much...You're too sensitive...You overreact to every- thing...You're too young to be this tired...You're tired because you're getting old...What now?...Everyone's got something; you need an attitude adjustment...buck up, that's life...What does your doctor say?...Your doctor said it's not Lyme so stop it...When did you get your medical degree?...You're really taking this Lyme thing much too seriously...It's getting you down...You're not yourself... Maybe you need antidepressants...Where could you have gotten Lyme?...Were you ever in Connecticut?... You didn't go camping...Did you see the tick?...When did you get bitten?...Oh yeah, I read that Avril Lavigne has it. They say she's getting better—why don't you find out what she's doing...Who is Yolanda Foster's doctor?...You're lucky it's not cancer...How about that Zika virus?...It could always be worse...Maybe you should just try eating like everyone else...You'd better take care of yourself...Toughen up...C'mon, stiff upper lip...You need to gain some weight...A little bit of fresh air and sunshine should do the trick...You're canceling our plans together again?...I wish you would just come out with us anyway; it can't be that bad...You'd better smarten up or your boss is going to fire you...You'd better get to work; you've missed too many days...I'm not going to listen to this constant complaining any- more...A headache again?...I'm so tired of your misery...

Quit your whining...It's always something...No one wants to hear it...The doctor said it's all in your head... You're blowing this way out of proportion...This, too, shall pass...I'm sure you'll be better soon...You need a hobby...Let's go shopping; that will make you feel so much better...Count your blessings...Everyone has problems you know...Have a piece of my chocolate cake; it will give you the pick-up you need...What do you mean you aren't having a drink?...You're missing the party next weekend?...Your friends are going to stop calling... You're just no fun anymore.

Clearly, these remarks are not helpful. Banal statements never are.

Try listening instead. Be empathic. Ask intelligent questions. Please stop judging and commenting, without being informed.

Know that chronic Lyme sufferers can feel different from one moment to the next. Symptoms can appear and disappear––without notice. Just because your friend is out and about, don't assume all is well. It likely means they've had a spurt of energy that minute––or that hour. It likely means that your friend is looking for that sliver of hope, that last tether to their former existence where they had fun, interests, hobbies, a life. It is likely that they are feeling desperate to re-enter the land of the living and get back to a world of 'normal' again––if only for a morning or an afternoon. And they might do this even knowing that the next day or so they'll likely pay a huge price for this unusual wave of activity.

Your friend might look great, but underneath that thin veneer is a crumbling mess of debilitating symptoms you cannot see. That's why chronic Lyme is referred to as an "invisible" disease.

There's a poster meme that says it perfectly. To the left it shows a Lyme sufferer looking "normal," with a caption that reads *On the Outside*. To the right of the poster, that same Lyme sufferer has an axe in her skull and an arrow through her head, a knife in her heart, barbed wire on her arm, with a caption that reads *On the Inside*.

So before you utter the words, "You look good," or "But, you don't look sick", stop and listen. Tune in to what your loved one is experiencing. Meet them where they are.

Understand that there is no quick fix or magic elixir. Trust that your Lyme sufferer has exhausted most resources and has likely read about every potential treatment protocol under the sun. Assume they are the experts on their own condition—because they *have* to be.

Appreciate that they are Googling daily and immersed in Facebook groups, Instagram, Twitter, and blogs; chatting with other Lyme sufferers around the world for comfort and information; asking questions, listening to what others have to say, comparing symptoms and treatment protocols; soaking up information in an attempt to figure out how to get better—if that's even possible.

Reach out. Let your loved one know you are there. Suggest real, concrete things you can do to help. Send in a meal. Offer to clean their house, get groceries, look after their kids, take them to a doctor's appointment. Read up on a new treatment protocol they have yet to research themselves. Watch the documentary *Under Our Skin* or *Ticked Off: The Mystery of Lyme Disease*. Offer to sit with them to help ease their loneliness and isolation.

And listen. Just listen. With presence of mind, openness

of heart, and loads of empathy.

Lyme is a miserable existence. It's extremely hard to cope with day after day, year after year—and you can't fix it.

Above all, if you really love that Lyme sufferer, stop diminishing and denying their reality. Become informed so they don't have to use up all of their precious energy trying to explain it to you. Make sure you read from sources that are credible—ones that give you the *real* chronic Lyme story.

Please know that Lyme sufferers are sufficiently tormented without having to explain themselves over and over again. Without having to justify or defend their daily affliction. This is a lonely and isolated journey. Many are left to fend for themselves. Their loved ones often act as if this medical nightmare is an inconvenience to them——perhaps a disturbance of their time and reality. They often do the bare minimum and give it about as much attention as the most trivial of matters.

Is it not enough of a burden that Lyme sufferers can't get their doctors to listen——let alone you, their family and friends?

I Discovered People Who "Get It"

At this point in our journey, with the connections that I'm making on Facebook, I'm beginning to feel a bit of relief in discovering like-minded people with similar experiences and sensibilities.

The light came on for me when I found Emily Reach White. I was enthralled. A bright and eloquent young woman with a degree in narrative medicine giving a brilliant presentation on what it's like to watch a loved one live with Lyme. In her TedxGreenville talk on "Invisible Illnesses and Incommunicable Diseases," Emily shares how she "watched in silence and shame as her dad struggled with chronic

Lyme disease for over ten years." After his death in 2007, she began to question: "What makes some diseases more culturally visible, and more culturally acceptable, than others?" She explains that "not all diseases are created equal."

In her blog, *Lyme: At Least It Isn't Cancer*, Emily nails it, speaking powerfully to Lyme as an invisible disease—a disease without cachet, without casseroles, without credibility, without global consciousness—and how simply crushing the invisibility of it can be. In her blog, she compares chronic Lyme disease to cancer in two ways: the similar physical and emotional devastation that both illnesses leave in their wake; and the starkly contrasting manner with which people respond.

I hope Emily's words help to validate and support you as they did for me, shedding light on the impact of this enormously under-recognized, widely negated, yet globally experienced disease. And once you've read her deeply resonating piece, I'm certain you'll want to read her other blog posts at http://www.mysickstory.com.

Here's what **Emily Reach White** has to say,

I probably won't make a lot of friends with this post— but I hope I don't make any enemies either. I hope that what I'm not saying is as clear as what I am saying.

I'm not saying that late-stage Lyme Disease is worse than Cancer. I'm not trying to make any comparison between the two diseases...as diseases. Both Cancer and Lyme Disease are devastating. Both wreck families. Both make victims unable to eat, unable to stay awake, unable to sleep, unable to work. Both involve excessive, invasive treatments that kill healthy cells. I have lost friends and family members to both.

But there are some notable differences—and those differences are all in how other people respond to the illness. How other people perceive the sick person, and the sick person's family.

If you have Cancer, or another sickness from the established disease Canon. The register of approved diseases. Diabetes or AIDS or Parkinson's or Multiple Sclerosis or Cancer. If you have Cancer, people will listen.

If you have Cancer, your health insurance will probably cover your treatment, at least partially...whatever you want that treatment to be.

If you have Lyme Disease, you will get letters from your health insurance company saying that they can't cover any of your treatment because the IDSA Guidelines don't recognize chronic or late-stage Lyme disease.

If you have Cancer, people will establish foundations, and run 5k's, and pass acts in Congress and wear ribbons and buy bracelets and pink things to raise funds for research—to the tune of billions a year.

If you have Lyme disease, no one will raise funds for research, or even believe that you have a disease. But you'll look around one Saturday and realize your 5-year-old daughter is missing...and you'll find her down the street, peddling her artwork and her trinkets door-to-door. To raise money for the family.

If you have Lyme Disease, you will go broke...while you're going for broke.

If you have Cancer, and you're a kid, the Make-A-Wish Foundation will arrange for you to meet your favorite celebrity or go to Disney World. And Hollywood will make movie, after movie, after movie about your story.

If you have Lyme Disease, and you're a kid, your gym teacher will tell you that you have to run the mile unless you can get a note from your doctor. Your teachers will fail you for missing too many days of school. And people will tell your parents that you're just going through a phase. That you just want attention.

If your dad or your mom has Cancer, people will organize workshops and therapy groups for you. People will tell you that it's OK to express your feelings.

If your dad has Lyme Disease, people will tell you that he doesn't love you. Let me repeat that and assure you that I do not exaggerate. If you're a kid, and your dad has Lyme Disease, well-meaning people will tell you that, if your daddy loved you more, he would get better.

If your husband has Cancer, ladies from your church will show up at your door with casseroles.

If your husband has Lyme Disease, ladies from your church, people in your own family, will tell you to leave him. Will call you an enabler. And you'll be too busy helping him crawl from his bed to the couch, or steadying him as he stands so that he can use the bathroom, or helping him finish his work so that your kids can eat to wonder what, exactly, you're enabling him to do.

If people ask you: "Is your dad sick?" And you say: "He has Cancer." Their eyes will well up. They'll squeeze your hand and offer to bring you dinner, put you on their prayer list. They'll say: "If there's anything we can do..." And they'll mean it.

If people ask you: "Is your dad sick?" And you say: "He has chronic Lyme Disease." They will look confused

> *for a moment. They'll say: "What?" And then they'll*
> *shake their heads, smile, and say:*
> *"Well...at least it isn't Cancer."*[84]

Then I was fortunate to come upon Kate Serro—an impressive young woman in her early twenties who withdrew from her undergraduate program to come home and look after her mother who is suffering from chronic Lyme. Kate created a riveting YouTube video called *"Lyme Disease Awareness: The View from a Daughter's Eyes."*

In this video—based on her personal experience—Kate pleads with loved ones to please believe in and take care of their Lyme sufferer. She makes a highly convincing argument, filled with real depth and true emotion. In her video **Kate Serro** says,

> *My mother has been suffering with this disease for over*
> *three years. And I haven't always been able to under-*
> *stand her, and I have sometimes become frustrated*
> *with her. Until I took the time to try to understand*
> *and research the facts for myself. I haven't been there*
> *for her, but now, I have never left her side. This is for*
> *those of you who do not support your family. You have*
> *no idea what they are going through until you actually*
> *try to understand. Here are some facts that you need*
> *to know; they are not crazy, they are not lazy, and it is*
> *not all in their head. The reality is that a highly evolved*
> *bacteria with lethal intent courses through their body*
> *with chronic Lyme disease. Literally dismantling their*
> *body in a malicious manner over an extended period*
> *of time until death comes. That's reality. All other*

claims are a true reflection of a person's inability to reason effectively. They are not stupid; they are under the influence. Within their brain resides a bacteria releasing deadly toxins that are directly interfering with the nerve relapses of their central nervous system. They are on a special diet. When they say they can't go out to dinner with you it's because they can't eat anything. My mom is 100 pounds because she cannot eat anything that won't make her sick. They are not ignoring you, they're reeling. They are most likely lying in their bed, or on the couch, in both a physically and mentally ailing state. Wondering time and time again why they have to be the "lucky" ones to have gotten this disease. Their aspirations have come to a standstill and their life now almost 100 percent revolves around restoring it. Also consider that in addition to the reeling, a person with Lyme disease is more than likely experiencing what is called "floating." And more than likely is exhausted in attempting to explain what they're going through to members of our species, when they themselves don't have all of the answers. I don't have Lyme disease, but I can't even imagine trying to explain to my family what is happening, and no one supporting me, or trying to understand. And I know that is what a lot of you guys are going through, and that's what my mom is going through. Yes, they had to leave their job, or drop out of college, or both. If a person with chronic Lyme can't even carry on a simple conversation, how does one expect them to delve into the untouched matters of the universe in their college courses or the physical demands of their job. The ultimatum to leave *college, or work, although it may be temporary, it is never taken lightly by the heart. I know for a fact my mom still cries about leaving her job every single day. Most importantly, stop saying "well, you look healthy to me." The truth is almost 100 percent of all of the visible evidence to determine how severe or ill a person with chronic Lyme is, resides within their interior. The debilitation can only be felt and truly understood by the person, themselves. Yes, they've been enduring it for many months, or even years. Hopefully by now you have made the rational decision to forget the ignorant notion that three weeks of antibiotics is all that is needed to remove chronic Lyme from the body. Treatment makes them feel worse. The idea that treatment for chronic Lyme causes a person to feel worse is almost counter intuitive, but only to the person's brain. The Herxheimer reaction can become so severe that it can actually kill them. For the record, the severity of their Herxheimer reaction is a direct cause and reflection of their mental and physical state that day. They don't have all of the answers. They're currently struggling for truth and answers, as they are not easy to find. Try not to make them feel like they owe you more than the truth. They're not bipolar, it's actually quite normal because their bodies have been biologically hijacked by a highly evolved bacteria with the intent to kill and seize their biological function. I'm not asking you to give them pity, I'm asking you to try to understand and support them, rather than judging them and walking away, out of their lives with no one to support them. And I'm so glad now, everything that I know, that I can be here for my mom, when no one else is. And I hope you share this video with your friends and loved ones if you are suffering with chronic Lyme. Because maybe this will help them understand, coming from a 22-year-old girl who dropped out of college to come home and take care of her mom. I'm currently working full time, and going back to school to finish my bachelors. Just take the time to understand, and stop pushing them away, and making them feel alone. Thank you for watching this video, I hope you share it.*"[85]

The Power of Being Seen

In one of the Bantu dialects of Africa, there is a word that is uttered daily. The word is *ubuntu*, which colloquially means "I see you."

Ubuntu is a philosophy, a way of life. It speaks to the oneness of all humanity, the connection we share—what you feel, I feel—empathy, compassion, a mirroring of our experiences.

In Sanskrit, the greeting *namaste* shares a similar sentiment. With our hands pressed together and held at the heart, and our heads bowed, we say namaste to one another, quietly declaring, "I honor the divine in you and the sacredness and equality in all humankind."

In both of these sayings, there is a great deal of sacredness and a profound understanding that, without you, I am nothing because we are all the same—all human beings on this journey called life—and we must respect and honor one another as we would honor ourselves, our children, our loved ones.

At the core, both ubuntu and namaste mean that my humanity is tied up with yours. We are one and the same—together we are whole.

So when you—my loved one, my friend, my neighbor, or a stranger—are suffering, I suffer, too. I feel your pain. I will do what I can to help. I know that I can only be whole and of service in my connection to you and to others. When you are hurting, I am hurting. When you are sad, I am sad. I feel your pain.

Nobel Peace Prize winner, cleric, and activist Desmond Tutu said,

Ubuntu speaks of the very essence of being human. We say "Hey, so-and-so has ubuntu." Then you are generous, you are hospitable, you are friendly and caring and compassionate. You share what you have. It is to say, "My humanity is inextricably bound up with yours. We belong in a bundle of life. A person is a person only through other persons.[86]

In our North American culture, concepts and sentiments like ubuntu and namaste are not woven into the fabric of our daily lives. We are conditioned to be separate, competitive, self-protecting, self-serving, isolated beings who connect on a more superficial level.

We celebrate winning, ego, what's mine is mine. We don't naturally or easily cultivate an experience of sharing, generosity, kindness, and love. We operate from a place of threats, fear, resentment, and competition.

Every day, I'm reminded how to value self and others above all else. How to worry less about materialism and focus more on spirituality—the very heart of who we are and what makes us human. How to practice graciousness, kindness, generosity, and not to be afraid of being vulnerable, hurt, or taken advantage of. How to practice active listening, gratitude, and empathy—for a richer, more connected, more meaningful life.

What, after all, is the meaning of life other than human connection and service? I practice this as a psychotherapist daily. I feel lucky and blessed that my vocation is my passion and that I am able to do what I love, in the service of others. Empathy is natural for me. It's what makes me tick—pardon the pun.

To be empathic doesn't mean being a saint. It just means you have both the interest and the ability to tune in deeply to others, to understand what they're feeling and what makes them who they are at the very core of their humanness.

What your Lyme loved one needs is this:

Empathy. Validation. Kindness. Caring. To be seen. To be heard. To be understood. To have someone, like you, stand in their shoes and truly get their suffering.

I urge you to practice empathy, even if it feels feigned, hard, or uncomfortable.

Don't let your fear of illness, your fear of being vulnerable, your fear of intimacy, and your fear of expressing difficult emotions stop you from reaching out in a meaningful way. Find your way into the heart, the pain, and the suffering of those with this chronic illness. Even if you can't heal them, rescue them, or save them from this disease, they will be forever impacted by your love and your efforts to share in their suffering.

And above all, believe them.

Writer and grief expert Megan Devine says, "Some things in life cannot be fixed. They can only be carried."

While I truly believe that Matt's illness *will* be "fixed" in good time, I also know that what he needs—what anyone needs when they're suffering—is to be carried in their pain and in their grief.

Trite, albeit well-meaning, remarks from others are more irritating and energy depleting than supportive. That's why this journey is a very lonely one. People just don't know how to be there. What to say. What to do. How to be helpful.

And, in fairness, this experience has caused many of us push others away. Because we are hyperfocused. Because we are living in an alternate universe and speaking a completely different language. Because we are seeing and understanding things that are dark and frightening that others in our world don't have to see or understand. Because we are trapped in this desperate search for answers and I, for one, have not had the energy to engage in small talk or talk about anything other than Lyme for quite some time.

Writing this book has been a great outlet for me. It has allowed me to make some sense of this madness. It has provided me with the power of connection and community with other Lyme sufferers, caregivers and advocates. It has provided us with resources and treatment protocols that have helped us and given us hope.

In turn, I hope this book will provide you with clarity, validation, and understanding—helping you to feel seen, heard, carried, and empowered as you read about our journey and about the journey of others just like you.

So many things about this global Lyme story are mad, crazy, insane, senseless, deranged, upside down, inside out, frightening, and preposterous. Writing *Lyme Madness* is by far the best thing I've done to ground myself. And at times I've had to stand my ground against the scrutiny of those in Lymeland who have wanted to knock me down.

This is far and away the best thing I've done to help us find our way out of this rabbit hole.

One page at a time.

5. DOCTORS FALL FROM GRACE

You're not the same as you were before. You were much more..."muchier." You've lost your muchness.

—ALICE'S ADVENTURES IN WONDERLAND

I have been disillusioned by the health-care system for decades.

That's not to say there aren't some stellar medical doctors out there. There are. And I have found a few of them in my time—but only with a great amount of drive and determination.

These special gems in a broken system are doctors who have their egos intact and their sense of curiosity nicely placed. They are the ones who think for themselves. Who practice with open minds and open hearts. They are doctors with true empathy—the real stuff, not the feigned "tsk, tsk, there, there", delivering platitudes style of caring.

They are the broad-thinking ones. The ones who admit what they don't know. The ones who say yes before they say no, and are willing to explore all kinds of possibilities with their patients.

They are the ones who practice responsibly but bravely, at the very edge of a system that rules them.

These are doctors who really listen, and who show their patients respect for their ideas, research, and intelligence. Doctors who try to understand the situation from their patient's point of view. Doctors who tap into their own intuition and medical training, rather than blindly abide by the party line. They are the true healers who don't adhere to groupthink.

And they are the ones who are NOT threatened by Google.

There is a well-known meme out there—on coffee mugs and posters. It's an arrogant inside joke among doctors at the patient's expense. It goes like this:

Please DO NOT confuse your GOOGLE search with my MEDICAL DEGREE.

As Beaux Reliosis of Bad Lyme Attitude Blog (BLAB) so correctly counters,

"PLEASE DO NOT CONFUSE YOUR MEDICAL DEGREE with the ability to think critically, understand science, solve complex problems, and treat people with dignity."

Beaux continues, "Twenty years and probably a hundred doctors...and I can count three mainstream medical practitioners who have validated my very real and debilitating illness."[87]

Beaux's experience reflects that of millions, including our own.

To doctors with medical degrees: How dare you confuse arrogance as a viable replacement for medical care? How dare you misperceive your disdain and invalidation of patients as a right that comes with your credentials? How dare you ignore a real and debilitating disease because you don't believe in it or have been conditioned to think that it doesn't exist?

Chronic Lyme disease is not a religion, a philosophy, or a cult. It is not something you "believe in." It is a real and devastating medical condition—with millions of sufferers who can personally attest to the daily misery it causes. We can also point to the hundreds of peer-reviewed journal articles providing scientific evidence to support it.

Yet Lyme sufferers are met daily by doctors who are disinterested and condescending at best, dismissive and cruel at worst, completely marginalizing this "patient group" and relegating them to a life of hell.

At least Google offers resources, research, guidance, and answers—more than we get from you, the ubiquitous medical doctor, whose very job it is to provide this, at the very least, and whose professional role is slowly but surely being rendered ineffectual with the proliferation of this disease.

Physician Peter Ubell, MD, says that much of what is broken about the medical system is that doctors are miserable in their profession.

Ubell explains,

...increasingly burdensome rules and regulations are making it hard to enjoy medical practice these days. Several decades ago, physicians largely practiced as autonomous professionals, governed by standards developed by their professional peers.

Physicians' jobs are becoming increasingly bureaucratic. This bureaucratization can draw physicians' attention away from the purpose of their work—making patients' lives better.[88]

In defense of patients who Google their illnesses and maladies, Dr. Joseph G. Jemsek, a Lyme-literate MD in North Carolina, said this:

Let's face it, some of our patients are as smart as we are, maybe much smarter than we are, and so they can do their own research with this tool. And they will get to the answers because they are highly motivated...and that is what a lot of patients with Lyme disease will do. If they have the money, the time, the interest, the support system, they will find a way to figure this out because they are not satisfied with what they're being told.

In his remarks to the North Carolina Medical Board, and in further defense of patients everywhere, Jemsek said:

Medicine is a profession, not a job. This is a lifelong educational obligation, is it not? We learn every day, and never do we have the opportunity to learn more than when the physician interacts with patients who do not fit the standard diagnostic box. It is a constant learning process, thank goodness, because I never want to work in an environment where we color by the numbers.[89]

Thank you, Dr. Jemsek. You're the kind of doctor I want in my corner.

Doctors without Heart

My personal skepticism of conventional medicine began when I was twenty-five and my father was dying of stage-four metastatic melanoma. It was a grueling three years of illness for him. And a nightmare for us.

My mother, my two sisters, and I had to battle the medical system every step of the way to make sure he got the best treatment, to ensure we were heard, and that my father was medically attended to in a way that was humane, caring, and helpful. We knew that nobody was going to be able to make him well. No one was going to make this dire situation better. But some reassurance and direction from a doctor, a suggestion on how to manage his pain better, some guidance on what to expect, a sense of support so that we weren't going through this alone, would have been nice. And not too much to ask for, we thought.

It was 1985, and all I can recall is a great deal of uncertainty, a great deal of sadness, a great deal of fear, and a deep and abiding loneliness because we felt so bereft and powerless on this journey. It felt like there was little direction or guidance. There was no reassurance that we had a group of professionals to keep us afloat.

In my father's final hours on this earth, he was in such unimaginable pain, like a caged, wounded animal, pacing, wincing, screaming, writhing—not knowing where or how to get relief from his cancer-racked body. We took him to the hospital emergency room late at night because we didn't know what else to do. Shouldn't some medical professional have anticipated this would happen at the end? Shouldn't they have forewarned and forearmed us with round-the-clock nursing care, with the proper pain meds—something so that we weren't drowning in grief, horror, and helplessness on our own?

Instead, on that last night of his life, we were forced to watch him writhe in indescribable pain, at home and in the emergency department, with a doctor barely attending to him. My last images of him were that of a helpless, powerless, broken shell of a man—frenetic, agonizing, thrashing, and struggling about, the lifeblood fully drained, all vitality gone, his organs shutting down. There was nowhere for him to escape the hideous and merciless pain that had taken over his body. This man, who was my father, who was my rock, was reduced to barbaric, subhuman suffering.

It's difficult enough to watch your father's life being violently taken from him. It's quite another to witness the inconceivable pain, impossible breathing, the deep, guttural moaning and groaning, and the unimaginable suffering that a human being can be forced to endure. With no palliative care.

Haunting. Terrifying. Traumatizing. I've been living with those images ever since.

Why was he treated in such an offhanded manner in those last few hours? Why did the emergency room staff not get on his case right away and manage his pain? Where were the doctors? Was the hospital understaffed? Why didn't they see him as a priority in his last few hours on this earth?

A week after he passed away, I took it upon myself (at the naive age of twenty-five) to write a letter to the president of the hospital, admonishing the medical staff for their inattentiveness, neglect, and poor treatment of my father. I remember getting a pro forma response in the mail offering nothing more than a sincerely insincere apology and a promise to look into the matter further. No follow-up ensued.

My next "doctors without heart" experience happened shortly after my father passed away, and I ended up with sciatica which was extremely painful and debilitating. I was on an eight-to-twelve-Tylenol-a-day regimen for eight months—just to manage the symptoms. Despite working with a chiropractor and a physical therapist, my lower back continued to deteriorate at the ripe old age of twenty-five, and I was reluctantly scheduled to have back surgery with *the* foremost Toronto back surgeon at the time. Before going ahead with it, however, I decided to get a second opinion as I believed any well-informed, intelligent patient should do.

When this big-shot surgeon with an outsized ego heard that I had sought the opinion of another orthopedic surgeon, he called me at home, scolded me, and outright refused to perform the surgery—followed by a loud click as he abruptly and angrily hung up on me. I was stunned and broken. In the end, he did me a huge favor. My back eventually healed on its own. His megalomaniacal savior complex saved me from a surgery I ultimately didn't need. While his self-aggrandizement kept him from being a truly great doctor, it ironically protected me in the end.

Then there was my "doctors without heart" journey in 2009 when I needed a hysterectomy because I had multiple uterine fibroids, was hemorrhaging every month, and had iron levels so low that my knees would often buckle without warning. All of my research pointed me in the direction of taking an approach less invasive than a full or even a partial hysterectomy for a better outcome. After consulting with several specialists—all of whom delivered some ridiculously insulting, meaningless, and ill-informed opinions, including one idiot doctor who told me to just have the full hysterectomy because my uterus was nothing more than a "rotten baked potato" (you can't make this up)—I was then fortunate enough to find a true saint of a surgeon, Dr. L. She agreed to perform a myomectomy—the removal of the fibroids— leaving my uterus intact. The previous doctors (other than two in the US) were simply reiterating the party line that any woman over fifty has only one option—a hysterectomy. Talk about groupthink. If you ask my friend Holly Bridges, author of *The UnHysterectomy*, you will see how *untrue* that party line really is.

There have been so many more of these experiences—— both large and small. Matt's chronic Lyme disease obviously represents "doctors without heart"—in spades. Getting the attention of the medical community at large remains a gargantuan work in progress—for us and for all Lyme sufferers. While we were lucky enough to eventually get some good medical care, there are hundreds of thousands, likely millions, of chronic Lyme sufferers who cannot say the same.

A Forced Sea Change

For decades now, we have put up with a medical system that is neglectful, dismissive, fragmented, herd-like, and broken. I can clearly see that with chronic Lyme disease, there is a forced sea change happening in the medical system. As sea changes go—slow, steady, trudging—it may take decades before we see any real progress, but I'm certain we are at the forefront of a paradigm shift in the way our healthcare system operates.

David Bornstein of *The New York Times* writes,

Medicine is facing a crisis, but it's not just about money; it's about meaning.

We often think of medicine as a science, and many doctors do come to think of themselves as technicians. But healing involves far more than knowledge and skill. The process by which a doctor helps a patient accept, recover from, adapt to, or endure a serious illness is full of nuance and mystery. [90]

In an article entitled, "Medical Fraud," published in the Canadian magazine *Vitality*, Helke Ferrie, who writes on the politics of medicine, and who is also the author of *Ending Denial: The Lyme Disease Epidemic*, says,

> *Nicolas Regush, well known for his investigative reporting on health issues for CBC radio and television, wrote the following observation shortly before his death in October of 2004:*

> *"There is no way to be nice about this. There is no point in raising false hopes. There is no treatment or vaccine in sight. There is no miracle breakthrough on the horizon. Medicine, as we know it, is dying. It is entering a terminal phase. What began as an acute illness reached the chronic stage about a decade ago and progression towards death has been remarkably swift and well beyond anything one could have predicted. The disease is caused by conflict of interest, tainted research, greed for big bucks, pretentious doctors and scientists, lying, cheating, invasion by the morally bankrupt marketing automatons of the drug industry, derelict politicians and federal and state regulators—all seasoned with huge doses of self-importance and foul odour."*

> *Later, in the same piece, Ferrie says, "Mainstream medicine is in an uproar, and it's the most prestigious and most decent people who are doing the roaring."*[91]

In an article entitled, "Has Drug-Driven Medicine Become A Form of Human Sacrifice?" Sayer Ji, founder of GreenMedInfo says,

We have entered an era where medicine no longer bears any resemblance to the art and science of healing. The doctor no longer facilitates the body's innate self-healing capabilities with time, care, good nutrition and special help from our plant allies. To the contrary, medicine has transmogrified into a business enterprise founded on the inherently nihilistic principles of pure, unbridled capitalism, with an estimated 786,000 Americans dying annually from iatrogenic or medically caused deaths.[92]

We need to get back to a time when doctors were true healers. When they had strict ethical standards and integrity. When doctors took the time to get to know a patient holistically—not just their charts or symptomatology. When doctors saw the bigger picture and could draw from disciplines other than just their own particular area of medicine.

A time when doctors were the embodiment of the very reason they were drawn into the medical profession. When they could tap into that original drive and passion for taking care of vulnerable human beings. A time when patients were treated like people, not case studies or numbers, were followed carefully, supported lovingly, treated respectfully, without doctors intellectualizing, defending, minimizing, or negating a medical issue just because it doesn't fit with their preconceived ideas. A time when a patient's symptoms and chronic suffering were not negated or referred on, but rather more fully investigated.

We need more doctors with curiosity, empathy, and, above all, courage. Doctors who are willing and able to move outside of their own particular scope of practice; who are willing to consider the falsities of the party line to help a patient. Doctors who care more about the patient's humanity and wellness rather than serving their licensing body, insurance companies, pharmaceutical reps. Doctors who recognize when something is not right and are willing to fight for something different. Doctors who think more for themselves, outside of the conventional medical box.

With the proliferation of lawsuits, restricted access, doctor burnout, insurance company complications, and the practice of defensive, hurried medicine, this may all sound like just a childish fantasy. If any of this could ever happen, however, it will be a time when doctors will rise up again as healers—and heroes—in the eyes of many, and perhaps recover the respect they've so clearly lost.

It will be a time when doctors adhere to their code of ethics and reassume their fundamental responsibilities of considering the well-being of the patient above all else, practicing with integrity, dignity, and respect, and providing appropriate and sufficient care, even when you don't "believe in" or fully understand the disease you're treating.

It will be a time when the patient is trusted and respected for their subjective experience above all else.

I'd like to hold on to this fantasy—just for a brief moment, please.

Specialization Doesn't Work

Medical specialization no longer works. The term itself is defined as knowing increasingly more about increasingly little, and focusing on a limited scope of services. It describes how doctors work in "silos," and are not trained to treat the whole person.

George Weisz, professor of social studies of medicine at McGill University, and author of *Divide and Conquer: A Comparative History of Medical Specialization*, traces the origins of modern medical specialization to 1830s Paris. From there it spread to Germany, Britain, and the US, evolving from a feature of academic teaching and research into the dominant mode of medical practice since the 1950s.[93]

Before 1850, the US had only generalist physicians, but as medical information was introduced, physicians increasingly segmented themselves on the basis of organ systems. We now have hundreds of specialty areas, with more ABMS [American Board of Medical Specialties] approved specialist roles being introduced annually.[94]

It is evident to me that chronic Lyme disease—as well as other multisymptom, multimorbid, multisystemic illnesses—have rendered the era of medical specialization a dysfunctional construct.

There are tens of millions suffering from complex chronic illnesses, including Lyme. The majority of healthcare expenses go to treat these chronic diseases. As more and more patients show up at their general practitioners' offices with chronic multisystemic diseases, a multidisciplinary, integrative approach to diagnosis, treatment, and healing is required. What we desperately need is a "Dr. House—style approach," with multifocused teamwork and a systematic and thorough workup using an exhaustive differential diagnostic approach—the process of weighing the probability of one disease versus that of another to determine patient's illness.

The very design of an isolated, compartmentalized practice of medicine—with narrowly focused specializations, such as neurology, endocrinology, rheumatology, ophthalmology, and the like—is what forces patients to run from one specialist to another, and yet to another, without ever receiving clear or definitive answers.

Generalists are too general and don't have the training, skill set, or resources to diagnose complicated illnesses. Specialists are instructed to see a patient through their idiosyncratically trained lenses and ultimately compartmentalize symptoms and illness.

Therein lies one of the major problems of our medical system when it comes to complex disease.

With multisystemic and chronic illnesses on the rise, sufferers require doctors to have a broad, complex, and highly nuanced lens to get the medical care they need. This truth is reflected in a study that was published in *The Lancet*:

Recently, a group of researchers in Scotland examined the healthcare usage of 1.7 million people—nearly a third of the country. Their findings, published in The Lancet, suggest that 23 percent of Scottish people have multi-morbidity, roughly the same percentage as in the United States, and that this percentage increases drastically as people age.

These patients, said to have multi-morbidity, see a different specialist acting in isolation for each condition. Additionally, because clinical care guidelines and randomly controlled research trials typically focus on patients with only one disease to avoid confounding variables, specialists rarely know how the treatment they administer interacts with other concurrent treatments. This fragmentation results in frequent adverse reactions to drug combinations, redundant or ineffective care, and overall poor health outcomes.

Our findings challenge the single-disease framework by which most health care, medical research, and medical education is configured.[95]

Groupthink and Herd Behavior

It happens everywhere. In corporations, institutions, religion, politics, and the like. People often readily adopt the thoughts, ideologies, paradigms of others, without relying on their own ideas and instincts.

Social influences are powerful. So are party lines and the propaganda machine. When an initial premise devised by the few at the top is filtered down through the ranks to the many, even if it is false, and even when it doesn't make sense, people tend to adopt what they learn and what they hear, conform to the status quo, without thinking for themselves. Even some of the more intelligent among us may have a very hard time straying from dominant, widely held beliefs.

Herein lies one of the reasons we have the global medical negation of chronic Lyme disease. This is one reason why the majority of doctors—as educated as they may be—will tell you that "chronic Lyme isn't real" or that it's "hard to catch, easy to diagnose, and easy to treat."

In his blog, cardiologist Dr. S. Venkatesan cites several examples of herd behavior in the medical system. According to Dr. Venkatesan, herd behavior is "a behavioral pattern where animals and humans in large numbers tend to behave in the same way at the same time without application of mind."

He describes how we see herd behavior in humans daily—in stock market crashes, street demonstrations, sporting events, and mob violence. Herd behavior tends to manifest in any large, highly managed institutional setting where people are often discouraged from thinking for themselves. Venkatesan says,

The practicing habits of medical professionals move symmetrically as a herd. When a top journal or an opinion leader utters something, everyone tends to move in that direction. If a herd leader says a particular treatment is great, every one will say yes. If he says nay, every one will say nay!

No one will really question the direction they move unless the correction occurs from within the herd. No external forces usually are effective.[96]

Russell Blaylock, a retired US neurosurgeon with some interesting views about medicine, wrote,

It pains me to see men and women who are brilliant physicians, dedicated to the art of healing, humanitarians who work tirelessly for their patients, shaking their heads in despair, wondering how much longer they can last in the private practice of medicine. Unfortunately, many have given up the struggle. They no longer dream of being able to preserve their independence, an independence they should know is necessary for the practice of the art of medicine.[97]

Unreliable Research

In August 2005, a landmark study was published in the medical journal *PLOS*, titled, "Why Most Published Research Findings Are False."

PLOS (Public Library of Science) is a nonprofit open-access scientific publishing project aimed at creating a library of open-access journals and other scientific literature under an open-content license. This publication has helped to liberate tens of thousands of research articles and advance scientific discovery as a pioneer of open-access publishing, using an effective and sustainable way to share the latest and best research with everyone.

The author of this landmark study, John Ioannides, boldly stated that,

> *There is increasing concern that most current published research findings are false... Simulations show that for most study designs and settings, it is more likely for a research claim to be false than true. Moreover, for many current scientific fields, claimed research findings may often be simply accurate measures of the prevailing bias.*[98]

When you read John Ioannides's essay in full online, you will see what a travesty it uncovers.

With such startling news—that the most current published research findings are false—what does this mean for the scientific community? Is the jig up? Has a ruse been uncovered? Will medical researchers now lose credibility? How do we know which publications and studies to trust and which are unknowingly skewed? Do medical school professors know whether the curriculum they are teaching is accurate? Are the prevailing standards of practice really safe for patients?

What do evidence-based double-blind studies actually mean?

This changes everything.

In a paper published in the *JAMA* medical journal, Charles Seife sheds even more light on the fraudulent research and conflicts of interest in the medical system. In summary,

- Clinical trial data determined to be fraudulent or mis-handled by the FDA is rarely excluded from research studies published in scientific journals.

- Fifty-seven clinical trials warranted significant action by the FDA.

- The fifty-seven trials Seife identified were, in turn, linked to seventy-eight research articles published in the peer-reviewed scientific literature.

- Ninety-six percent of these articles failed to mention the violations identified by the FDA inspection.

- Two-thirds of medical research is sponsored by drug companies, and industry-sponsored trials are more likely to report favorable results for drugs because of biased reporting, biased interpretation, or both.

- Just as research misconduct and fraud are often not reported, conflicts of interest in academic research are rarely disclosed.[99]

Says Dr. Richard Fried, a physician at The Kimberton Clinic in Pennsylvania,

Some years ago, Marcia Angell, editor-in-chief of the prestigious New England Journal of Medicine (NEJM), "shocked" the medical world with an extraordinary apology. Despite the Journal's explicit policy of disqualifying doctors with a financial conflict of interest from writing reviews of new drug treatments, this policy had been violated 19 times over the previous three years. (NEJM, Feb. 24, 2000). More recently, the same journal revealed, in a survey of hospital review boards that watchdog experiments on patients, that one in three members takes money from the very companies whose drugs and medical devices are being studied. (NEJM, November 30, 2006).[100]

Dr. Richard Horton, current editor in chief of *The Lancet*—considered to be one of the most well-respected peer-reviewed medical journals in the world—says,

The case against science is straightforward: much of the scientific literature, perhaps half, may simply be untrue. Afflicted by studies with small sample sizes, tiny effects, invalid exploratory analyses, and flagrant conflicts of interest, together with an obsession for pursuing fashionable trends of dubious importance, science has taken a turn towards darkness.[101]

Ego, Arrogance, and Greed—Before Patient Care

In my personal experience with doctors over the years, it seems that ego, arrogance, power, and greed often outrank drive or desire to provide quality care. There is a well-known aphorism in medicine: "Mistakes don't kill patients. Egos do."

Some two thousand years ago, Hippocrates said that the fundamental quality of a doctor is to accept his limitations and ignorance. Every physician should aim only at removing the suffering of the patient. Historians also tell us that the success and kudos that Hippocrates enjoyed did *not* go straight to his head. Rather, it drove him to try to improve medical therapies to offer better, longer-lasting, or permanent cures.

In a study entitled "Brief Report: Physician Narcissism, Ego, Threats and Confidence in the Face of Uncertainty," the authors say, "A healthy ego is an important part of overall psychological resilience. However, when faced with an ego threat, individuals with high but unstable self-esteem may be prone to maladaptive behaviors aimed at bolstering or safeguarding their self-image. The medical field, which tends to select individuals who are high in self-confidence yet exposes them to situations characterized by great uncertainty and high stakes, might be fertile ground for behavior patterns of this type." [102]

All I know is that we spent tens of thousands of dollars on medical care while chasing Matt's diagnosis. How can it be that we were unable to get answers? These doctors had no problem charging us for their time, ultrasounds, MRIs, and medications. Only to leave us hanging—without direction, answers, or care.

To those top NYC doctors that Matt consulted with over a period of eighteen months in order to get to a diagnosis, all of whom offered spurious answers to his severe and chronic suffering, I have this to say:

No, it wasn't just a matter of dehydration or low blood sugar.

No, it wasn't just a matter of anxiety or depression.

No, it wasn't just a matter of stress.

No, it wasn't just a matter of a migraine condition.

No, it wasn't just a matter of craniosacral imbalance.

No, it wasn't just a matter of high-reverse T3 mimicking hypothyroid-like symptoms.

No, it wasn't just a matter of a weak Krebs cycle.

No, it wasn't just a matter of allergies.

No, it wasn't just a matter of taking amitriptyline and hoping the symptoms would dissipate.

To what do we attribute this long, arduous string of medical misdirection, this unconscionable series of diagnostic blunders?

Was it pure disinterest and inattention to Matt's story—not taking a very detailed account of his symptoms, jumping to conclusions, not digging deeper, doing little to no differential diagnostic work? Was it about ego, greed, power? Was it groupthink and herd behavior, mimicking what you've been told, without reflecting outside of the box? Was it the knowledge that you might get your hand slapped, or worse, by your regulatory board for treating Lyme? Or was it just sheer negligence?

Tell me, *why didn't chronic Lyme hit your radar?*

To all of those doctors who were willing to waste Matt's time, send him down the wrong diagnostic and treatment path countless times—causing him to become more and more frightened, and his condition to worsen with each passing week and month—and take our money gladly, *we'd like a refund, please.* Even more invaluable to us and to the millions of Lyme sufferers in kind would be some recognition that you bombed!

Chronic, systemic, mysterious diseases like Lyme create great discomfort with doctors and their egos. For the most part, doctors don't like to be challenged by their patients. They don't appreciate being stumped, one-upped, or called out by the layperson. They are uncomfortable not having answers. I've experienced this countless times.

It's a shame that doctors don't realize their patients' anger and frustration comes from being roadblocked as they fearfully search for answers to their illness.

Understanding their patients' high emotional response is part of a doctor's job. It would behoove doctors to not take it so personally. Or mock their patients for delving further.

In a recent article posted by the CBC, Canadian Megan Duczminski recounts how "she will never forget the moment when, lying in a hospital bed and waiting for treatment, she overheard residents outside her door talking about her case."

> *"They were laughing. They were saying 'Oh, she thinks she has this symptom, too? And she thinks she has that symptom, seriously?'" she said. "They were ridiculing me."*

> *Duczminski, 29, said she's spent close to two years in and out of hospital seeking respite from a myriad of symptoms, ranging from headaches to partial paralysis, only to get conflicting diagnoses, ridicule or both.*

> *Duczminski had unsuccessfully searched for answers since the first symptoms appeared, including going to doctors in the U.S. who now say she has Lyme disease.[103]*

Such a tragically common experience for Lyme sufferers.

In the meantime, please hear Jennifer—a Toronto Lyme sufferer who had just come back from the US, where she had round two of five traumatic days of painful IV antibiotic treatment. When she returned home, she needed some blood work done, and walked into a downtown medical clinic. The doctor's ignorance and arrogance caused her to turn to the only defense she knows—sarcasm driven by palpable rage.

To start, I love how walk-in clinic doctors make me feel like a criminal—like I am doing something shady and it's the biggest snub to our province's incredible medical system.

How dare I question it and go elsewhere for treatment? We are so "advanced" here—how could I go elsewhere?

I have to defend myself and my choices to them, like I am doing something illegal. I'm not asking them to give me heroin. I am asking for bloodwork because I am on abx. It's pretty simple. I got a condescending and sideways look from this little punk genius because I asked for bloodwork.

He asked how I came to my diagnosis. I said I was bored on a Thursday night and needed the thrill of coming up with a WebMD diagnosis just to stump him. He stopped listening and walked out of the room with the requisition.

When he came back, he asked in this self-righteous tone, "So why didn't you just get treatment here? You can't find anyone here?" I responded with, "Clearly not, are you offering?" The answer was an outright "No."

As if I didn't think of getting treatment in my own province where I live?

His last line and stupidest comment by far was, "But you're better now, right?"

Oh ya, 100%. I'll be running an ironman in two weeks. The fact that my muscle spasms have lasted two full days now and I am shaking like a Parkinson's patient is no big deal. I'm going to have to buy plastic dishware at this point because I drop everything, but yes I am feeling much better after my one round of IV antibiotics that you know of.

Idiot...

And when I asked for a cardiologist referral, he asked casually if I have ever had a stress test, and I said, "Yes, it's called life."

To all the medical doctors who are this stupid and this arrogant, I know you can't see my pain just like I can't see your stupidity until you open your mouth...and no I'm not better.

The Toxicity of Big Pharma

What happened to the Rife machine invented by Royal Raymond Rife after it was discovered to heal cancer and other diseases way back in the 1930s? What happened to the orthomolecular branch of medicine that claimed significant health benefits by administering megadoses of vitamins after it was discovered by Dr. Abram Hoffer and double Nobel Laureate Dr. Linus Pauling in the 1950s? What happened to the discovery that turmeric has healing potential in over one hundred different types of cancers?

There are so many examples—just like these—of non–Big Pharma discoveries with tremendous healing properties that somehow got shelved before they fully reached the public domain.

Meanwhile, it is clear that conventional medicine—driven and strong-armed by Big Pharma—often doesn't work. It can be dangerous, costly, and highly ineffective. Will antibiotic resistance and pharmacological toxicity mark a shift in the power held by Big Pharma, with chronic Lyme at the helm of this decline?

Dr. John Regan Virapen is a former Eli Lilly and Company executive who after thirty-five years with the business decided to quit and speak out about Big Pharma's profit motive, and how these companies ultimately benefit from sustaining rather than healing chronic, lifelong, symptomatic diseases.

In *Death by Medicine*, authors Gary Null, PhD, et al. report, "Over 700,000 Americans die each year at the hands of government-sanctioned medicine, while the FDA and other government agencies pretend to protect the public by harassing those who offer safe alternatives."

"Something is wrong when regulatory agencies pretend that vitamins are dangerous, yet ignore published statistics showing that government-sanctioned medicine is the real hazard."

The authors continue, "A definitive review of medical peer-reviewed journals and government health statistics shows that American medicine frequently causes more harm than good."[104]

While long-term antibiotic treatment is the first line of defense for chronic Lyme sufferers, most are all too aware that Big Pharma and conventional medicine do not provide the answers they need for healing, and some pharmaceutical protocols have, at times, even proven harmful.

Let's look at Cipro, for example—a fluoroquinolone antibiotic used to treat bacterial infections like Lyme. When I learned that my son was given Cipro last summer, I was horrified. Here's why:

While the FDA requires that all medications warn users of potential side effects, Cipro actually comes with a *black box warning*—the strictest warning label for prescription drugs or drug products required by FDA when there is reasonable evidence of an association of a serious hazard with the drug.

Has your doctor ever told you about this FDA black box warning before prescribing Cipro to you? Or Levaquin or Avelox, for that matter?

If not, why not?

Why aren't doctors informed? And if they are informed, then why aren't they informing and warning *us*?

As reported on WebMD:

The new warnings apply to fluoroquinolones, a class of antibiotics that includes the popular drug Cipro. The FDA has told companies that the drugs must now carry "black box" warnings alerting doctors and patients that the drugs can increase risk of tendinitis and tendon rupture in some patients.[105]

What this article doesn't explain is that the lawsuits pending—and there are thousands—are making claims for the drug's possible connection to peripheral neuropathy, a type of nerve damage that is something far more debilitating than the aforementioned description of ruptured tendons.

According to the description of the condition on Mercola.com, "Peripheral neuropathy is nerve damage in the arms and/or legs, characterized by 'pain, burning, tingling, numbness, weakness, or a change in sensation to light touch, pain or temperature, or sense of body position.'"[106]

Just watch some of the YouTube videos on this to understand the horror that Cipro can create. Do a Google search on Cipro, FDA black box, and YouTube, and watch firsthand accounts of people who have suffered permanent damage from this antibiotic.

Or listen to Lisa Sikes, a Lyme sufferer I met on Facebook who was eager to share this:

> I took two pills of Cipro in January of this year and have not been able to walk since. There are thousands with severe injury from this class of drug. I believe that those who took these antibiotics in the course of treating Lyme may have been injured, but didn't recognize the drug side effects due to the Lyme herx. I share this in hopes that we can warn the Lyme community about these drugs. I have dealt with Lyme for 13 years and never had the tendon pain and weakness that I have from this drug. It put me in a wheelchair.

> Yes! Please share it, I feel we must be responsible for getting the word out as a community because the FDA does NOT have our best interests at heart and are failing to protect us. I especially feel that Lyme patients are vulnerable to the side effects. So please do put a warning out!"

It's interesting to note that Johnson & Johnson is now facing an $800 million RICO lawsuit over accusations of mislabeling, misbranding, and downplaying the harmful side effects of its own fluoroquinolone antibiotic—Levaquin—for the company's financial gain. This after thousands have been injured.[107]

Yet—every single day—doctors are still prescribing these drugs to uninformed patients like you and me.

Only recently did we learn that Dr. Margaret Hamburg, former commissioner of the FDA, was charged in a federal lawsuit "with conspiracy, racketeering and colluding to conceal deadly drug dangers—under the federal Racketeer Influenced and Corrupt Organizations law (RICO) law. The amended RICO lawsuit was filed on April 11, 2016 in the US District Court in Washington DC on behalf of eight plaintiffs who claim they have suffered severe harm by ingesting the drug, Levaquin whose deadly risks were concealed to protect financial interests."[108]

It's about time someone pays a price for these crimes against humanity.

The Vaccine Debate

The great American cartoonist Charles M. Schulz once said, "There are three things I have learned never to discuss with people... Religion, Politics, and The Great Pumpkin." If he were alive today, he may have considered an even more contentious lineup of topics never to broach: "Religion, politics...and vaccines."

There is no debate more inflammatory or polarizing than that of immunization.

On the one hand, we have Big Pharma and other stakeholders who are obviously provaccine, and whose standard argument centers around herd immunity and the eradication of disease. "Look at polio," they say. "Where would we be without that vaccine? It has eradicated this disease from most regions worldwide."

With a diametrically opposed point of view, we have the antivaxxer movement, consisting primarily of parents who refuse to inoculate their children due to vaccine injuries and justifiably demand freedom of choice. It is led by such notables, to name a few, as American osteopathic physicians Dr. Sherri Tenpenny and Dr. Joseph Mercola, Mike Adams of Natural News, and, of course, Dr. Andrew Wakefield and Del Bigtree, the director and producer, respectively, of the newly released US documentary *Vaxxed: From Cover-Up to Catastrophe*, alleging a cover-up by the Centers for Disease Control and Prevention of a purported link between the MMR vaccine and autism.

There is a whole spectrum between these two opposing factions. Those who may not oppose immunization altogether but would also like to make informed choices as to how and when to vaccinate their children. Those who are not against herd immunity but rather resist herd mentality. They will argue that they have a right to do their own research, to carefully assess the individual health of each of their children before deciding to vaccinate, to decide whether each vaccine and the current vaccine schedule suits their needs, whether to delay or opt out of certain shots altogether. They reasonably submit that it's undemocratic to have vaccines mandated. Some parents, for example, feel that they should have the right to opt out of or simply delay administering those particular vaccines where the potential adverse outcomes of the shot may seem more ominous than the disease itself. This is especially the case as today's vaccine schedule consists of upward of seventy vaccines, a huge increase from my era when we were given no more than five or six throughout our childhood and teenage years to consider.

The history of immunization dates back hundreds of years. From Buddhist monks who drank snake venom and Edward Jenner who discovered a vaccine for smallpox, to Louis Pasteur who created vaccines for anthrax and rabies and Jonas Salk (killed-type vaccine) and Albert Sabin (oral, live, attenuated vaccine) who were responsible for the eradication of polio, vaccines have been part of our medical world for eons.

And the debate is not new.

As stated by Inmaculada Melo-Martin and Kristen Intemann in a 2014 *Perspectives On Science* journal article, "Many have argued that allowing and encouraging public avenues for dissent and critical evaluation of scientific research is a necessary condition for promoting the objectivity of scientific communities and advancing scientific knowledge. The history of science reveals many cases where an existing scientific consensus was later shown to be wrong. Dissent plays a crucial role in uncovering potential problems and limitations of consensus views. Thus, many have argued that scientific communities ought to increase opportunities for dissenting views ..."[109]

Those who have contested vaccines have been well documented over the years.

Dr. James. R. Shannon, former director of the National Institutes of Health, once said, "The only wholly safe vaccine is a vaccine that is never used."[110]

Leonard Scheele, the Surgeon General of the United States, addressing an AMA Convention in 1955, said, "No batch of vaccine can be proved safe before it is given to children."[111]

Sir Graham S. Wilson, a noted bacteriologist, said,

"Vaccines, of one sort or another, have conferred immense benefit on mankind but, like aeroplanes and motor-cars, they have their dangers...It is for us, and for those who come after us, to see that the sword which vaccines and antisera have put into our hands is never allowed to tarnish through over-confidence, negligence, carelessness, or want of foresight on our part."[112]

Before you judge my own dissenting view, know that I am *not* an antivaxxer. My kids both had the scheduled vaccines as children and teenagers. Nor, as I've stated before, am I an immunologist, a microbiologist, or an analytical chemist.

What I am is a deeply concerned mother who has been forced to dig deep in order to understand the mechanisms of my son's chronic illness. And I am clearly a chronic Lyme disease advocate. If that should put me in the same category as an antivaxxer, then so be it.

I have been warned not to discuss vaccines because it is a topic that is so complex and so highly inflammatory. As such, I will keep this discussion brief and contained to our personal experience.

At the heart of the vaccine debate is the list of ingredients used. The main ingredient in most vaccines is the antigen, the killed or weakened germ (a.k.a. flu bacteria for the flu shot), which causes the body to create specific antibodies or sensitized T cells. Apart from antigens, vaccines include adjuvants which are designed to induce an immune response to the antigen, produce a higher amount of antibodies, and provide longer protection; antibacterial agents, to prevent contamination during the manufacturing process; and preservatives and stabilizers to help maintain quality during storage at different temperatures.

It is the preservatives and stabilizers in vaccines that are often a source of great concern for parents and patients and at the same time widely defended as perfectly safe by the manufacturers and other stakeholders.

One of these preservatives is thimerosal, a mercury-based neurotoxin that is used in the flu vaccine to prevent any growth of bacteria, fungus, or germs that could contaminate the vaccine.

The research that I've come across, along with our own personal experience, makes me question whether vaccines—filled with adjuvants, antibacterial agents, contaminated microorganisms like mycoplasma, and poisonous treats such as mercury, aluminum, fungi, and mold—may be one of many triggers responsible for expressing a long list of conditions in some people, including chronic Lyme.

While we don't know how Matt contracted chronic Lyme disease, I have to wonder if it is possible that thimerosal—an organic mercury compound and a preservative in my son's flu shot that he received in October of 2012—may have been the catalyst, *not the cause*, for Matt's chronic neurological immnunosuppressive illness. I repeat: the catalyst, not the cause. Or was it the aluminum phosphate, the fungi, the formaldehyde, the mold?

According to PublicHealth.org, "Today, no vaccine contains Thimerosal except the influenza vaccine, and Thimerosal-free alternatives are available."[113]

It was the influenza vaccine that Matt had in October 2012. One week later, he began to feel ill and wondered whether he had been subjected to a "bad batch." He did not have the thimerosal-free alternative. He didn't know there was such a thing or a need for such a thing. Nor were we at all aware that his immune system was already highly compromised.

So here's my plea to the medical profession.

Shouldn't there be a protocol for assessing the health of a patient's immune system before administering vaccines?

Shouldn't doctors be made more aware of the potential for the serious immunosuppression that vaccines can cause?

Shouldn't vaccine makers be spending more time and energy training their public servants—a.k.a. doctors—to inform patients of the ingredients in vaccines, to communicate the potential side effects other than a sore arm, and to assess the immune health of their patient before jabbing them?

Again, it was Dr. Thomas Rau of the Paracelsus Clinic in Switzerland who made it crystal clear for me. In his video, he says that not every tick bite will contribute to inflammation and that the Borrelia bacteria are not the only enablers of the disease. In this video that unlocked the mystery for me of how Matt and so many others may have contracted chronic Lyme, Dr. Rau reveals how vaccines threaten human health—in a way most of us may have never considered.

In his research, Dr. Rau discovered the difference between those who healed on their own from those who could not. Those who could not heal on their own also had viruses—in fact, 100 percent of them had underlying viruses and toxicity that added to the stress of the immune system.

Dr. Rau's research led to other revelations. He determined that specific vaccine viruses were also cofactors: tick-borne meningoencephalitis vaccine, hepatitis B vaccine, *flu vaccine*, Coxsackie vaccine, and the Epstein-Barr virus (EBV) vaccine.

At the heart of the vaccine dispute is the potential harm created by fungal-viral synergy and injecting live vaccines into immunocompromised hosts. Fungi are well known to suppress the immune system and reactivate viruses.[114]

It is the way in which vaccines can affect our immune system, possibly causing dysregulation and the inability to respond properly in the face of illness, that is of most concern.

What I understand is that due to vaccines, and the fungal-viral synergy it can create, the immune system may become suppressed and multiple herpesviruses (EBV, CMV, HHV-6, to name a few) can be reactivated. Due to immuno-suppression, you may not even produce antibodies to these herpesviruses. You may also become susceptible to all kinds of opportunistic infections which can result in Post-Sepsis Syndrome, or immunoparalysis.

Now back to thimerosal. From mad hatter syndrome in the late 1800s, to pink disease in the first half of the twentieth century, to the Iraqi grain incident in the early 1970s, humans have learned time and again of the debilitating neurological and physical damage that mercury can cause. Then why and how did it end up in our vaccines?

Thimerosal is listed on the box of the flu vaccine. It is added to the flu shot to safeguard against contamination of the vial. While no specific set of symptoms will show up definitively as mercury poisoning, symptoms can range from tremors, headaches, and cognitive dysfunction, to muscle weakness, loss of fine motor control, vision impairment, and damage to your organs. Some of the very same symptoms experienced with neurological Lyme.

Everyone is exposed to mercury in some way—fluorescent lighting, fever thermometers, novelty items, electronic gadgets, dental fillings, and certain types of fish. The question as to whether mercury is toxic has never been up for debate. And it's not so much about the possibility of exposure but rather whether the mercury is ingested or injected straight into your bloodstream, the amount that is consumed or transmitted, how your immune system will handle this poison, and whether your body can eliminate it without devastating effects to your immune system.

We know that mercury can contribute to the dysfunction and downregulation (or suppression) of your immune system. And mercury, it seems, is the preservative of choice for many vaccine manufacturers. The real problem lies in not being told by our doctors who administer the vaccines that this is the case, and then receiving this poison via a vaccine without knowing how or if your body can manage its potentially disastrous aftermath.

The documentary *Trace Amounts: Autism, Mercury and the Hidden Truth* explores the origin of the use of mercury in vaccines and exposes the continued greed-based decision to keep mercury in the vaccines through several decades.

Trace Amounts is the true story of Eric Gladen's painful journey through mercury poisoning that he believes resulted from a thimerosal-loaded tetanus shot. His discoveries led him on a quest for the scientific truth about the role of mercury poisoning in the Autism epidemic.[115]

The New York Times reported that a ban on thimerosal might "devastate public health efforts in developing countries," which prominent doctors and public health officials claim as the reason why there continues to be a strong push for the addition of thimerosal to vaccines:

> ... *a proposal that the ban include thimerosal, which has been used since the 1930s to prevent bacterial and fungal contamination in multidose vials of vaccines, has drawn strong criticism from pediatricians. They say that the ethyl-mercury compound is critical for vaccine use in the developing world, where multidose vials are a mainstay.*

Banning it would require switching to single-dose vials for vaccines, which would cost far more and require new networks of cold storage facilities and additional capacity for waste disposal, the authors of the articles said.[116]

Apart from the toxicity that the flu shot potentially transmits, it has been reported that it may not really do the job it's meant to do. Affirming the flu shot's lack of efficacy and its potential dangers, Dr. Mercola, a board-certified family doctor, writes in his blog,

"Despite the fact that last year's (2014 to 2015) flu vaccine was a major flop with an abysmal 18 percent effectiveness rate, the US Centers for Disease Control and Prevention (CDC) publicly expressed unreserved confidence in this year's (20152016) vaccine ... Unfortunately, instead of warning the public that annual flu shots may carry unknown risks and cause effects that are not well understood, public health officials continue to promote them as a panacea for influenza prevention. To say this is misleading is a vast understatement.[117]

CBC News also recently reported that "People who receive flu vaccines year after year can sometimes show reduced protection, an effect that Canadian infectious disease specialists say muddies public health messages for annual flu vaccine campaigns."[118]

The debate about the efficacy, safety, and potential damage caused by the flu shot (among other vaccines) wears on. It is a debate that centers around the interests of Big Pharma and other stakeholders, which rationalize their actions based on their duty to public health both here and in developing countries, versus the health and vitality of so many who are immunocompromised and negatively affected.

Just to reiterate, my understanding about Matthew's case of Lyme disease—which we had to determine ourselves, and which mirrors the experience of so many others—is that he was perhaps bitten by a tick at summer camp as a teenager, or at his university where Lyme is highly endemic. We don't know. He never saw the tick, the bull's-eye, or the bite, which is the case for most chronic Lyme sufferers. So the jury is still out on that theory for us. But what we know now—and did not know then—is that his immune system was highly compromised due to the Lyme bacteria and retroviruses such as EBV that lay dormant in his system.

The flu shot, it seems, due to fungal-viral synergy and the mercury additive, was the *Stealth Bomber* that finished him off, taking his already-weakened immune system to an all-time low of shutdown mode.

It was just one week after the flu shot that his cascade of acute and varied symptoms appeared—sending us on this mad, crazy, unsupported medical journey to try to understand what was making him so ill.

Can I prove it unequivocally? Of course not. But with all of the research that I've collected from a multitude of sources—along with Matt's carefully detailed chronology of his symptoms—my own personal analysis points directly to the flu shot as the trigger that expressed his disease.

To make matters worse, Matt was required to get several more vaccines in order to receive his US green card that he had been so anxiously awaiting for six years. There was no option if he wanted to continue his life in NYC—get these shots or leave. Mandatory vaccinations, even for the immunosuppressed.

So that's our vaccine story.

I certainly understand and empathize with the antivaxxer platform now.

Please keep in mind that most mothers who are anti-vaxxers were once mothers who blindly vaccinated their children—that is, until their children were irrevocably harmed. In the reporting period from November 16, 2014, to February 15, 2015, there were 117 adjudicated cases of vaccine injuries and deaths in vaccine court, primarily due to the flu shot.[119] These cases were purported to result in Guillain-Barré syndrome, a disorder in which the body's immune system attacks part of the peripheral nervous system, and one of the many conditions that Lyme is known to imitate.

In conclusion, I have to believe that antivaxxers are no "crazier," no more conspiratorial than Lyme activists, or even AIDS activists in the '80s, for that matter. I'm certain that if we were all better informed or personally affected, this group would grow exponentially. At least until such time as the pharmaceutical industry becomes more accountable to those who are vaccine injured and routinely tests for those whose immune systems are compromised and may be adversely affected.

The Advent of Narrative Medicine

Hippocrates, the father of modern medicine, dedicated his entire life to understanding and researching health, medicine, and the human condition. He once said: "It is more important to know what sort of person has a disease than to know what sort of disease a person has."

One bright light in this depressing, stagnant, and too often dysfunctional medical world we live in is the introduction of narrative medicine in colleges, universities, medical schools, and professional development workshops.

Since the 1970s, in response to the growing disheartenment among doctors and patients alike—where it was clear that medicine had become far more about treating problems rather than people (i.e., the cancer patient in room 243, the heart patient in room 456)—narrative medicine was slowly introduced to help doctors open their eyes, stretch their minds, and exercise their hearts to something beyond the clinical picture of illness.

This newer branch of medicine was introduced to promote a deeper understanding between the doctor and patient, to give the patient a way to construct some meaning and context for their illness, to provide doctors with analytical clues that could aid in a more accurate diagnosis, and to encourage a more holistic, whole-person approach to medicine.

Rita Charon, an internist with a PhD in English literature, was the pioneer of narrative medicine. She was responsible for encouraging more than half of North American schools to include it in their core curriculum.

The purpose of narrative medicine, Charon hoped, was to teach empathy and to prevent further doctor and residency burnout—which the medical system's construct so often promotes.

Dalhousie University was the first university in Canada to introduce such a course. Known as HEALS—Healing and Education through the Arts and Life Skills—the program offers visual arts, narrative, music performing arts, and the history of medicine with the intention of offering new ways to make a significant difference in the lives of the very ill.

In 2004, The Heartbeat Project was introduced by then-president of the College of Family Physicians of Canada, Dr. Rob Wedel, along with Dr. Ruth E. Martin.

The Heartbeat Project's mandate has been to collect

and publish a book of stories that had "awed, encouraged, moved, inspired, provoked, troubled, humbled or worried us" in the course of their family practice careers.

The project received a warm welcome among the medical community.

Narrative medicine stands on the shoulders of many of the master healers who understood the healing power of the arts. Maimonides wrote *Art of the Cure*, among dozens of other similar treatises. More modern-day works include *Bedside: The Art of Medicine* by cardiologist Michael Lacombe and *Narrative Medicine: Honouring the Stories of Illness* by Rita Charon.

Classics such as psychiatrist and author Victor Frankl's seminal work *Man's Search for Meaning* is an example of man's ability to survive and even thrive through story, as he creates meaning out of atrocities through the written word. The great writers throughout history are clearly driven to write not for fame, glory, or ego, but for the purpose of healing, sharing, connecting, and telling their story. The ill and the suffering are discovering that this process works for them as well.

What we know in psychology, in particular, and in medicine, in general, is that there is nothing more healing than the opportunity to tell our story—and to be heard and supported by others in the telling. Our stories—written, expressed aloud, and truly heard—connect us, bond us, comfort us, help us to feel less isolated, less alone. They help us to feel like we are part of the human experience and can help others along the way.

Recurring themes in stories about the human condition, with illness or not, always include love, belonging, community, safety, freedom, family, listening, relationships, and the universal need to be seen.

In my psychotherapy practice, I've witnessed the indescribable destruction caused by childhood emotional trauma—and adult trauma—ultimately transformed into a positive life force, simply by encouraging clients to tell or write their stories. I've seen the deepest heartbreak overcome with the expression of the spoken and written word. I've seen depression and anxiety ameliorated by the client putting pen to paper—journaling, writing personal prose, poetry, and the like. And I've been privileged enough to hear the magic, experience the beauty of the soul, and come face-to-face with the true spirit of those who have found the courage to tell their stories.

Anatole Broyard, an editor and author who died of prostate cancer, wrote:

> *Physicians have been taught in medical school that they must keep the patient at a distance because there isn't time...or because if the doctor becomes involved in the patient's predicament, the emotional burden will be too great. As I've suggested, it doesn't take much time to make good contact, but beyond that, the emotional burden of avoiding the patient may be much harder on the doctor than he imagines...A doctor's job would be so much more interesting and satisfying if he simply let himself plunge into the patient, if he could lose his own fear of falling.*[120]

I'm all too aware that nothing is more healing than being able to tell our story, explain the complexities, write about our suffering—and have somebody hear us.

Just recently, I posted a Facebook image on my Lyme Madness page. It read, "There is tremendous healing power in being heard and validated. It's a matter of survival." This post had a reach of more than 2,500 people and forty-two shares in less than a day. The message hit a nerve. We need to be heard.

How hard is it to let patients tell their stories and actually listen? Isn't that a doctor's job at the very least?

Moving Toward Functional Medicine

We finally have an emerging health-care model that is making great strides with patients who are frustrated and fed up with not finding answers to what ails them in the offices of conventional doctors.

Functional medicine, or integrative medicine as it is also known, is a systems-driven, science-based approach to practicing medicine, and not just a lifestyle approach, as its mainstream critics would have you believe. The whole person is addressed—including a patient's biochemistry, physiology, genetics, and environmental exposures—when looking for the root cause of a specific medical issue or set of symptoms.

In contrast to conventional medicine, functional medicine addresses the underlying root causes of a disease, including such factors as toxins, allergens, microbes, nutrition, and stress. When it comes to more complex, multisystemic diseases, there seem to be far more answers to healing with this approach.

While functional medicine is still in its infancy, it may be one of the answers to the necessary sea change that we are hoping for—driven primarily by a growing number of patients who are not getting the answers they need in the allopathic system.

A few of the more high-profile doctors who practice functional medicine are Dr. Mark Hyman, Dr. Joseph Mercola, and Dr. David Perlmutter, who you may want to check out online. There's also Lissa Rankin, MD, an integrative medicine physician, author, speaker, artist, and founder of the online health and wellness community OwningPink.com.

According to the Institute for Functional Medicine, the practice is guided by six core principles:

- An understanding of the biochemical individuality of each human being, based on the concepts of genetic and environmental uniqueness

- Awareness of the evidence that supports a patient-centered rather than a disease-centered approach to treatment

- Search for a dynamic balance among the internal and external body, mind, and spirit

- Familiarity with the weblike interconnections of internal physiological factors

- Identification of health as a positive vitality, not merely the absence of disease, emphasizing those factors that encourage the enhancement of a vigorous physiology

- Promotion of organ reserve as the means to enhance the health span, not just the life span, of each patient[121]

Great Hope in Biological Medicine

Biological medicine, which originated in Europe, is a medical model that, much like functional medicine, looks at the root cause of the patient's illness, rather than approaching illness with symptom management only. Rather than treating the diseased organ—heart, liver, kidney, etc.—biological medicine approaches each patient as a whole and integrated energy system that will balance, heal, and maintain itself if looked after properly.

Unlike the allopathic medical model, which is designed to make you feel better but not necessarily to restore your overall health, biological medicine treats the underlying dysfunctions and unhealthy state of your body that has allowed the disease to grow and flourish. The treatment protocols are customized to address each patient's medical needs on an individualized, highly personalized basis using hematological, metabolic, genetic, and other tests, as well as an in-depth interview and examination. The protocols range from ozone therapy, cryotherapy, IV therapy to colon hydrotherapy, light therapy, naturopathic medicine, and more in an effort to restore the body's natural functions. The order in which these protocols are administered is also a key factor to successfully improving the patient's health and well-being.

It's important to note that *biological medicine*—a medical model designed to eliminate toxins, activate the body's defense mechanisms, rebuild immunity, resume balance, and address chronic illness—is not the same thing as *biologics*, which can be summarized as "a wide range of products such as vaccines, blood and blood components, allergenics, somatic cells, gene therapy, tissues and recombinant therapeutic proteins."[122]

The Promise of Energy Medicine

When we speak about energy medicine, the term is broad and far-reaching. It includes everything from the ancient practices of Reiki, meditation, homeopathy, acupuncture, chi gong, and yoga, to the more modern-day application of pulsed electromagnetic fields, sound waves, light waves, vibrational frequency, and transcranial direct-current stimulation—all designed to reduce pain, inflammation, stress, circulation, oxygenation, and more.

Many medical healers on the world stage——including Dr. Deepak Chopra, Dr. Jon Kabat-Zinn, Dr. C. Norman Shealy, Carolyn Myss, PhD, Dr. Judith Orloff, and Dr. Christiane Northrup, to name a few——are influential proponents and teachers of these energy practices and are responsible for introducing them to the mainstream of the Western world.

Healing technology—which began to surface with the Rife machine in the 1930s—includes everything from far-infrared rays, amethyst crystals, ONDAMED, bioresonance such as MORA and Bicom, low-level lasers, BioMat, Oasis Pro, and the like. This technology comes in all shapes and sizes—handheld, home use, and the larger, more expensive versions you might find in the clinic of a practitioner (likely a naturopath, homeopath, or an osteopath) who may practice this form of healing.

According to one source,

> *Physicists at Arizona State University say they have developed a method to calculate the exact frequency that it would take to shake a virus to death, according to an article published in the journal* Physical Review Letters. *Researchers have discovered that when viruses are bombarded with laser pulses of the right frequency, they shake apart. This arises from an inherent characteristic of all objects called a "resonant frequency," which is the frequency at which an object naturally vibrates.*[123]

In an article published on Oprah.com, Dr. Erin Olivo explained in detail the promise of energy medicine:

When we talk about energy, we are really referring to two kinds of energy fields: veritable energy fields, which can be measured, and putative energy fields, which cannot be measured with our current technology. Veritable energy fields include things like vibrational energy (sound), and electromagnetic forces such as visible light, magnetism and monochromatic radiation (lasers).

Most frequently, the term energy medicine refers to techniques that involve the putative energy fields. Although it has not yet been able to be measured by conventional methods, therapists who work with this type of energy claim that they can see it with their own eyes or that they can sense it with their hands or bodies.[124]

Before anyone rolls their eyes at this, imagine yourself in a place where conventional medicine cannot help you. You are chronically ill, doctors have turned their backs for the most part, and you are desperate to get well. Wouldn't you take a leap of faith and try almost anything that shows a modicum of promise?

For those who are exceptionally wary about this field of medicine, I suggest you read anything and everything by Professor Jim Oschman—author of a groundbreaking series of articles on "healing energy" published in the *Journal of Bodywork and Movement Therapies*, and now developed into two books: *Energy Medicine: The Scientific Basis* and *Energy Medicine in Therapeutics and Human*

Performance. These books explore the physiology and biophysics of energy medicine.

Dr. Oschman's work will convince even the most skeptical scientists, as he has the academic credentials to back up his theories, including degrees in biophysics and biology from the University of Pittsburgh, work in major research labs around the world, including Cambridge University in England, Case Western Reserve University in Cleveland, Ohio, the University of Copenhagen, Northwestern University in Evanston, Illinois, and served as a staff scientist at the Marine Biological Laboratory in Woods Hole. He has written many scientific papers published in the world's leading journals. He was president of the New England School of Acupuncture, and received a Distinguished Service Award from the Rolf Institute. He continues his research and writing in Dover, New Hampshire, where he is president of Nature's Own Research Association.

From everything I've read and from all that we have experienced, I am utterly convinced that energy medicine is the answer to healing and the "wave" of the future. It will require a complete paradigm shift in our thinking and belief systems before it can take hold. It will require a leap of faith, but I am convinced it's a leap worth taking.

As conventional medicine continues to fail us, as Big Pharma continues to put questionable ingredients into our vaccines and make decisions that don't serve us well, as the true nature of scientific research becomes more transparent and less effective than we have believed all these years, energy medicine may eventually prove to be the best shot we have at healing what ails us.

I can already see the positive effects that the Rife machine is having throughout this stretch of Matt's healing journey.

An interesting side note is this text message I received from Matt:

Mom—I thought you'd appreciate this. I was at the doctor's office today and she asked me in front of another Lyme patient, "What is your current protocol?" and I responded "I am using a Rife machine." The other patient asked "What is Rife?" And the doctor said "It is a type of frequency device. I would offer it but I don't want to lose my license and I am not up for the fight; however, if I had Lyme I would definitely use one myself."

Lose her license if she offers her patients Rife treatment? Madness!

Matt also shared with me that the doctor proceeded to show him an old, wooden Rife machine from the early 1900s that she had on display in a glass case—a gift from one of her patients.

Most recently Matt is the proud owner of a rented low-level laser as a new healing protocol, programmed with frequencies specific to his symptomatology. For more on this, I suggest you read Dr. Norman Doidge's book, *The Brain's Way of Healing.* This has restored some renewed hope for us.

Things Are Shifting

Here's some good news on the medical front. *The Washington Post* recently reported,

Robots are not coming to kill us. They are coming to save our lives. Literally...And it's finally starting to happen, and not a minute too soon.

If you've ever gone to a doctor with an odd set of symptoms and realized that your doctor has no clue what they signify, you too might have wished he had access to some heavy computing power. Those medical mystery stories you've read are one long saga of the tragedy of unfindable medical information.[125]

We haven't just read those medical mystery stories. We are living it. And it's never been clearer to me that medicine has lost its cachet as a result of its incompetence and, even more so, by turning its back on the sick and infirm when it doesn't serve the medical powers that be.

Medicine, as we know it, is dead. There is a sea change happening—a revolution of sorts because we're mad as hell—*sick* as hell—and we're no longer in awe of doctors or waiting for them to rescue us. They can't and they won't. We know more about Lyme than they do. And their arrogance and disinterest has killed our respect for them. It's madness.

Let's bring on more energy medicine, functional medicine, narrative medicine, frequency technology, and the like. Let's replace doctors' arrogance and ineptitude with computer technology that can cross-reference information to navigate the complexities of chronic, multisystemic illness.

It's happening. Medicine is facing a crisis, and a necessary paradigm shift. Lyme, coinfections and other chronic illnesses, are at the forefront of this massive change in direction. With every breakdown, a breakthrough is sure to follow. It's just a matter of time.

My Head Is Spinning

My many life experiences facing inept, disinterested, cavalier, uncaring medical doctors are unfortunately being further validated with this Lyme battle. And what a battle this is!

My private logic has always said, "You're on your own. No one is going to rescue you, so you'd better figure this out for yourself."

This lifelong belief has been affirmed time and time again. Now, sadly, it is being fully realized with this Lyme madness medical experience. Over the course of my life, I've been conditioned to expect doctors not to listen, and for them to be dismissive, arrogant, disrespectful and autocratic in their approach. This time they've proven me right at every turn. And no, this fact certainly does not make me happy or gleeful. I wish it were not the case.

I have fought several other medical battles in my life. These battles were all-consuming and maddening because doctors weren't listening. But each one of the battles I've fought pales by comparison to this Lyme battle.

There are some great doctors out there, but to find them is much like finding needles in a haystack. These are the doctors who think for themselves, who do not follow the pack. They are the ones who listen, who are empathic, who do not lead with ego—but rather with humility, humanity, compassion, and courage.

The medical system is broken, and in the case of chronic Lyme disease, we've been completely abandoned.

No one can argue otherwise.

I'm alone with my research, reading about the broken medical system, thimerosal in vaccines, Lyme wars, Lyme theories, Lyme conspiracies, and the deeper underpinnings of this Lyme madness.

My head is spinning. No one is listening. Few want to hear about it.

The story just gets more and more overwhelming as each new layer is revealed.

It's all too much to carry by myself.

And, I'm afraid, we're just getting started.

6. WELCOME TO THE LYME WARS

"The question is," said Alice, *"whether you can make words mean so many different things. "The question is,"* said Humpty Dumpty, *"which is to be master—that's all."*

—THROUGH THE LOOKING-GLASS

Regardless of who originally coined the term "Lyme Wars"—the scientific community, the traditional press, the alternative press, or someone else—it has stuck.

Sadly, this ugly war wages on.

As in all wars, there are good guys and bad guys, theories and conspiracies, right and wrong, underdogs and heroes. As the Lyme Wars continue to escalate, there are ever more layers to examine, people with fresh perspectives, and a political and medical system that feels highly suspicious.

What other conclusion can there be when examining a disease that affects tens of millions, yet supposedly doesn't exist? Either the sufferers are crazy or the medical and political systems are tainted. You decide.

In all of my research on chronic Lyme disease, I have yet to be able to simply answer the question, "Why is there so much controversy?" The best answer I can come up with, albeit wholly unsatisfying, is, "Follow the money." That is usually the case with most controversial issues. It's often about power and ego as well.

As in all wars, there are countless casualties. Mother, fathers, children, sisters, brothers, friends, loved ones—millions who are suffering without proper medical intervention. People who have lost everything—their health, their livelihoods, their savings, their relationships, their will to live.

The issues that drive the Lyme Wars must be settled before we lose more lives. It's been more than forty years since we first acknowledged an outbreak of this disease in the US. It's time to settle the score—if only we understood what the score was.

What Is Under Dispute? *Everything!*

In a 2003 PubMed article titled, "The Lyme Wars: time to listen," authors Raphael B. Stricker and Andrew Lautin say,

Lyme disease represents a public health threat of major proportions. The murky science and acrimonious politics of Lyme disease have created barriers to reliable diagnosis and effective treatment of this protean illness.[126]

In a 2014 *PLOS* journal article, Raphael B. Stricker and Lorraine Johnson "propose[d] the need for an HIV/AIDS-style 'Manhattan Project' to combat this serious epidemic that threatens the physical and mental health of millions of people around the world."[127] An idea that might bring the attention so desperately required to finally address this real and escalating threat—a threat that is being so widely ignored.

As Michael Specter points out in his January 2015 *New Yorker* article, "A New Front in The Lyme Wars," "Nobody disputes the existence, the danger, or even the rising incidence of Lyme disease. It is an infection caused by the bacterium *Borrelia burgdorferi*."

What is in dispute, however, is an endless number of factors, including:

- Whether to even acknowledge that this disease in its persistent form exists
- How many people are really suffering from it
- What to call it
- Calling it something else altogether, like chronic fatigue or fibromyalgia
- Whether to refer to it as chronic Lyme, late-stage Lyme, post-Lyme disease syndrome, or persistent Lyme
- Where it can be contracted
- How it can be contracted
- How, if, or why it persists
- How to best diagnose this disease
- How to best treat it

As you can see, very little is agreed upon.

In a forty-five-page letter to New York congressman Chris Gibson, Kenneth B. Liegner, MD—a board-certified internist with additional training in pathology and critical care medicine—states,

> *Unfortunately, thus far, the Federal government's response to Lyme disease has been woefully inadequate. While CDC is composed of many fine individual physicians and scientists, denial of the existence of*

chronic and seronegative Lyme disease by CDC, as an agency of government, has harmed many in New York State and elsewhere.

In the same letter, he implores state legislators to,

Listen to your constituents who have been bearing the brunt of ignorance, bias and discrimination surrounding Lyme disease. Who will be next to be told their care is "experimental," "not medically necessary" or "not a wise use of scarce resources"?

Liegner also says,

Physicians who have cared for persons with chronic Lyme disease have faced harassment at a minimum and for some, their careers have been ruined. Researchers who have seriously dedicated themselves to the scientific study of chronic Lyme disease in humans and/or animals have often found themselves attacked or marginalized. To persist in their researches would have resulted in virtual career suicide and some have been forced, by exigencies of survival, to leave the field.[128]

Who's at War?

There are primarily two factions at war: the medical establishment, and Lyme sufferers and their supporters worldwide. Let's take a closer look at each.

The medical establishment—the CDC, IDSA, Big Pharma, and other stakeholders:

The medical establishment is a powerful force.

"The medical industrial complex as it is increasingly referred to is even bigger and more powerful than the military industrial complex. Its turnover is massive. A small group of companies that make medically-related machines and drugs and sell health services, is responsible for fully a third of the $600 billion spent on the nation's health in 1989."[129]

The medical entities responsible for overseeing Lyme disease—the Centers for Disease Control and Prevention (CDC), the Infectious Diseases Society of America (IDSA), and other political drivers—claim that Lyme is *hard to catch, easy to diagnose, and easy to treat.*

To this day, the CDC maintains that Lyme disease is a rare, self-limiting illness localized to well-defined areas of the world. They say that Lyme disease is hard to catch and easy to cure because the infection is rarely encountered, easily diagnosed in its early stage by distinctive clinical features—and in more advanced stages by accurate commercial laboratory tests—and effectively treated with a short course of antibiotics over two to four weeks.[130]

According to the stakeholders keeping chronic Lyme disease in the shadows,

Advocacy for Lyme disease has become an increasingly important part of an antiscience movement that denies both the viral cause of AIDS and the benefits of vaccines and that supports unproven (sometimes dangerous) alternative medical treatments. Some activists portray Lyme disease, a geographically limited tick-borne infection, as a disease that is insidious, ubiquitous, difficult to diagnose, and almost incurable ...The relations and actions of some activists, medical practitioners, and commercial bodies involved in Lyme disease advocacy pose a threat to public health.[131]

ILADS and all chronic Lyme sufferers worldwide:
The International Lyme and Associated Diseases Society (ILADS) is a nonprofit, international, multidisciplinary medical society dedicated to the appropriate diagnosis and treatment of Lyme and associated diseases. The group—along with hundreds of thousands, likely millions, of suffering patients worldwide—counters the medical establishment with its own facts: that Lyme is difficult to diagnose and difficult to manage and heal, with the possibility for a cure still up for grabs.

In stark contrast to the views of the IDSA and its supporters, the real threat to public health is a growing pandemic that is being denied, cajoled, negated, invalidated, and rationalized out of existence, even though the CDC just recently admitted there are 300,000 new cases in the US per year, a big jump from their original long-standing number of 30,000.

If they truly believe that the antiscience, invalidated, unorthodox treatment methods we are seeking are so dangerous, then what are they waiting for? We'd gladly welcome an effective treatment method for what ails millions.

What most Lyme sufferers and supporters will agree to is that, contrary to the IDSA's so-called evidence-based, peer-reviewed scientific opinions, the *real* threat to public health is not the alternative approaches. The ongoing threat to global public health is a medical and political system that denies the very existence of a disease that is affecting the lives of millions, if not tens of millions.

Madness!

The Great Divide

Here are a few of the key arguments that form "the great divide" between conventional medicine and those who suffer from and advocate for medical support of chronic Lyme disease.

The Rash

- **"Conventional" Thought:** About 70 to 80 percent of Lyme disease patients present with a characteristic bull's-eye erythema migrans (EM) rash.
- **What Lyme Sufferers Know:** The bull's-eye rash appears far less often than established medical doctors would have you believe. One reliable source says that it can show up in fewer than 26 percent of Lyme disease patients. And when it does appear, it may present in an atypical way and not necessarily in a bull's-eye pattern.

The Treatment

- **"Conventional" Thought:** Those in the established medical field claim that the early stage of Lyme disease is easily treated with a two- to four-week course of antibiotics.
- **What Lyme Sufferers Know:** Early Lyme disease often goes undetected because we don't see either the tick or the EM rash. Furthermore, the Lyme disease spirochete disseminates quickly, thereby making it resistant to treatment even in the early stages.

The Tests

- **"Conventional" Thought:** Most doctors believe that ELISA is the preferred method to diagnose Lyme disease due to its "sensitivity, adaptability to automation and ease of quantitation."

- **What Lyme Sufferers Know:** The Lyme ELISA consistently misses at least 50 percent of Lyme disease cases due to the assay's insensitivity and variability with antibiotic treatment. The CDC and Western blot diagnostics were originally developed for surveillance of Lyme disease, and not for diagnostic purposes.

The Doctors

- **"Conventional" Thought:** Specialists, including infectious-disease doctors—the very medical professionals who we would imagine would be our go-to support for chronic Lyme disease—tend to adhere to the CDC and IDSA guidelines in diagnosing and treating Lyme.
- **What Lyme Sufferers Know:** These guidelines—written years ago by a panel of researchers and clinicians—do not conform to current standards of evidence-based medicine. Community-based providers who actually witness and deal with the clinical nightmare we know as chronic Lyme disease on a daily basis have rejected the CDC/IDSA guidelines because they don't work. Instead, they offer more advanced and reliable testing methods, along with a more informed and thoughtful clinical diagnosis. Lyme sufferers are forced to seek out "Lyme-literate" providers because the conventional thought leaders have failed them, offering no more than the pejorative statement that "it's all in your head."

The Vaccine

- **"Conventional" Thought:** The Lyme disease vaccine was withdrawn due to lack of public interest.
- **What Lyme Sufferers Know:** The Lyme vaccine LYMErix was withdrawn in 2002, four years after it was first introduced, in response to a class action lawsuit involving hundreds of patients who claimed they developed a "Lyme-like" illness after receiving the vaccine.

The Science

- **"Conventional" Thought:** Chronic Lyme disease does not exist. Rather there is an ever-growing cult of conspiracy theorists who live in a pseudoscientific echo chamber and seek out doctor after doctor until they can find a quack who will validate their delusional beliefs.
- **What Lyme Sufferers Know:** There are seven hundred peer-reviewed articles citing chronic infection associated with tick-borne infection[132]... and millions of people suffering who will gladly provide their subjective truths and anecdotal evidence.

The Media

- **"Conventional" Thought:** Traditional media tend to echo the same Lyme disease rhetoric as the medical-industrial complex, if they even choose to cover this disease at all.
- **What Lyme Sufferers Know:** We must dig deep and depend on our own research and critical analysis to get to the truth of the Lyme Wars.

In the documentary *Under Our Skin*, pathologist and Lyme researcher Dr. Alan MacDonald says: *"The CDC does not want chronic Lyme disease to have a foothold as a legitimate medical entity in the United States or elsewhere in the world."*[133]

Lyme-literate doctor Joseph G. Jemsek says: *"The sins committed are so great and so ugly that it can't be negotiated out. So, [CDC's] lie is too big to confess at this point."*[134]

In reference to the far outdated and wholly ineffective but firmly planted, immovable IDSA Lyme treatment guidelines, Jenna Luche-Thayer, former senior adviser at the United Nations who has also worked on many US government federal projects and is highly studied in US statutes and laws, says, "Given my previous experience, I find CDC's lack of attention and action regarding Lyme Corps' appearance of preferential treatment to be highly irregular."[135]

Without a doubt, there is something very wrong here. The CDC continues to support a set of guidelines that are keeping people from getting well. Why?

When faced with a chronic illness that is denied by the medical community at large, when faced with a chronic infectious disease that the infectious-disease doctors refuse to acknowledge and treat in any reasonable way, when faced with a government and medical system that fails to address the problem, then, please tell me what are intelligent, abandoned, ill patients supposed to think and what on earth are they supposed to do?

They look for answers elsewhere.

They seek out open-minded physicians who can help them achieve a decent to good clinical outcome. Certainly there are dangers that exist. The free market can and will undoubtedly take advantage of desperate, vulnerable people.

But for chronic Lyme sufferers, it is far more dangerous and debilitating to wait for the CDC and the IDSA to get around to actually acknowledging and treating this disease—a disease that is growing exponentially and affecting so many. It's been more than forty years. How much longer will sufferers have to wait? And what will it take for the powers that be to acknowledge this disease and its global devastation?

The way in which we solve complex problems is often in small steps, with small, meaningful actions. This truism worries me, as Lyme sufferers can't wait. We need to take big steps, all with meaningful action—now.

Deaths from Chronic Lyme

In a 1994 AP press release, Dr. James Olson of the CDC claimed, "Nobody dies from Lyme disease."

Please tell that to Karen Forschner, Rosanna Magnotta, and the family of Emmy-winning producer-director Scott Brazil. Tell that to Tara Geraghty and her twin children, Brynn and Callen, whose husband and father, respectively—David A. Geraghty, fifty-three, of Cumberland, Rhode Island, who was originally misdiagnosed with ALS—died on December 22, 2015, after a two-year battle with chronic Lyme disease. Tell that to so many who have lost loved ones to Lyme.

I'm sure they would wholeheartedly disagree with the notion that nobody dies from this disease. Their devastating losses tell them so—and tell the rest of the world so as well.

In an abstract for "A Review of Death Certificates Listing Lyme Disease as a Cause of Death in the United States," Lyme disease was listed as an underlying or multiple cause of death in 114 death records during 1999 to 2003. Upon review, only one record was consistent with clinical manifestations of Lyme disease. This analysis indicates that Lyme disease is rare as a cause of death in the United States.[136]

Are deaths from chronic Lyme disease not recorded because it suits the powers that be, keeping it consistent with a "hard to catch, easy to diagnose, easy to treat" disease? Or is it because there is no correlation? I believe the former to be true.

Judy Stone, an infectious-disease specialist experienced in conducting clinical research and the author of *Conducting Clinical Research*, says in *Forbes* magazine that Lyme deaths from Lyme inflammation are likely worse than we thought. According to Stone,

> *How much heart involvement is there with Lyme? Based on cases submitted to the CDC, only 1.1% of patients had carditis. I suspect the real number is substantially higher, given that I've seen several patients with it and based on other reports in the literature, which often cite a 4-10% incidence of carditis.*[137]

The author of an article on owndoc.com claims that the case fatality of Lyme disease is nearly 100 percent. Says this author,

> *The definition of "case fatality rate" (often confused with "mortality rate") of an illness is the percentage of people who die while they are still not cured of that illness. That implies that the CFR is an imprecise metric, it encompasses deaths due to the disease and deaths due to other causes. 3rd stage Lyme in the CNS is, contrary to what the medical establishment claims, incurable with currently available treatment. All that can be done is slowly reverse the symptoms, and only when proper*

oral or IV antibiotic treatment is administered for as long as symptoms persist. The patient usually remains more or less ill for the remainder of his or her life.

I think it is more accurate to state that when left untreated, late-stage (chronic) neuroborreliosis will eventually kill the patient.[138]

Those Who Have Lost the Battle

It has become impossible to track deaths from Lyme disease. People are literally dying at the rate of several a day now. And hospitals and coroners are not reporting Lyme as cause of death.

A Lyme group Facebook member posted the results of his own survey of deaths due to Lyme disease:

Six years ago, I did an unscientific survey of obituaries I had published on Lymeblog.com and found that suicide was the 2nd leading cause of death for people with a Lyme disease diagnosis.

The number one cause of presumed cardiac arrest would indicate heart block being the causative agent. Heart block is one of the most common symptoms of tertiary Lyme (final stage, neurological). Heart block means that the signal telling the heart to beat is blocked from reaching the heart. This causes irregular heart beats in many Lyme patients.[139]

The Blogspot owndoc.com lists more than five hundred chronic Lyme deaths. The author says,

The theory of unexplained neurological syndromes

being caused by neurospirochetoses is taboo in the medical world, in spite of the overwhelming evidence for it, and the lack of any other credible explanation ... spin doctors employed by the US government say that over 99% of coroners were wrong when they listed Lyme as a contributing cause of death.

In spite of the fact that their deaths are "whitewashed," the list of Americans who died as a direct consequence of their neuroborreliosis is ever growing.[140]

And remember that, in 1994, Dr. James Olson of the CDC said, "Nobody dies of Lyme Disease."

Here are some real stories of real people who have, in fact, died of chronic Lyme.

The *Poughkeepsie Journal* reported on the tragic death of seventeen-year-old Joseph Elone, who died suddenly after having been sick for about a month with flu-like symptoms. Early in his illness, the young man tested negative for Lyme disease. After he died, health officials initially suspected tick-borne Powassan virus. That has since been ruled out and it has been determined that Joseph, in fact, had disseminated Lyme disease. So far, however, that has not been named as a cause of death.

The following remarks are from New York State Lyme activist Jill Auerbach, who lives in the same county as Joseph's family:

They have dismissed Powassan encephalitis and found that Joseph was suffering from disseminated Lyme disease which invaded his heart. While they should find out if there were any extenuating circumstances to expand diagnostic measures, it is already two months since he died. That makes it appear that they are searching for reasons other than Lyme disease to blame as the cause of his death. Wouldn't it have been nice if they (the doctors) paid as much attention to him while he was ALIVE and prevented Joseph from dying.[141]

Emmy-winning producer-director Scott Brazil, whose television shows included *The Shield* and *Hill Street Blues*, died at age fifty of respiratory failure due to Lou Gehrig's disease and Lyme disease complications.[142]

In another case, three people literally dropped dead from Lyme carditis. NBC News reported, "One was found dead in a car that veered off the road. Two others collapsed and died suddenly without warning. The two men and a woman were young, aged 26 to 38, and had not been treated for Lyme disease. And no one suspected an infection until an astute pathologist readying heart tissue for a possible transplant noticed something wrong."[143]

In a 2013 CNN Producer Note, Dr. Daniel Cameron, an epidemiologist and past president of the International Lyme and Associated Diseases Society, said there is growing evidence that Lyme disease can lead to serious and sometimes fatal psychiatric symptoms. "There have been chronically ill Lyme disease patients who have been suicidal. Whether psychiatric manifestations including suicidal ideation are due to an infection or the poor quality of [life] has yet to be determined."[144]

The deaths, losses, tragedies, and slow, merciless stripping away of people's lives does not get the media attention you would expect. Chronic Lyme has all the makings of media sensationalism—denial, suffering, corruption, conflict, more suffering, conspiracy, and even death. Yet the media only seems to cover the surface story and only more so in recent months.

If people are dying of chronic Lyme, then why isn't this being reported with greater urgency? If, in fact, suicide is a growing cause of death from Lyme disease, then why aren't we talking about this at all? Why is it so difficult to find statistics on those who have died? Who, if anyone, is studying this?

Whose heart is breaking daily from the growing list of casualties caused by this invisible, neglected, woebegone disease? I know mine is. And I know all too well that there are many more broken hearts out there.

Where is the heart of the CDC, the IDSA, Big Pharma, the insurance industry?

If any of these organizations actually had a heart, they couldn't keep pretending that their actions and inactions are justifiable. How do they sleep at night knowing they are withholding information, skewing treatment guidelines, and ignoring the sick?

In the world of psychology, we call this behavior *sociopathic*. In a more esoteric realm, we might refer to it as *evil*.

Children Being Taken from Families

In an article in *Psychology Today*, author Pamela Weintraub, who wrote "Cure Unknown: Inside the Lyme Epidemic," reported on a disturbing trend:

> *Call them the Munchausen mothers. A growing number of women stand accused of deliberately sickening their children for attention from doctors. In an era of patient advocacy and hard-charging moms, there's no end in sight to this hotly contested diagnosis.*

When children suffer complex, or controversial, or confusing illnesses, when symptoms are amorphous or vague, parents can be accused.[145]

In Colorado, a young boy was removed from his family home and his father was incarcerated over a Lyme disease disagreement. According to an article by Christina England,

Greg and Jasmine Eckenrode's story began in July 2014, when they took their fifteen-year-old son Max, who suffers from Lyme disease, to Denver Hospital in Colorado, as he was suffering from severe stomach cramps and vomiting.

Without having a full set of medical records, the physician in charge of Max's case allegedly decided that Max was not as ill as his parents were saying and instead they were over-medicating him. Without vital reports and lacking the information required, according to Max's parents, the "ill-informed physician" reported the family to Child Protective Services (CPS), portraying Mrs. Eckenrode as a mother suffering from Munchhausen Syndrome by Proxy (MSBP).[146]

Families Are Crumbling

People and families are going broke just trying to get well. In a 2015 study of one hundred self-reported patients, the annual financial impact of Lyme disease (including health-care expenses and lost wages) averages a total of $53,000 per patient.[147]

There are hundreds, if not thousands, of GoFundMe crowdfunding sites like that of the Gack family. In their

GoFundMe photo, they look like a perfect family—blond, blue-eyed, beautiful. All eight members of this family—mom, dad, and six kids—are battling chronic Lyme disease, transmitted sexually and congenitally.

There are so many families just like this—families who are falling apart, losing their savings, and struggling to stay afloat. In their GoFundMe profile, they explain their devastating circumstances due to Lyme:

> We are a family of 8 all fighting Lyme disease. Our medical bills are overwhelming and at this point we can't afford treatment for the kids. 4 of the 6 kids are very symptomatic and struggle in areas of food sensitivities, neurological issues, painful muscles and joints and seizures. We are currently trying to finish treatment for Amy (mom) but the treatment is costing close to $1,000 a week plus all the supplements for her and the kids and the high grocery bills due to the strict diet she has to be on. Amy has had Lyme for 36 years but wasn't properly diagnosed until 2013.[148]

Doctors Are Being Taken to Court

Are we living the McCarthy era all over again?

One of the most head-shaking, crazy-making outcomes of the maddening politicization of chronic Lyme disease is that doctors who are on our side—those trying to support Lyme sufferers in their illness—have been stopped cold in their tracks.

McCarthyism—the practice of making accusations of subversion or treason without proper regard for evidence—is back in town. Let's call it *Lyme Madness* for now.

As is clear by now, the majority of doctors and researchers

say Lyme disease is difficult to catch and easily treated with a round of antibiotics.

But a small group of doctors know otherwise—that this disease is actually *very* easy to catch, *very* difficult to diagnose, and the infection is persistent, wreaking havoc on millions worldwide. The debate is intense, and very few doctors in the mainstream are willing to speak publicly about it.

Do you blame them? It's a lose-lose situation. When this small group of medical Lyme warriors acts in the best interest of sufferers, they often get pummeled. It's that simple.

The doctors who humanely attempt to treat Lyme beyond the IDSA twenty-eight-day guidelines are faced with medical board prosecutions and costly lawsuits. These medical soldiers—who are on the front line every day of the week, fighting for Lyme sufferers everywhere—are some of the biggest casualties of this ongoing war.

It might be of interest to note that Lyme sufferers will not name their Lyme doctors on Facebook for fear of reprisal. You'll notice that I've referred to most with only an initial. We are a very protective bunch—for obvious reasons.

Sadly, Lyme doctors represent a very small army—one with limited resources and limited power. The few doctors who care enough and who are brave enough to step up immediately feel the oppression and dominance of the Lyme cabal, which is made up of a select few representatives from government agencies, the insurance industry, and Big Pharma.

Dr. Joseph G. Jemsek has been dragged through this war and has lived to tell about it.

In April 2006, the North Carolina Medical Board (NCMB) charged Joseph G. Jemsek, MD, with unprofessional conduct that involved inappropriately diagnosing and treating ten patients with Lyme disease. At the time, the Jemsek

Clinic—located in Huntersville, North Carolina—was said to be the largest private HIV/AIDS clinic in the Carolinas.

The NCMB charged Dr. Jemsek with offenses ranging from unsatisfactory lab evidence, lack of clinical evidence of efficacy of IV antibiotics, lack of informed consent regarding his methods of diagnosis, and so on and so forth. In August 2006, the board issued a one-year "suspension with stay" that allowed Dr. Jemsek to continue practicing medicine if he complied with stipulations that had been set at the NCMB meeting in July.

The board did not relent. In April 2008, the board issued a letter of concern that Dr. Jemsek had treated purported Lyme patients with hyperbaric oxygen. The letter also noted that Jemsek had failed to properly supervise three nurse practitioners with the result that they received public reprimands.[149]

Because of this ongoing battle, Dr. Jemsek was forced to file bankruptcy, foreclose on his office building, and he almost lost his house. He lost almost everything. But, before long, Dr. Jemsek emerged even stronger—reopening his clinic in Washington, DC.

In an interview with Lyme sufferer and activist Tina J. Garcia, Dr. Jemsek said,

Here's the ugly fact and the ugly truth: **This disease is a TSUNAMI.** *The disease is so prevalent and it's affecting so many decision-makers and their families, that this will force the change. And I predict that in the next year or so we're going to get some big names involved. Congressmen and CEOs are being affected, and I've seen doctors and their patients for this illness, so it's bound to happen. And at some point somebody with some outrage will step up and there will be questions* *answered. I think the film* Under Our Skin *has done more than anything before it, or anything that may come, to change the consciousness of America about Lyme disease. We all get comfortably numb with what's going on, but not for long, and we can't be indifferent and ignore it anymore.*[150]

Dr. Charles Ray Jones was also taken to task for treating children with chronic Lyme. The creators of the documentary *Under Our Skin* posted an update on Dr. Jones:

Dr. Charles Ray Jones, a 79-year-old Connecticut pediatrician, has treated more than 10,000 children with Lyme disease over the course of his career. In addition to seeing patients six days a week, Dr. Jones has spent the last four years and hundreds of thousands of dollars defending himself against state medical board charges of "inappropriate" treatment of children with Lyme and other tick-borne diseases.

Because of generous donations to his legal defense fund, [Dr. Jones] has been able to continue treating desperately sick children during the four years of legal proceedings. Feeling the pressure of the 37% increase in Lyme disease cases from 2006 to 2007, Dr. Jones's office is averaging three new patient calls a day, in addition to training new Lyme-literate pediatricians through the Turn the Corner Physicians Training Program.[151]

I personally know a Lyme sufferer who would be lost without Dr. Jones, as he treats her three young daughters. Imagine if you *and* all three of your kids had this disease.

Without Dr. Jones, she would be even more anguished and overwhelmed than she already is. And yet his practice was almost shut down forever.

In a formal letter dated September 14, 2010, addressed to the members of the Institute of Medicine (IOM) Committee Panel for "Lyme Disease and other Tick-borne diseases," Kenneth B. Liegner, a New York State Lyme-literate doctor, boldly said, "Physicians who have cared for persons with chronic Lyme disease have faced harassment at a minimum and for some, their careers have been ruined. Researchers who have seriously dedicated themselves to the scientific study of chronic Lyme disease in humans and/or animals have often found themselves attacked or marginalized. To persist in their researches would have resulted in virtual career suicide and some have been forced, by exigencies of survival, to leave the field."

To further explain the madness and drive home the point that the medical community has turned its back, Dr. Liegner continued, "Laboratories that test extensively for Lyme disease, including use of direct detection methods such as PCR, have found themselves subjected to concerted smear campaigns and harassed."

Doctors everywhere—in the US, Canada, and elsewhere—are being shut down, threatened, harassed, bullied, taken to court, and stripped of their licenses and practices. Laboratories, too, are being harassed and defamed. All because they are listening to us and doing their best to support Lyme sufferers. Madness!

We in the Lyme community are very grateful to Dr. Liegner for his clear understanding and support of Lyme sufferers. He is a rare breed indeed. In the very same letter addressed to the IOM committee members, he made a summation that powerfully, pointedly, and perfectly describes the madness. His carefully crafted words are a clarion call to the medical field to wake up. With the following passage, Dr. Liegner has greatly served the Lyme community by validating our collective experience.

This is a quote worth repeating:

"In the fullness of time, the mainstream handling of chronic Lyme disease will be viewed as one of the most shameful episodes in the history of medicine because elements of academic medicine, elements of government and virtually the entire insurance industry have colluded to deny a disease. This has resulted in needless suffering of many individuals who deteriorate and sometimes die for lack of timely application of treatment or denial of treatment beyond some arbitrary duration."[152]

Another Mother's Voice that Must Be Heard

Beaux Reliosis (note the clever moniker) is an important voice in the Lyme Wars. She and ex-Pfizer analytical chemist and LYMErix whistleblower Kathleen Dickson—who are closely aligned in this battle—are two of the Lyme activists whose work I admire most. (Much more on Kathleen to come.)

As Beaux tells us, she is

...a 20-year survivor of Lyme disease, or, more accurately, relapsing fever borreliosis. For 18 years, I accepted it and lived with it, until my daughter was diagnosed with congenital Lyme. In the past year I have transformed from complacent, timid and uninformed, to activist research junkie with a mission. My mission

is to get the Lyme criminals prosecuted so the millions suffering can be properly diagnosed and treated. I will not stop until that happens.

Like all of us in Lymeland, Beaux is angry—angry that people are losing their lives, their livelihoods, their loved ones—and no one is listening. She is angry that celebrities are deflecting from the real issues—the crime that is Lyme.

Beaux is one of the most prolific and articulate Lyme activists that I've had the pleasure of speaking with. I urge you to read anything and everything she has written.

Here is an excerpt from two of her more recent blogs at Bad Lyme Attitude Blog (BLAB):

I am livid about a 22-year-old mother losing her life to Lyme, and her baby daughter losing the one person who would, without question, throw herself in front of a speeding train to save her daughter. That's what mothers do. And now this child has no mother. Doesn't that make you FURIOUS?

I am angry about celebrities flitting from gala to gala in the name of Lyme research. Note to celebs: the research on the basic disease mechanism is all wrapped up in a neat little package, right here. I am angry about the time that is wasted in proportion to dollars spent by wealthy people with Lyme disease. Tick tock, tick tock. How many more lives will be lost in the name of annual awareness galas?

People say it's not healthy to be so angry. You have to be positive or no one will listen. I say NO. I am ?!&$@ pissed *off and you should be, too. It's not about rainbows and bunnies and unicorns, unless the unicorn has skewered the bunny and cooked it in the pot on the other end. Look at what being positive and complacent has gotten us for 20 years: dead friends and a damned quilt.*

STUFF HAPPENS WHEN PEOPLE ARE ANGRY ENOUGH TO MAKE IT HAPPEN. Where is the anger? Where is the outrage? Where is the activism?

This is a war. It will not be won with gentle hugs or doctor protection bills. It cannot be won by supporting anyone who denies the undeniable science of the disease. IT WILL BE WON by those of us who are MAD AS HELL about our sisters and brothers being tortured to death. I refuse to let this continue another 20 years, or 10, or even 5. I intend to get this done.

In this blog post, Beaux pleads with someone, *anyone* (including whistleblower and documentarian Michael Moore) to listen:

Whoever has a conscience, please help. An estimated 30 million people are suffering from debilitating illness, shamed, blamed and unable to get treatment because our government does not want us to know the source of the autism pandemic.

You inject a fungally-contaminated vaccine, along with a live, attenuated virus into a child, and the child gets the disease instead of the protection. What happens when you hypervaccinate thousands of soldiers who end up mysteriously disabled? What happens when you push a Lyme disease vaccine that uses the very same antigen that causes the disabling symptoms of Lyme disease?

Immunosuppression with reactivated viruses and subsequent opportunistic infections. Chronic mold exposure? Think black mold. We were all pretty hyped up about black mold removal a few years ago, right? The result is immunosuppression with reactivation of latent viruses plus opportunistic infections of all sorts.

Bad stuff, right? Do I have to say it again? The result is immunosuppression with reactivation of latent viruses plus opportunistic infections of all sorts. Starting to sound like AIDS, right? OF COURSE they don't want us to know that Gulf War Syndrome, ME/CFS, Fibromyalgia, Lyme disease, HIV and autism share a common mechanism. Fungal immunosuppression, chronic reactivation of herpesviruses and opportunistic infections leading to the "Great Imitator" diseases.

These government criminals will stop at nothing to destroy the lives of U.S. Citizens, children, and especially those who dare to speak out about these unspeakable crimes. In fact, it seems, they'd like to retract the disability insurance of one of our prominent activists, in the hopes that this person will die destitute, and the incriminating data will simply go away.

In the Lyme world people are dying, two or three a week. If it's not from their illness, it's because they couldn't take the ABUSE any more. FROM DOCTORS: ridicule, shame, blame, retaliation, ignorance, lack of care, lack of empathy, denial of treatment, psychiatric diagnoses, i.e. we create our illness using our own magical brains. FROM INSURANCE PROVIDERS: denial of illness, denial of coverage, ridicule, shame, blame, red tape and paperwork that's difficult even for healthy people. FROM OUR OWN FAMILIES AND FRIENDS AS A RESULT OF THE DOCTOR/INSURANCE VICTIM-BLAMING: disbelief, mistrust, divorce, shunning, ridicule, isolation, retaliation for being disabled and unable to do normal activities. FROM OTHER INSTITUTIONS: denial of disability insurance, denial of unemployment insurance, denial of sickness by employers, bankruptcy, homelessness. FROM ANYONE IN A POSITION TO QUESTION OUR PARENTAL RIGHTS: investigations by DCF, accusations of child abuse, neglect and "Munchausen's," government-mediated kidnapping of our sick children, criminal charges of child abuse for the crime of trying to get treatment for our sick children.

A complaint was filed with the USDOJ in 2003. The complaint stated that research fraud committed by CDC officers led to the fraudulent adoption of a "new" Lyme disease case definition so that the aforementioned Lyme vaccine could be fraudulently qualified. FRAUD, FRAUD, FRAUD. And they meant to profit from it, as evidenced by the multiple patents owned by said fraudsters, by marketing diagnostic devices and test kits. RICO AND FALSE CLAIMS.

We are OCCUPYING THE USDOJ starting June 1. We DEMAND JUSTICE for all those who are denied care, denied treatment, denied of a physical illness that is killing us. We humbly ask for assistance in making TRUTH prevail. The truth will save our children.[153]

7. THEORIES AND CONSPIRACIES

If I had a world of my own, everything would be nonsense. Nothing would be what it is because everything would be what it isn't. And contrary wise, what is, it wouldn't be. And what wouldn't be, it would. You see?

—ALICE'S ADVENTURES IN WONDERLAND

There is no better example of a global travesty, perversion of justice, and medical wrongdoing than the manipulation and lies surrounding chronic Lyme disease.

The author of owndoc.com says:

What I call fraud can be more accurately described as a mixture of ignorance, cowardice, deference to authority, intellectual laziness and greed. No massive Lyme conspiracy, just ordinary human behavior. There are conspiracies involved as well, but they remain limited to a silent understanding between peers here and there. The medical system protects itself and that is only natural.[154]

I have spent months trying to understand this madness. While I'm determined to make some sense of the political complexities surrounding this disease, I also realize that so many have been trying to unlock this mystery for decades now, to little or no avail.

Here I will share with you some well-documented theories and conspiracies. These theories, posited by experts, will have you shaking your head, as I shake mine. All have merit and possibility. All are interconnected. The full truth is still waiting to be fully unveiled.

As you read this chapter, I ask you to hold two important concepts front and center:

• The psychological tactic known as *gaslighting*

• The psychological underpinnings of what it means to be a *conspiracy theorist*

As I mentioned in the introduction, *gaslighting* is a powerful form of psychological manipulation and mental abuse in which information is spun and twisted to make the victims doubt themselves and their own experiences. The goal is to override a person's reality and thus instill confusion, anxiety, and helplessness, all wrapped in a power play for some higher gain.

It's also important to deconstruct the term *conspiracy* to understand how Lymeland was created. A conspiracy suggests that two or more persons or organizations have conspired to cause or cover up an event or situation typically regarded as illegal or harmful. Perhaps conspiracies abound here simply because some people and/or groups are driven to enforce and retain their position of power, control, and personal gain—at the cost of many. Not too far fetched as theories go.

The simplest way to keep a conspiracy in play, or a cover-up fully covered up, is to turn the table on the victims, make them the crazy ones, spin, turn, and twist information so the abuser remains the sane one, the reasonable one, the omnipotent god, the hero who keeps his power while the victim remains victimized by being shamed, minimized, discredited, and ridiculed endlessly. As you can see, gaslighting and conspiracies are clearly intertwined.

And it's all orchestrated so very elegantly with falsified definitions, doublespeak, untrue but well-rehearsed party lines such as, "Lyme is hard to catch, easy to diagnose, and easy to treat," or, "There, there, my dear—it's all in your head. Go see a shrink."

Say this often enough, condition doctors to believe this is true, and you've got an entire medical industry turning its back on millions suffering.

The prevailing, persistent denial of chronic Lyme disease, causing millions to suffer needlessly, leads us all to speculate, think, theorize, and keep an open mind because we are desperate for answers. Desperate to understand why this is happening. Without the transparency that we need, and that we may never get, conjecture and conspiracies are really all we have.

When you understand the infrastructure of this massive medical denial, the so-called conspiracy theories begin to sound reasonable and sane, if not greedy and cruel. Much saner, in fact, than the actual denial of this disease itself.

One of the driving forces behind this book is my need to make sense of this madness. I hope this chapter offers, at the very least, some food for thought and helps to clarify, in part, the "why" of this crazy, life-altering, cynical-making, maddening, dizzying, exhausting, exasperating, and very dark experience.

Theory or Conspiracy #1: Patents and Profits

The Lyme outbreak in 1975 occurred just before the rush to profit in the early 1980s, when researchers and scientists were given the green light to patent their findings. All the more reason to follow the money.

In 1980, the US Congress passed the Bayh-Dole Act—also known as the Patent and Trademark Law Amendments Act—which gave intellectual property rights for research findings to institutions that had received federal grants. This meant that discoveries and inventions from public funds could be patented and licensed, initially to small businesses, with exclusive rights of royalties given to the grantee.

The Bayh-Dole Act of 1980 permitted universities, small businesses, and nonprofit institutions, using federal funds for research, to produce an invention and to retain the title on any patent issued for such inventions. The creation of this act may have been borne out of noble intentions. But ultimately, it allowed for a medical system in which corruption could flourish. Where profit would take precedence over the public good.

Many researchers consulted for the private sector, creating strong corporate ties. Naturally, lead scientific researchers came to favor certain companies when licensing out the patents, which would promote unfair competition and skewed research. Many university researchers created ties to private industry, with some researchers jumping on the entrepreneurial bandwagon and heading up companies of their own.

Scientists struck deals with venture capitalists. By the mid-1980s, there were hundreds of new companies with academic scientists as officers, board members, or consultants. The commercialization of biological techniques occurred at an accelerated rate, causing scientists to become more focused on reaching desired goals, at all costs.

By 1983, every large chemical and pharmaceutical company had made a multimillion-dollar investment in biotechnology, and established major funding partnerships with universities.

Thus, the era of scientific conflicts of interest was born.

In her book *Deadly Monopolies*, Harriet A. Washington—the award-winning author of *Medical Apartheid*, explores contentious and commercial-driven issues in modern biomedical research caused by the marriage between Big Pharma and universities. Washington begins with the Bayh-Dole Act, which she says led to a purely profit motive—robbing universities of their independence and seizing control of medication design, costs, and medical journal articles.

In this profoundly disturbing read, Washington shows us how Big Pharma became a $310 billion industry by selling excised tissues without permission, patenting human genes that were found to be linked to diseases, and even conducting research on uninformed trauma victims and suspicious drug trials in third-world countries. All the while bankrupting first-world patients and ignoring many third-world diseases.

In an article entitled, "How the Medical Industry Profits from a Broken Patent System," reporter Mytheos Holt says:

> As negotiations over patent reform continue to crawl along, sometimes at a pace that would make a snail jealous, one of the big sticking points across both sides is the issue of how to handle pharmaceutical patents. To hear both sides tell it, the issue varies wildly in terms of importance, with the industry claiming the future of medicine hinges on how it's handled, and their

opponents dismissing this as simple fear-mongering by rent-gobbling crooks.[155]

In her 2008 *New York Times* article "When Academia Puts Profit Ahead of Wonder," author Janet Rae-Dupree, who writes about science and emerging technology, tells us,

In the past, discovery for its own sake provided academic motivation, but today's universities function more like corporate research laboratories. Rather than freely sharing techniques and results, researchers increasingly keep new findings under wraps to maintain a competitive edge. What used to be peer-reviewed is now proprietary. "Share and share alike" has devolved into "every laboratory for itself."

In trying to power the innovation economy, we have turned America's universities into cutthroat business competitors, zealously guarding the very innovations we so desperately want behind a hopelessly tangled web of patents and royalty licenses.[156]

Theory or Conspiracy #2: The Vaccine IS the Disease

In response to growing reports of Lyme disease cases in the United States—from 1982 to 1996, by thirty-two times—SmithKline Beecham (now GlaxoSmithKline) developed LYMErix, the first and only licensed vaccine against Lyme. It was licensed in 1998.

The licensed product was a recombinant vaccine containing an outer surface protein A (OspA) from the *Borrelia burgdorferi* bacteria. Given in a three-dose series, the vaccine had an unusual method of action: *it stimulated*

*antibodies that attacked the Lyme bacteria in the tick's gut
as it fed on the human host, before the bacteria were able to
enter the body.* This was purported to be about 78 percent
effective in protecting against Lyme infection after all three
doses of the vaccine had been given.

So unlike most vaccines, which are designed to transmit
antibodies to fight a germ, LYMErix was designed to immunize the disease's vector—the tick. When administered, it
made the human recipient a walking canister of tick spray
made of OspA/Borrelia. Now, imagine what that might do
to one's immune system. Turn it off, perhaps?

Or, as LYMErix whistleblower Kathleen Dickson suggests, "Carpet bomb the immune system by shedding toxic
fungal antigens. The infection becomes stealth or undetected by the immune system and the immune system has
no antibodies to remove the foreign antigens [OspA] or to
fight infection [Borrelia]."

By 2002, SmithKline Beecham had withdrawn LYMErix
from the market, and Pasteur Mérieux Connaught decided
not to apply for a license for its own Lyme vaccine candidate, despite having already demonstrated its efficacy in a
Phase III clinical trial.

The sanctioned story is that LYMErix was withdrawn due
to extensive media coverage of "vaccine victims," falling sales,
and ongoing litigation, but that it was always a viable, safe,
and cost-effective public health intervention "to prevent the
most common tick-borne infection in the United States."[157]

Today there are no vaccines available to prevent Lyme
disease, and it is unlikely that any will be licensed in the near
future. The inauguration and then subsequent withdrawal
of the Lyme disease vaccine has lasting implications for
future vaccine development and use.

Between December 28, 1998, and July 31, 2000, 905 reports were made to Vaccine Adverse Events Reporting System (VAERS) about adverse events. Sixty-six were classified as serious—resulting in a life-threatening illness, hospitalization or lengthened hospitalization, or disability.

Despite these challenges, the authors conclude that "Lyme disease is a serious illness and those who live in areas where it is spreading deserve a vaccine."[158]

So began the doublespeak, false reporting, and under-reporting of the effects of LYMErix and chronic Lyme. The two are closely intertwined.

Ultimately, I am told, *the vaccine itself made people as sick as an infected tick bite.*

SmithKline Beecham insisted the reports of adverse effects were minimal.

Andrea Gaito, MD, and a founding member of the International Lyme and Associated Diseases Society (ILADS) reported she had thirty-five patients with problems stemming from the vaccine, including rheumatoid arthritis-like presentations. Reports Gaito,

What I have found, is that people with Lyme who become asymptomatic may, upon vaccination with LYMErix, experience a retriggering of symptoms. Those who never had symptoms of Lyme disease, meanwhile, will, upon vaccination, experience the symptoms of Lyme disease.

The introduction and failure of the LYMErix vaccine was a nail in the coffin for the medical industry. SmithKline Beecham worked hard to keep its failure small, using confusing language to keep the FDA and Physicians in

the dark. They tried to shift the blame from the vaccine to the patient with statements such as "the possibility of a severe rheumatologic, neurologic, autoimmune adverse event is inherent in Lyme disease."

The company did not inform physicians that the adverse events can result from LYMErix, completely apart from the disease. GPs in the US were kept in the dark about the life-threatening side effects of LYMErix.[159]

It is clear that the researchers and doctors who developed the Lyme vaccine had a vested interest in showing the world that it worked. Those who had had the vaccine and showed symptoms of late-stage chronic Lyme were denied any validation of their suffering by their doctors because it would prove that the vaccine, in fact, didn't work.

Here, it seems, we may have an important factor in the widespread denial of chronic Lyme.

Reenter Kathleen Dickson, ex-Pfizer analytical chemist and LYMErix whistleblower who has also been called the "Cassandra of Lyme" because of her prophetic gifts and her unique ability to see the real picture of Lyme disease that, to this day, no one in power is willing to believe.

For decades, she has been fighting the powers that be in this Lyme War. She has been active since the beginning of the outbreak, and she knows all the details and players from the start, including Karen Forschner, Polly Murray, and the other chronic Lyme disease pioneers.

Kathleen is one of the boldest, most prolific, and dogmatic Lyme fighters I've come across. Her website—ohioactionlyme. org—is chock-full of the most detailed, well-documented information. Her site reads like the best-ever Arthur Conan Doyle whodunit—if you are able to keep her mountains of research and the who, what, when, where, why, and how clear in your mind. The sheer amount of data Dickson makes available to the world is truly mind-boggling.

With hundreds of scientific articles backing up her claims, Dickson explains everything, from when things first got derailed to how a certain prominent university defrauded the government, to who owns the patents, who are the perpetrators of the falsified Lyme case definitions, how LYMErix caused neurological Lyme, and much, much more.

Dickson has filed human rights complaints to the UN in Geneva and has served the United States Department of Justice with five criminal charge sheets that read like rap sheets for the most criminally insane members of society. In these charge sheets, Dickson implicates the big guns, including specific members of all three organizations—with decades of falsifying research, defrauding the public, and causing mayhem and destruction for millions.

One of her many mantras: "Cowards are despicable, and that is all the United States has. Cowards and stupid people, which is the same thing—willful ignorance."

Some might call her crazy. Others call her a mad genius. Often, it's a fine line. Let's keep the concepts of gaslighting and conspiracies in mind when we think of Kathleen's difficult journey to get heard. She has been unduly punished for her dog-on-a-bone tenacity.

In 2003, she was involuntarily committed to a psychiatric hospital, labeled a danger to herself and others, and had her kids taken from her—all because she and her children have neuropsychiatric Lyme and she tried to go after the big guns. She clearly presented a threat to someone, and she hit a nerve—or two. And still, Kathleen keeps on trucking at a faster and more ferocious clip than ever before.

Dickson has no qualms about naming the bad guys, which she has done publicly on her site and in her criminal charge sheets. For the clearest explanation to date, watch her video—"*Cryme Disease: The Lyme Cryme Against Humanity. TRUTH from the LYMErix Whistleblower*"—which she produced along with her associate Beaux Reliosis. Be sure to also watch the rest of the Lyme Cryme video series on YouTube.

Dickson knows it was all happening around 1999, when, as she told the FDA, she began hearing about LYMErix victims, claiming they felt they had contracted Lyme again. This made no sense to Dickson and she began what would become a fifteen-plus-year investigation and dogged fight to uncover the "Lyme Crymes," as she calls them.

She wrote and presented a thirty-page report to the FDA. She explained what happened at Dearborn—a watershed event in Dearborn Michigan, the second National Conference on Lyme disease testing where Lyme disease was officially redefined—and included pages from the Dearborn booklet proving it was not, in fact, a consensus conference. She cautioned that the LYMErix vaccine was never really a vaccine, never proven, and the testing was bogus. She also cautioned that OspA (transmitted by both a tick and by LYMErix) was causing immunosuppression and the reactivation of a dormant infection.

Dickson says, "I didn't know how right I was at the time since nowhere could you find the structure of the OspA online." It wasn't until 2005 that she did find it in a Korean chemistry journal not listed in PubMed.

"If ILADS really wanted to help," Dickson says, they would be asking, 'What is OspA?' They've never bothered to ask."

In January 2001, Kathleen Dickson blew the whistle at the FDA, exposing Dearborn, how OspA causes immuno-suppression, and that LYMErix was not a vaccine.

To summarize her findings, which are micro-detailed and overwhelming, there are really only two things that Dickson needs people to know: "that the testing was falsi-fied to sell a vaccine; and this fungal toxin vaccine caused the exact same disease (chronic neurological Lyme disease) that was thrown out at Dearborn," she claims.

Dickson continues,

You (Lyme and Lymerix sufferers alike) are victims of a Holocaust and we are trying to arm you. You are not going to mind if we say, "Shut up and learn how to use this TRUTH weapon." Are you? Also, the Truth is the only positive "healing energy" force. You already know this. (You feel better already knowing that some people know exactly why you are not getting better, and that there is a group of people dedicated to getting the perps busted.)

What we are going to find is that [a certain prominent University], by not reporting the adverse events to LYMErix (or bothering with these patients at all), missed the common link to all chronic, devastating and deadly illnesses: ALS, MS, cancer, CFIDS/FM, Leukemia, what was wrong with the HIV vaccines, etc. and that link was OspA/(Pam3Cys).

OspA is a fungal (mycoplasmal) antigen that turns off the immune system through various mechanisms. This allows common latent viruses of all kinds to become un-latent. The latently infected cells do not autokill as they should when the common latent viruses start replicating (the normal mechanism of immunity), and the fungal Pam3Cys antigen OspA, turns off antibody production against similar antigens.

IF LYMErix [Lyme vaccination] gave people the same disease we know of as chronic neurologic Lyme, then what is the disease? The Cryme IS the Disease. The Cryme was that they claimed that OspA was a vaccine when it was the very thing responsible for causing this AIDS-like illness.

It was said, at the time that LYMErix was still on the market, that this vaccine, via its claimed mechanism of disinfecting ticks with human antibodies (yes, if you can believe it), that LYMErix would turn humans into walking canisters of tick disinfectant, when in fact, LYMErix turned people into walking cesspools of disease.

The same is true for Chronic Lyme. Chronic Lyme victims' immune systems are "overwhelmed"- a term used by a [certain CDC officer], when describing what antigenic variation in spirochetes does to humans (US Patent 6,719,983).

This is a term you want to remember in case you hear it again: "overwhelmed" immune system means "turned off." Turned off is the complete opposite of an "inflammatory" or "autoimmune disease."

Dickson is clearly a force to be reckoned with. She is brilliant and seems to understand the intricacies about Lymeland better than anyone. And, as is often the case, the maddest of all hatters among us are ultimately recognized as the greatest of heroes in the end.

I've been trying desperately to understand Dickson's theories and the science behind them for a very long time now. I'm still not fully clear. However, I am convinced that she gets it better than most.

When I told her I was writing a book on Lyme, she admonished me as she is wont to do, saying:

We've done the personal stories routine and it didn't work. Don't distract people with nonsense. It's cruel.

JUST try to get them to focus on what they need to know: what is the cryme; and how is it true that the cryme (saying OspA was a vaccine) is the disease? Because the vaccine itself actually CAUSED the sepsis or septic shock outcome as a fungal toxin that suppresses the immune system.

OspA is the Great Detonator of this AIDS-like disease, and everyone who has Lyme disease has LYMErix disease since they are all exposed to tons of shed OspA. Lyme is the Great Detonator of latent viral infections. So, it's not Lyme. It's what Lyme reactivates via immunosuppression. I sure wish we all could just start telling the story right, and quit with the sensational nonsense.

In summary, Dickson says:

You will never understand Lyme Disease or Chronic Fatigue or Fibromyalgia unless you understand how the OspA (fungal, TLR2/1-agonist) vaccine [LYMErix], caused the same disease and how they admitted it in their patents and at the FDA meetings. They literally said, and I am quoting them, that LYMErix caused a multi-system disease indistinguishable from Chronic Neurologic Lyme disease and protean (meaning many different) manifestations—just like Chronic Lyme.

How can I convince everyone not to write ridiculous nonsense about Lyme?

Spirochetes do not live in colonies in vivo and therefore do not hide under "biofilms," preventing antibiotic success. The reason spirochetal diseases (spirochetes are not bacteria—they are technically their own phylum, like fungi and viruses) are incurable is because they shed fungal endotoxins which ruin the immune system and cause what is known as post-SEPSIS-syndrome, with numerous reactivated viruses like AIDS.

Dickson is by far the most definite of all the scientists and activists I've come across. The powers that be, you can imagine, want desperately to shut her down. They've tried. Oh, how they've tried.

In addition to Dickson, who refuses to back off, the powers that be have also had their hands full with other activists along the way, including Lisa Masterson and Elena Cook of the UK, Tina J. Garcia of the US, Huib Kraaijeveld of Amsterdam who wrote *Shifting the Lyme Paradigm*, and Canadian Helke Ferrie who wrote *Ending Denial: The*

Lyme Disease Epidemic—just to name a few.

"Lisa Masterson, one of many outspoken critics of the Lyme Crimes in the UK, was bagged and put in a mental hospital for speaking out about the altered Lyme tests that show a false negative to prove an ineffective vaccine. She was forced to become silent about the crimes in order to be released from torment and abuse."[160]

Theory or Conspiracy #3: The Dearborn Definition

At Dearborn, Michigan, in 1994, the medical powers held a second national conference on the serological diagnosis of Lyme disease.

The primary chasm in these decade-long Lyme Wars is the definition of Lyme—arthritis (bad knee Lyme) versus chronic neurological, systemic, AIDS-like, immunosuppressive, recurring fever Lyme. There is a very BIG difference between the two.

Lyme activists like Dickson maintain that the medical powers were all too aware that if they changed the case definition and testing methods, and narrowed it to arthritic symptoms only, then much to their benefit, chronic Lyme could not be found.

"If you can't find Lyme disease," says Dickson, "then you can't find vaccine failure, right?"

This new, falsified 1994 nonconsensus "Dearborn case definition" said only people with late, HLA-linked, autoimmune-linked Lyme arthritis could have a "case" of "Early Lyme."

So, then, what about the other 85 percent of people who were formerly considered Lyme cases—the neurological type? Says Dickson, "They were thrown out with the vaccine-failure and vaccine-caused adverse events cases. Only about 15 percent of the population have the arthritis HLAs, which means Lyme disease will be missed in 85 percent of the cases—this was the crime."

"No one knows exactly why," she continues. "Dearborn was obviously not a consensus conference. It could be that because the CDC officers who ran the Dearborn conference were also owners of multiple patents that would be commercially worthless if it was known that 85 percent of the victims of Relapsing Fever, especially this new one with the abundant Outer Surface Protein A (OspA), which is a fungal antigen and is immunosuppressive for the other 85 percent, rarely produced any antibodies other than band 41 or the anti-flagellar antibody for any length of time."[161]

As Lyme sufferer John Coughlin so aptly said: "You can not fix something unless you know what it is you are trying to fix. If I listened to the ignorance from medical professionals and didn't stay the course, I would probably be dead by now for sure or in a wheelchair."

Lyme sufferer and activist Jerry Seidel said: "I am surprised that so many people describe the Dearborn criteria and the people involved with it with very weak words. Words like bias and conflicts of interest. Using those weak words is like accusing a mass murderer of giving someone a booboo."

Dickson filed a Racketeer Influenced and Corrupt Organizations (RICO) Act and fraud complaint with the US Department of Justice in 2003. For more than ten years, there has been a total failure by the USDOJ to prosecute this crime and protect US citizens.

With Dickson at the helm, and armed with her criminal charge sheets, activist patients are now organizing and mobilizing with national efforts to #OccupyTheUSDOJ.

Says Dickson,

Though we are extraordinarily ill, we have passion and truth on our side. We also have all the necessary research and documentation to prove this crime. Those responsible will be prosecuted. We will get justice.

This is one of the biggest corruption cases in U.S. history. It involves medical research fraud, and organized crime between government agencies, academia, and the health care industry. Everyone's assistance in bringing attention to our movement has the potential to help millions of people suffering needlessly all over the world.

How many years will [these perpetrators] get?

Allow me to share a little tidbit. There are RICO and False Claims Act laws on the books for a reason. It is not a novel idea that crooks who defraud the government should be charged with "defrauding the government." And RICO means organized crime, as in, there is an "enterprise," established to commit crimes, or an organization who coordinated the crimes. In this case, Lyme, CFIDS, Fibro, Autism, GWI—it's all about the CDC staff working on behalf of their own personal profit and on behalf of the corporations who sell vaccines. That is it. Simple. It's simple profiteering made to look like "government policy."

Another Activist's Viewpoint

Wendy Woodhall, a Canadian Lyme activist and founder of a Lyme support group in Waterloo, Ontario, agrees with most of what those in Lymeland believe.

Given that Woodhall has been struggling with Lyme for years, as have her two children, she knows this disease and the politics very well. She believes she transmitted Lyme to her two kids through nursing. This is the cause of her greatest heartbreak.

Woodhall presents with a calm and logical style. She concurs that 80 percent of the doctors on the IDSA board had conflicts of interest with pharmaceutical companies, university funding, and insurance, and that doctors covered up the findings to covet profits.

Says Woodhall,

No one in the IDSA wants to admit they were wrong.

This is where the anger, the rage, the madness is coming from...They have so much power.

In Connecticut... the governor—Richard Blumenthal—created a task force to look into the IDSA guidelines. A whole new group of doctors were assigned to this task force. They disagreed with the original findings, saying that chronic Lyme DID exist but that document was never signed into law for whatever reason.

As Canadians, we follow the United States. We wait for them to take the lead—we have no medical minds of our own. We've got cutting-edge research and researchers of our own, if only we were free to explore where they would lead us. Once you say you have chronic Lyme, all bets are off. No doctor will talk to you.

Did you know that veterinarians and dentists are treating

people for Lyme? Under the table of course. Isn't it insane that your dog can get inoculated and treated for this disease, yet you can't? Something is very wrong with that.

There are remarkably deep layers of secrecy and protection for the medical powers that be. Subsequently, we have to protect our doctors—the ones who do support us in our illness. We don't post LLMD's names anywhere. It all has to be done in a quiet, hush-hush manner. What we have been through to get treatment has been a life-and-death struggle. I can never get disability and I can never get insurance for my kids or myself.

It's a travesty.

Beaux Reliosis provides one of the clearest explanations of the controversy to date:

Recent research has confirmed that chronic Lyme is an acquired immune deficiency disease. When we all start speaking this language maybe something will change.

Personal stories, non-profits, protests, complaining about the guidelines get us nowhere because this is a criminal matter. CDC officers who were involved in the development of the Lyme vaccine literally changed the disease definition to exclude neurological cases when the vaccine trials revealed that the vaccine caused the same disease.

In fact, they knew before the trials even started that the antigen they used in this fake vaccine was the same fungal-type toxin that is shed by spirochetes, causing a post-sepsis-like, permanent down-regulation of the immune system. The fact that the "vaccine" caused the same disease tells us that chronic Lyme is not about spirochetes. They knew this, marketed LYMErix anyway, and to do so, they changed the disease definition so neuro-Lyme and LYMErix victims could not get diagnosed.

The DOJ so far has refused to prosecute... Meanwhile we are stuck with the phony case definition and "activists" are screaming about changing the diagnostic & treatment guidelines.

Guess what? As long as the case definition says Lyme is an arthritic knee only, the guidelines will always be geared toward treating that hyper-inflammatory outcome instead of the AIDS-like outcome that 85% of us have.[162]

Theory or Conspiracy #4: Plum Island and Operation Paperclip

Nazis, Operation Paperclip, Lyme and biological warfare, Plum Island and Lab 257, Osama bin Laden and terrorism—oh my!

If by now I haven't convinced you that Lymeland is a mad, crazy, insane world where nothing is clear and everything is dark, scary and mind-boggling, I'm going to stretch your mind even further with this last theory/conspiracy—that Lyme is being purposefully used as a biological warfare weapon, right in the heart of the good ol' USA.

It sounds mad, I know. You may need to catch your breath here—before you venture into this theory that is both outrageous and, at the same time, well documented.

I suggest, as was suggested to me, that you start by reading

Lab 257: The Disturbing Story of the Government's Secret Germ Laboratory, by Michael C. Carroll. Then read Rachel Verdon's *Lyme Disease and SS Elbrus*. Two of the most fascinating findings in my madcap adventures down this rabbit hole.

Michael Carroll spent seven years researching and writing *Lab 257*. A native of Long Island and an avid outdoorsman, Carroll is now general counsel of a New York–based finance company. He lives on Long Island and in New York City.

In *Lab 257*—a book about the biological warfare lab located on Plum Island, just a short ferry ride from New York City—Carroll skillfully argues that the real world of science is hands down more riveting, maddening, and incredulous than science fiction.

We learn that Plum Island, which is strictly off limits to the public, is also covered with beaches, cliffs, forests, ponds—and the deadliest germs on earth. Many of the rich and famous who summer in the Hamptons, just minutes away from this mysterious and forbidden island, have no idea that it exists or what it's all about.

Carroll tells us that with his book and his long investigative journey, the mystery of Plum Island—the focus of many dark conspiracy theories—is all about to change.

Lab 257 "reveals the stunning true nature and checkered history of Plum Island. It shows that the seemingly bucolic Plum Island, on the edge of the largest population center in the United States, is a ticking biological time bomb that none of us can safely ignore."

Carroll's book takes readers...

...deep inside the secret world of Plum Island and learn startling revelations, including virus outbreaks, biological meltdowns, infected workers who are denied

treatment by the government, the flushing of contam-
inated raw sewage into area waters, and the insidious
connections between Plum Island, Lyme disease, and the
deadly 1999 West Nile virus outbreak.[163]

Dr. Willy Burgdorfer once worked in a biowarfare lab as a military epidemiologist. Is this perhaps the reason he was not permitted to be interviewed by *Under Our Skin* producer and director Andy Abrahams Wilson without having an official government escort? Burgdorfer died shortly after breaking the silence on the heated controversy, so we may never know the full story.

Rachel Verdon's *Lyme and The SS Elbrus* examines how "the US Health Department remained silent for over half a century on the advancement of these tick borne plagues, the American Intelligence Community opened the doors to Nazi Paperclip scientists and Dragon Returnees 'from Russia with Love' to fight the Cold War, totally compromising our national security."[164]

Verdon's biography reads,

Verdon was born and raised in Glastonbury just a few miles north of Old Lyme, Connecticut, where Lyme disease was first diagnosed in the 1970s. After a life-time of poor health and the tragic deaths of eleven next door neighbors involving suicides, drugs and autoim-mune diseases going back as far as the 1950s, she was prompted to investigate their cause. Once diagnosed with 'chronic borreliosis,' the Lyme spirochete, by Dr. Paul Lavoie in San Francisco in 1987, it became appar-ent to the author this was not a brand new disease of the 70s. The resulting seventeen-year investigation for

> *the origin of Lyme disease has uncovered a scandalous collaboration between the Nazis and the Soviet Union in biological warfare through World War I and World War II.*
>
> *Truth is the biggest weapon in a world of liars, murderers and thieves. The vectors of disease, drugs and poverty are rats; the furry ones, political ones, and medical ones. Let the rat wars begin!*[165]

As far as page-turners go, both of these stories have all the elements of a great mystery thriller. Both are confounding, jaw-dropping, and verifiable.

This theory/conspiracy—that Lyme disease has been created and distributed by a US government biowarfare lab—located a stone's throw from the first outbreak site of Old Lyme, Connecticut—is confirmed and validated by many other sources as well.

Other sources have documented that the nefarious history of Plum Island began after World War II when Erich Traub, a Nazi sympathizer and German biological warfare expert, joined the team. The Germans had a particular attachment to using bioweapons technology, and it seems that Traub had operated a germ warfare lab on an island in the Baltic Sea. According to an article by Barbara Andrews, editor in chief of The Dog Press website,

> *Either the U.S. Army knew nothing about migratory patterns or, as is more logical, Army researchers knew exactly what they were doing. Plum Island is on the Atlantic flyway that runs from the Florida coast up the eastern seaboard to Greenland. A million birds rest*

on the island before flying on to the Connecticut River estuaries in Lyme. It is possible but doubtful that the Army also overlooked the fact that deer regularly swim between the island and the mainland. In fact, Plum Island researchers believe the deer and birds were recognized as vehicles for distributive test.[166]

In her interview, Kris Newby told me that when filming her documentary *Under Our Skin*, they were not afraid to ask the tough questions. They knew, however, that if their line of questioning went down the biowarfare path, all of their funding would come to an end.

A US Lyme activist told me a personal story that also makes Plum Island feel mysterious and verboten. She said,

My father-in-law had a colleague who was a pathologist on Plum Island for many years. When my father-in-law called him to talk about chronic Lyme and gather more information to help me with my Lyme diagnosis, the pathologist colleague abruptly said, "Lose my number. Don't ever call me again!"

In an article about Lyme disease and Plum Island, Smaranda Dumitru reported this:

"I don't know if Lyme came from Plum Island," said April Ferguson, a chief strategy officer for a Hudson Valley policy-oriented think tank, "but it's weird that no one wants to talk about it, doctors are scared to treat and diagnose it, [and] the government doesn't talk about it."

Ferguson represents Lyme patients pro bono as an attorney. She considers the government's attitude towards Lyme very strange. ... *"Lyme disease is taboo and I don't understand why," she said.*[167]

And last, but certainly not least, there is a very interesting interview with Patricia Doyle, PhD, that I encourage everyone to read. Doyle is a recurring guest on the Jeff Rense broadcast show. On the Rense website, you can read the highlights from the show, where Doyle takes us on a journey back to Operation Paperclip and to proven tick research on Plum Island dating back to the 1950s.

Doyle quips, "I wondered how lone star ticks from Texas would get to my backyard in NY. The ticks had some help, i.e. germ scientists...and Plum Island?"[168]

Operation Paperclip is explained quite simply in this excerpt from an article by Laura Schumm:

In a covert affair originally dubbed Operation Overcast but later renamed Operation Paperclip, roughly 1,600 of these German scientists (along with their families) were brought to the United States to work on America's behalf during the Cold War. The program was run by the newly-formed Joint Intelligence Objectives Agency (JIOA), whose goal was to harness German intellectual resources to help develop America's arsenal of rockets and other biological and chemical weapons, and to ensure such coveted information did not fall into the hands of the Soviet Union.[169]

Didn't the Nazis do enough damage in the Holocaust during World War II? The US brought them to Plum Island to wreak more havoc on the human race? Now we learn that the Nazis, along with some US officials, are responsible for yet another holocaust—chemical warfare causing the first major US outbreak of chronic Lyme disease, too?

It's all just too much to fathom.

In the *Atlantic* in 2014, staff writer Olga Khazan explores the idea of "scientists [...] creating new and incurable diseases in labs" and wonders if it's reasonable.

"That worries people like Marc Lipsitch and Alison P. Galvani, two epidemiologists who write in a *PLOS Medicine* editorial today that creating these types of new infectious agents puts human life at risk. They estimate that if 10 American laboratories ran these types of experiments for a decade, there would be a 20 percent chance that a lab worker would become infected with one of these new super-flus and potentially pass it on to others," Khazan reports.

"The concern is that you're making something that doesn't exist in nature and combines high virulence for people with the ability to transmit efficiently," Lipsitch told Khazan.[170]

Could this have been the case with the bacteria for Lyme, causing the original outbreak in Lyme, Connecticut, in the early 1970s? Many are purporting that this is, in fact, the case.

What Lyme Denialists Say

In case the above theories and conspiracies seem like too much to wrap your head around, I thought I'd share with you some of the inane things uttered by the medical community's top Lyme denialists over the years, demonstrating that medical bigwigs have pushed us all too far, forcing us to dig deep, and prove them wrong, even at the risk of sounding conspiratorial.

In a journal article entitled "On the reception and detection of pseudo-profound bullshit," the authors say,

> *Although bullshit is common in everyday life and has attracted attention from philosophers, its reception (critical or ingenuous) has not, to our knowledge, been subject to empirical investigation. Here we focus on pseudo-profound bullshit, which consists of seemingly impressive assertions that are presented as true and meaningful but are actually vacuous.*

In the article's introduction, the authors submit:

> *There is little question that bullshit is a real and consequential phenomenon. Indeed, given the rise of communication technology and the associated increase in the availability of information from a variety of sources, both expert and otherwise, bullshit may be more pervasive than ever before.*[171]

I have to wonder if the authors of this journal article know about the decades-long dissemination of tall tales throughout the world of Lyme.

Here are just a few carefully paraphrased Lyme statements, uttered by some of the most prominent Lyme disease denialists—most of whom have a stake in the ground, a personal interest in keeping Lyme nonexistent or at the very least thought to be *"hard to catch, easy to diagnose, and easy to treat"*—providing no doubt that there's something very wrong in Lymeland:

Lyme disease is really no more than an arthritic condition...Lyme disease is easily treated...Lyme sufferers are far more anxious than they are sick...Lyme disease resolves itself in time, without any medical treatment... Lyme disease is just a nuisance condition that simply requires a trip to the doctor's office on occasion...If you get bitten and a rash develops over time, take a week or two of antibiotics and you'll be just fine...It is just not as big a deal as most people think or say it is...Tick-borne infections are limited to a select few geographical areas; nothing to be concerned about, we've got it contained...If you do get sick, it is easily cured...Lyme disease is just a matter of dealing with the aches and pains of everyday life; after all, who doesn't feel tired and have sore knees at times?...There is simply no evidence of persistent infection...Lyme disease is rarely fatal...We offered a vaccine, a few people complained, we took it off the market and look, they're still complaining... LYMErix failed solely because of some negative media hype...This whole Lyme thing is blown so far out of proportion...Antiscience Lyme advocates are, in fact, the real danger...They are living in a pseudoscientific echo chamber, whining about their fatigue and headaches, looking for attention...Lyme sufferers would rather invest in snake oil treatments than adhere to the real science...Lyme sufferers are crazy, and for some reason they keep harassing us—the very scientists who understand this disease best.

Lyme Madness in a Nutshell

So, as I see it, there have been several building blocks erected and sustained all these years by the powers that be, which have ultimately resulted in this experience we know as *Lyme Madness*:

- Weave an anti-chronic Lyme tale based on falsehoods and misinformation telling the world for forty years now that there is no such thing as chronic Lyme disease, that Lyme is geographically limited and therefore hard to catch. And that if you do catch it, it is merely a nuisance condition that can be easily diagnosed and treated.

- Change the definition of chronic Lyme from an "immunosuppressive, post sepsis, relapsing fever" (or OspA/borreliosis) to that of a simple arthritic condition.

- Tell and retell this story at an enormous cost to the public's health and welfare in order to protect the interests of major stakeholders in Big Pharma, government, insurance companies, and academia, thereby warding off potential lawsuits, maintaining lucrative patent holdings, and making tidy profits from the 350-plus conditions that chronic Lyme is known to imitate.

- Categorically deny the validity of more than seven hundred peer-reviewed evidence-based scientific articles citing that chronic Lyme does indeed exist.

- Render Lyme sufferers powerless by ignoring their pleas, by mocking their subjective truths and anecdotal evidence, using derogatory terms like *antiscience, pseudoscience* and *quackery*, while paying homage to "pure" evidenced-based science only, the results of which may at times be skewed.

- Ignore the fact that there are 700 evidence based journal articles validating the existence of chronic Lyme.

- Never admit to the fact that millions are suffering, as it would bankrupt the system by forcing insurers to make large payouts for medical treatment and disability coverage.

- Continue the academic debate about chronic Lyme year after year, detracting from the devastation of this medical condition, so that little progress is ever made.

- Continue to use a two-tier testing method that has an extraordinarily high rate of false negatives.

- Tell patients there is no Lyme here, ticks don't cross the borders, states, oceans, or travel across continents.

- Make sufferers feel like they're crazy, malingerers, hypochondriacs, try to convince them that it's all in their head, send them to a psychiatrist, and call it a day.

- Use medical and political doublespeak, such as post-treatment Lyme disease syndrome, to confuse sufferers, obfuscate the wrongdoings of the medical community, offload the responsibility, and blame the victims for their suffering.

- Keep people sick and infirm so they won't be strong enough to fight back, and perhaps this whole mess will eventually go away.

- Expropriate the licenses of physicians who dare to treat Lyme sufferers, or at the very least take them to court for years on end, exhaust their resources, and wipe them out entirely.

- Show tons of empathy for those with the Zika virus, shed a few tears on national TV, and pour mega-dollars into this newly spread disease so that the CDC looks like it actually has a heart.

- Get all media, politicians, doctors, insurers, and the public at large to believe that Lyme is no more than a little nuisance condition that is "hard to catch, easy to diagnose, and easy to treat."

Now that, my friends, is how the medical community so elegantly creates *Lyme Madness!*

If you are still asking "Why?", simply follow the money. Always follow the money.

This may seem conspiratorial. Impossible to digest. A touch cliché, perhaps.

But it's far more plausible than the impossible notion that millions of once healthy, active individuals, the world over, are faking their illness, suffering daily beyond the pale, and are participating in some kind of mass delusion that they are sick because they have nothing better to do than to become housebound, infirm, isolated, and penniless, and are looking for some kind of perverse attention with no perceivable payoff.

May I remind you of the foretelling by Aldous Huxley, humanitarian and author of *Brave New World*. In his iconic novel about a futuristic society set in the year 2540 AD, the individual is sacrificed for the state, and science is used to control and subjugate.

In a 1961 lecture to the California Medical School, Huxley said,

> *There will be within the next generation or so a pharma-cological method of making people love their servitude, and producing ... a kind of painless concentration camp for entire societies, so that people will in fact have their liberties taken away from them but will rather enjoy it, because they will be distracted from any desire to rebel by propaganda, brainwashing, or brainwashing enhanced by pharmacological methods.*[172]

What Now?

What do we need to settle this battle? And, more impor-tantly, how are we going to get people well? The controversy is so complex and so many years in the making.

As I continue my research, there are so many twists and turns.

I've learned that my son's illness is *not* necessarily about spirochetes and persisters and biofilms, but rather a condi-tion of immunosuppression, or an acquired immune defi-ciency, and OspA—with all the opportunistic infections, ret-roviruses such as EBV, and relapsing fevers that Lyme and LYMErix sufferers have fallen prey to.

I've learned that it may have all begun with Operation Paperclip, Nazi Erich Traub, and biowarfare on Plum Island in New York in the 1950s—a stone's throw from where my son lives in NYC? And was it orchestrated by the US government?

As if that weren't enough, is it possible that the madness was perpetuated further with an alleged toxic vaccine that was supposed to inoculate against but, in actual fact, may have caused chronic Lyme?

And can it be true that the definition of chronic Lyme was changed in order to sell this very vaccine, making the rabbit hole even deeper?

Is it possible that the very people who are supposed to be on our side, who are supposed to represent and care for us, are, in fact, the bad guys and the perpetrators in this upside-down, inside-out, twisted mad world of Lymeland?

I am *waking up* now as Alice once did. I now understand the saying "curiosity killed the cat." Sometimes it's better to shut your eyes, plug your ears, close your mind, and never mind what's not yours to mind. But this maddening position on Lyme as taken by the medical community at large became my business, whether I chose it or not.

Like Alice, I feel like a child who is playing with grown-up, dangerous, even explosive stuff that I'll never be fully equipped to defend against or fully comprehend. Unlike Alice, however, I cannot as easily accept the strangeness and madness that surrounds me. I've learned far more than I was prepared to know and the world, as such, has become a much darker place.

Before this story ends, my only job is to determine how we're ever going to get out of this never-ending, crazy-making, dangerous trap of a rabbit hole. A rabbit hole that has exposed us to the underbelly of life—the ugly, stark, cold truth, which has revealed that very few in the corporate, political, and medical world truly have our best interests at heart. I am not learning this for the first time. But the sociopathy is more profound, perverse, and pervasive than I had ever understood.

The politics of Lyme seem fouler, darker, more evil, and more parasitic than I could ever have imagined. I truly wish I could unsee it all.

8. OH, CANADA, SHAME ON YOU

No wonder why you're late. Why, this watch is exactly two days slow.

—ALICE'S ADVENTURES IN WONDERLAND

We, in Canada, are at least twenty years behind in our understanding of chronic Lyme disease. If we look at the US, the UK, Australia, and the like—and realize how deeply their proverbial heads are buried—then we have to take a good look at "the true north strong and free" to see how far behind we are as well.

We actually deny the existence of this disease outright. We don't admit that we have a problem here. We have muzzled our scientists for years. We have a completely faulty testing method. We don't allow our conventional medical doctors to treat it with antibiotics beyond twenty-eight days. We take our doctors to task and annihilate them outright if they try to support the sick and frail who may be suffering with Lyme.

Here is an amusing and horrifying anecdote.

A young woman I know—suffering profoundly with chronic Lyme and coinfections, which she was able to confirm by a doctor in the US—walked into a Toronto medical clinic to have a doctor or nurse administer an intramuscular shot of penicillin.

Her prescribing doctor is in New York City because there are next to no doctors in all of Canada (except for naturopaths in British Columbia, which is an even longer distance for her) who are entitled to and willing to prescribe antibiotics to chronic Lyme sufferers beyond the twenty-eight-day IDSA guidelines. In the US, some doctors get away with it as long as they keep a low profile and aren't somehow "outed" by a disgruntled colleague or patient. In Canada, few doctors have had such luck.

The doctor on duty at this medical clinic agreed to give her the Bicillin injection, but he was puzzled and wary. He asked the young woman about her condition. It was apparent from his body language and tone that he'd never heard of chronic Lyme. He was curious and flummoxed.

As they were finishing up, he looked at her and, without a hint of irony, he asked the young woman: *"So, apart from Lyme, are you healthy?"*

Only "Lymies," as Lyme sufferers are called, would really get the unintended, twisted humor in this doctor's question. When I posted this incident on Facebook, one UK Lyme sufferer told me she "was laughing like a drain!" It's good to find some humor in all of this—even if it's terribly dark.

To be clear, in case I haven't been already, when you're suffering from a multisystem, immunosuppressive, non-HIV, AIDS-like post sepsis disease, you *cannot* be healthy *apart* from chronic Lyme.

When you have chronic Lyme, it has infected and affected every cell, every organ, every synapse, every nerve, every inch, every fiber of your being.

This was probably the most ridiculous question a doctor could ask.

And yet he did. Right here in my fair city.

Oh, Canada. Surely, you can do better than this.

Lyme in Canada—a Dismal Mess

For any one suffering from Lyme in Canada—and there are tens of thousands—what we have is a medical standoff and an underground Lyme treatment network that sees Canadians travelling to the US and paying upward of $50,000 for treatment. All Canadian doctors who are vocal about treating chronic Lyme have been shut down.

—JIM WILSON, PRESIDENT OF THE CANADIAN LYME FOUNDATION[173]

If any doctor in Canada—and I assure you, there will be plenty of doctors on your Lyme journey—tells you that it's contained in the northeastern United States, that Lyme is impossible to contract here, that it is grossly overdiagnosed and highly overtreated, that there are so few real cases in Canada, by now it should be clear that you must not, should not, cannot believe what you're hearing.

If you hear anything to this effect from doctors, insurers, politicians, the media, or your neighbor down the street, boldly ask them to stop.

The story we hear in Canada is FALSE!

It's frustrating and confusing, to say the least. Our expectation in this country is that we are able to rely on our doctors. That we have an accessible health-care system where we are invited to openly consult with our medical professionals. Trust what they say. Believe in their care.

Is this wrong? Have we been fleeced? Sold a bill of

goods? With chronic Lyme, we cannot rely on a thing they say. All trust is lost.

The standard patter of all infectious-disease doctors here is that "Lyme is rarely seen in Canada and easy to treat if you do have it."

Canadian Lyme expert Dr. Ernie Murakami says, "If there are in fact 300,000 cases of chronic Lyme disease reported in the US, you must multiply that by 10, so it's closer to 3 million. Canada is always 10 percent of that for any disease or infection, colds, viruses."

Based on these suppositions, when I do the math, that's an estimated 300,000 cases of chronic Lyme disease right here in Canada.

Yet they tell us that chronic Lyme disease doesn't really exist here.

Due to climate change and vector expansion, some experts predict that 80 percent of the Canadian population will be exposed to deer ticks by 2020.[174]

Yet they tell us that chronic Lyme disease doesn't really exist here.

Evidence suggests that Canada's Lyme testing methods are flawed. False negative test results are common, especially in the early stages of Lyme. It takes time for antibodies to develop, so early tests often miss the bacteria. Contrary to bureaucratic statements, late-stage Lyme disease antibody testing is much less accurate. Just because we don't have stable and reliable diagnostic tools to confirm Lyme, it doesn't mean it doesn't exist.

Yet they tell us that chronic Lyme disease doesn't really exist here.

There is not one infectious-disease doctor in Canada—from coast to coast—who will treat Lyme beyond the twenty-eight-day IDSA guidelines for fear that they will be reprimanded and have their licenses revoked by the Royal College of Physicians and Surgeons.

Yet they tell us that chronic Lyme disease doesn't really exist here.

According to CanLyme, nearly 100 percent of Canadian doctors have become victims of the College witch hunts—simply for diagnosing and treating Lyme disease outside of the "appropriate" guidelines. In contrast, physicians, in general, are investigated by their College less than 2 percent of the time.

It is widely known among Canadian doctors that if they don't follow the limited twenty-eight-day IDSA protocol for treating Lyme—even though these are supposed to be just guidelines, and not legally enforced—they will pay a price. They are all too aware that if they don't toe the line, they will likely be targeted.

The tides began to turn recently when an internist who became a target for treating Lyme outside of the "appropriate" IDSA guidelines appealed the College's decision to the Health Professions Appeal and Review Board in Ontario. The decision to impose punitive measures was overruled.

Here in Canada, our knowledge is skewed. Our understanding is limited. Our testing is flawed. Our doctors are disinterested, brainwashed, afraid. Our treatment is inadequate at best, and nonexistent at worst.

And YES, chronic Lyme disease absolutely, unequivocally, undoubtedly, without question DOES exist here. And the number of cases is growing exponentially.

CBC reports,

Up until recently, most experts didn't think it was possible to get Lyme disease in Canada. Now with climate warming, ticks—specifically, the kinds of tick that spread Lyme disease—are catching a ride much further north on the backs of migratory birds. A 2012 study shows that they've been infiltrating Canada for the past 20 years and cases of Lyme disease in Canada are skyrocketing. In the documentary Ticked Off: The Mystery of Lyme Disease, *we learned that as temperatures warm, the tick's range is expected to keep expanding dramatically over the next 20 years when 80 percent of Canadians east of Saskatchewan will live in at-risk areas.*[175]

So why do we, in Canada, follow the insufficient and poorly constructed US-driven IDSA guidelines? Why don't we think for ourselves and set our own rules? What are we afraid of? Why are we so behind in our understanding and treatment of Lyme? Why do we deny its very existence here outright? Why are the Colleges so punitive when a doctor sticks his or her neck out to treat patients?

It seems that the US—which also greatly underreports, underdiagnoses, and undertreats chronic Lyme—has a slightly more open mind and a greater willingness in some states to "allow"—and I use that term loosely—doctors to treat the disease with long-term antibiotics. And that's not saying much. Believe me.

I only point this out to make it clear that while the US—and many other countries worldwide—are doing a profoundly inadequate job of dealing with this disease, Canada is performing even more shamefully.

Again, not to give the US too much credit—because they are just as culpable of neglect and abandonment of chronic

Lyme sufferers, and are equally punitive of their Lyme doctors. At least they just recently and reluctantly increased the number of cases reported each year from 30,000 to 300,000. In the Lyme world, we are pleased that "official" Lyme numbers are now being reported with greater accuracy, but we are skeptical as to why now.

Due to our justifiable skepticism, most of us in the Lyme world saw this reported increase as a big red flag rather than good news. When the CDC revised its numbers in August of 2013, it seemed suspicious. Why now? Why such a big jump? This wasn't news to Lyme sufferers. Anyone in Lymeland already knew this more realistic number of cases was somewhat closer to the truth. Where were these new numbers coming from and why were they being reported suddenly?

In Canada, we're still waiting, of course. Waiting for the Public Health Agency of Canada (PHAC) to fess up. Waiting for someone with authority and power to be more honest in their reporting and reflect what is truly happening in this country of ours.

Instead, we have doctors saying no to patients and showing them the door. We have doctors telling patients they're wrong, crazy, and have no business Googling uncertain sources. We have doctors writing opinion pieces stating that chronic Lyme is far less of a problem than non-hockey-related skating injuries.

With the number of cases predicted to escalate in the next several years, this ill-gotten medical behavior, this false party line, and editorial pieces of this nature seem pretty absurd to me.

There is clearly a chasm—an impossibly wide chasm—between what is true and what doctors, medical stakeholders, and the media are actually saying is true.

There seems to be little to no interest in chronic Lyme in this country. There is certainly no urgency in coming to the aid of those suffering here. In fact, PHAC has reported 833 cases since reporting began in 2009. They are only off by tens of thousands, depending on which source we believe.

Anne Kingston's May 2014 article in *Maclean's* magazine "The Truth About Lyme Disease" quotes Dr. Geoffrey Taylor, physician and chair of PHAC's Canadian Nosocomial Infection Surveillance Program, as saying that the rise from 128 cases in 2009 to 315 in 2012 is concerning.

First, these numbers are grossly underreported, and yes, the closer guesstimate of 30,000 to 300,000 cases per year is "concerning," keeping in mind that our numbers are typically 10 percent of US cases.

In the same article, Dr. Taylor then defends current protocols: "Based on what the evidence shows us, physicians in Canada are doing the best job they can," he says. US lab tests for Lyme are "invalidated," he says, noting that "post-treatment Lyme disease syndrome," the term given to those who experience symptoms after being treated with short-term antibiotics, requires research: "We don't know what's behind it," he says. "It could be the immune system; it could be a number of factors. That's typical when new diseases are emerging."[176]

Chronic Lyme disease is *not* new. And yes, it affects the immune system. Please stop calling it post-treatment Lyme disease syndrome—thereby abdicating all medical responsibility. By calling it this, it implies that *"we, your doctors, treated your illness with antibiotics for twenty-eight days. We can't understand why you're still sick. Let's call it post-treatment Lyme disease syndrome. Then we're off the hook. It's your problem now. Our job is done. We don't know how to help you any further, so it must be all in your head. Go see a 'shrink.'"*

Is this really the best we can do?

Stop invalidating a real disease and real people who are suffering right now, in real time. We know it requires research and we know you don't know what's behind it. What have you done and what are you currently doing to figure it out? That's all we care to hear. That's all we want to know.

Jim Wilson, president of CanLyme, says that Canada's incidence of chronic Lyme is seriously underreported. In fact, he says that his organization gets 3,000 new inquiries a year.

Numbers matter. When officials report unrealistically low statistics, they diminish the severity of the impact, causing great bitterness, loneliness, abandonment, and confusion. The denial, the invalidation, and the negation is crazy-making.

The powers that be are telling us one thing, and we're experiencing another. Everywhere we turn, every Facebook group we belong to, every sufferer we speak with, knows that chronic Lyme disease is real. That it's affecting many. That it's ruining lives. That it's debilitating, destructive, degrading, and deflating.

Canadian Lyme sufferers are all too aware that we have a very high rate of false negatives in our diagnostic methods, a false negative rate of 62 percent, in fact, using our country's "gold standard" ELISA test. Yet infectious-disease specialists here keep insisting that they *must* practice evidence-based medicine, which is code for following the guidelines as set out by the Infectious Diseases Society of America (IDSA), thereby not recognizing and treating those who don't pass muster using our unreliable testing protocols.

Canada's Bill C-442—the new federal initiative intended to create a framework for preventing, assessing, managing, and treating Lyme disease in this country—was passed in Senate in December 2014 because Health Canada finally recognized, in theory, that these very same so-called evidence-based IDSA guidelines are flawed. Yet infectious-disease specialists in Canada keep insisting, to patient after patient, day after day, that they must practice evidence-based medicine and follow the guidelines as set out by the IDSA. Guidelines that are flawed and wholly ineffective.

The US National Guideline Clearinghouse (NGC), a public resource for evidence-based clinical practice guidelines, has just recently delisted the IDSA Lyme disease guidelines due to their lack of evidence-based medicine, replacing the IDSA guidelines with the far more humane and efficacious ILADS guidelines as followed by US Lyme-literate doctors. Yet doctors in Canada keep insisting—every day—that they must follow evidence-based medicine—that is, the IDSA guidelines.

Not only are our doctors not treating Lyme sufferers, because they insist on using so-called evidence-based IDSA guidelines as their guidepost, they are also "warning" us every day that we must question and beware of US Lyme-literate doctors. Doctors here are maligning their credibility, diagnostic, and medical skill set, refusing to sign Ministry of Health Out of Country Approval papers, thereby denying Lyme sufferers access to affordable care, and, even worse, they are clearly telling Lyme sufferers that their complaints must be primarily psychological in nature. "Go see a shrink" seems to be the best they can offer.

The cognitive dissonance that is created by being told the opposite of what we know to be true leads to unequivocal outrage, helplessness, and utter madness—a madness that chronic Lyme sufferers refuse to succumb to. This is the gaslighting that Lyme sufferers are experiencing every single day. A campaign of misinformation and misdirection that is unconscionably harmful, as it prevents Lyme sufferers from getting the care they need, leaving them to suffer in silence, or break the bank traveling to the US for decent and reasonable care.

Infectious-disease doctors, along with the lion's share of the medical community in Canada, are not listening. And they are doing more harm than they realize by their widespread negation of this horrid disease. Lyme sufferers are having to go it alone and seek whatever help they can find, not in Canada and against the current medical tide.

Lyme sufferers are sick. Sick and tired of their illness. Sick and tired of the fight. To borrow an iconic line from the 1976 film *Network*, which struck a chord with people everywhere: *We're mad as hell and we're not going to take it anymore!*

Pushing the Lyme Agenda Forward

One of the most notable Canadian politicians advocating for the support of this disease is Elizabeth May, leader of the Green Party of Canada. She introduced a private Member's bill known as C-442, which would make it possible to recognize, diagnose, and properly treat Lyme disease in Canada.

Elizabeth May's private Member's bill, C-442—the Federal Framework on Lyme Disease Act—was passed unanimously at third reading by the Senate the morning of Friday, December 12, 2014. The private Member's bill called Lyme a "national crisis" and proposed a "made-in-Canada strategy" to deal with it. Since then, the bill has received Royal Assent by the Governor General and is now law.

Sounds promising, I know. However, there have been no tangible outcomes to date. Despite a "unanimously supported" call to action for better diagnostic and treatment protocols and a Canadian Lyme conference that has already taken place, we are still waiting for something of significance to happen.

On a provincial level, Michael Mantha, a New Democratic Party member of provincial parliament of Algoma-Manitoulin, went to Queen's Park to fight against Lyme disease, asking the government to do something more to help patients. Not surprisingly, the provincial government has yet to act. On November 27, 2015, MPP Michael Mantha asked the Minister of Health for an explanation of what has been done for Lyme patients and their families a year after all three parties agreed to develop a Lyme strategy for Ontario.

It's all so politically mired and slow and trudging; the result of these efforts seems to be nothing more than doublespeak, delays, and dismissiveness.

Also at the helm of Lyme advocacy is the Canadian Lyme Science Alliance (CLSA)—an organization that unites scientists and clinicians in the quest for a more comprehensive understanding of Lyme borreliosis, promoting evidence-based medicine.

The CLSA's current initiative is a petition requesting sound science-based policy from the Federal Framework on Lyme Disease (Bill C-442). They are asking for an inclusive, interdisciplinary, and transparent review of Lyme disease policy in this country, as well as high-quality unbiased research to resolve outstanding issues in the biology, health, and human impact of this disease.

And, of course, there's Jim Wilson—president and founder of the Canadian Lyme Disease Foundation (CanLyme). For more than twenty years, Wilson has been networking with Lyme victims and providing information. It all began when he contracted Lyme disease in 1991 in Dartmouth, Nova Scotia, and his daughter contracted Lyme disease in 2001 in the Okanagan Valley of British Columbia.

With a background investigating medical malpractice and legal liability matters, Jim provides unique insight into medical research from a perspective of conflict of evidence.

There is no humanity in medicine. We have a medical hierarchy that prevents us from making progress. The infectious disease community exists without a conscience. They're guided by the CDC, the IDSA and Big Pharma—all of whom need puppets to enforce their dogma. The infectious disease docs are those puppets.

I believe that what's happening in the medical community is criminal from a moralistic perspective. In good science, you're not supposed to prune research to what you think it should be. The IDSA referenced 400 research studies out of 20,000—over half of them are written by IDSA members themselves, and their friends.[177]

Wilson sees the government's "action plan" as preemptive. "They know what's coming down the pipes," he says. According to Health Canada, there were five hundred reported cases of Lyme in Canada last year, up from 128 in 2009, when the agency started keeping track. At a hearing into Bill C-442 in May, an infectious-disease specialist claimed Lyme "will affect more than 10,000 Canadians per year by the 2020s." Wilson believes we're at 10,000 Lyme cases annually now. He expresses concern that no infrastructure is being built to deal with the mounting numbers: "We're talking billions of dollars in healthcare and other tax dollars of social assistance [for people disabled by Lyme]," he says.[178]

In an interview, Jim told me,

With regard to research, we need to do human tissue study and find out how prevalent Lyme is. We need to determine how many people have Lyme who may have been misdiagnosed with MS. There is research going back to 1911. There's a 1957 Times *magazine article naming the spirochete. By 1960, the entire medical paradigm changed, creating a drug to manage symptoms and not cure the disease.*

What we have is a very corrupt and broken system. Dr. Klempner's leading study clearly demonstrates that one of the problems with the guidelines and scientific research is that it all leads to the proliferation of the false belief that chronic Lyme doesn't exist. We know it does. Without question. We also know that Lyme is being studied as a biowarfare weapon.[179]

Another powerful force in the Canadian fight against Lyme disease is Rossana Magnotta, whose husband, Gabe, died on December 30, 2009, of Lyme carditis. After witnessing her own family's struggle with Lyme, Magnotta clearly knows firsthand how frustrating, exhausting, and life-changing Lyme disease can be.

I was unable to reach her in person. However, on her website, her personal message to the Lyme community reads, in part, as follows:

With Gabe's illness, we didn't have answers from anyone for a very long time so we learned first hand the difficulties Canadians face in receiving an immediate, accurate diagnosis and ongoing care. There was nowhere for us to go in Canada that could understand and help us. After a 7-year battle, Gabe passed away.

This is not an isolated case. It's a story I hear again and again. For more than seven years, I have been inundated with calls from people who are frightened and just beginning their frustrating struggle to find answers and proper treatment for their loved ones.

... the real answer today is to establish a central place in Canada where people can go to get real help and end their frustrating and hopeless struggle. The G. Magnotta Foundation for Vector-Borne Diseases will focus on this mandate by raising funds to establish a facility dedicated to Lyme Disease research that will lead to better testing and treatment. It will also support studies and activities necessary to properly address this growing health crisis that affects all Canadians.[180]

Wendy's Lyme Story

Wendy Woodhall, who I briefly introduced you to in Chapter 7, is a long-time Canadian advocate for Lyme disease. She's driven to do the hard work that needs to get done because of her own suffering and that of her two children—James, seventeen, and Elyse, fourteen—both of whom have Lyme as well.

Says Wendy:

My family and I have done a lot of advocacy work in our locale. I founded the Waterloo Region Lyme Disease group. My family participated in a documentary three years ago but when they tried for government funding—they got denied.

My 73-year-old dad is running the distance across Canada on his YMCA track in Waterloo, Ontario to raise awareness for Lyme disease and treatment funds for James. On my website there is a video of him and my son, James. He hasn't been well enough to go to school all last year and struggled in the first half of this year, finally being unable to continue the second term. He is in constant pain from LD. The video is amazing and has been shared in Europe, Africa, South America, the Middle East, North America, Asia, and the UK, and I would love it if you would take a look and share it forward. He is doing this for all of us Lyme warriors. He is amazing.

Wendy was sick for years before realizing what was causing her health to deteriorate to the point of near death. She has put it all together and understands now that it all began when she was hiking in the mountains of South Korea at the tender age of twenty-seven.

Her health decline came in stages—first with a flu-like illness. Then—after she had her son in Bahrain in 1998—when she fell down the stairs back in Canada, pregnant with her daughter, Elyse, her fatigue and systemic pain worsened.

Wendy continues with her story:

The timelines are difficult to remember. I know that I fell ill, my pain, fatigue and emotional balance worsened. I was trying to juggle it all. Then I got pregnant with Elyse and my health declined further—fainting, fits of paralysis, astronomical pain and worst of all, a loss of cognitive function and memory. I gave this disease to both my kids through nursing. That is my biggest regret.

Elyse was extremely anxious from a young age—teachers were telling me it was all normal but I knew that it was clearly more than separation anxiety. From the moment she became verbal, she complained about pain in her legs and in her head. Anxiety and sleep got worse. She had constant crying jags—terrified all the time, well out of proportion.

The doctors said it was a generalized anxiety disorder.

In the meantime, my memory issues got so severe, I couldn't remember my students' or their parent's names. I felt like I had Alzheimer's and I was losing chunks of my mind. I had air hunger—I couldn't breathe. And the pain was getting worse which was inconceivable.

Things crashed. I had to quit work. I was a recluse. I was barely getting the kids on the bus. One day I fainted in front of the house and many of my neighbors, ones I didn't even know, ran to help the kids and I. I fainted in the grocery store, and I had to ask the cashier to not call the paramedics, and in the chair at the hair salon while getting a shampoo. I once fainted at the back of the public library and 4-year-old Elyse somehow dialed my mum and when she arrived Elyse was just sitting beside me and I was still unconscious. Nobody had found us in all that time. That probably traumatized her forever. Both my kids have PTSD from events like that happening throughout their childhood.

The paralysis was always there. I felt so weak so much of the time, I'd lie down on the floor and I couldn't shout or move. I'd lie there until it passed.

My parents had the kids a lot. I was on a lot of heavy-duty painkillers. I had to get off of Fentanyl once, by myself, because I didn't qualify for the addiction clinic. I said "Screw it—I'll do myself." By the time I was finished, I weighed just 80 pounds.

They kept telling me it was fibromyalgia, but I said, "I'm getting worse, and I thought you weren't supposed to get worse with this." You buy that stuff when you don't have other answers.

I had to be in a wheelchair—I couldn't drive anymore. I was bedridden. I couldn't remember words like rug, chair, toothbrush. I couldn't get a sentence out.

I was so irritable, and I had so many emotional outbursts—I knew I was dying. I wanted to scream, "Don't you people know I'm dying? I'm not going to be here a year from now, and don't you people get it. HELP ME!!!"

I didn't have the brain capacity to research and log on.

I was still fighting to drag myself down to dinner. I had no memory left. I had been tested at a 132 IQ previously and was in the superior intelligence range. And I couldn't make a sentence.

I was a recluse. I wasn't speaking to anyone about it.

My general practitioner sent me to a chronic pain specialist. She was amazing—tried every which way to test and to try to figure out what was going on. My GP cared a great deal—she put me on beta blockers for tachycardia, sent me to immunologists and neurologists.

Then the whole left side of my esophagus went into a hard ball and I couldn't swallow. It was becoming more and more frequent. I went to emergency—and after a half hour of sitting there, it let go.

I had my hymns written for my funeral service. I wrote letters to my kids. I told my husband how I wanted to be buried.

Then one day my dad saw an article in the paper and said, "WENDY, THIS IS YOU!!!"

In 2008, I met Dr. B., an infectious disease and internal medicine specialist. He told my dad, "I think it's Lyme, but I don't know because the tests are crap." I want people to know that doctors are not the enemies—their hands are tied. They [the College] have shut down every doctor who has tried to treat with antibiotics for more than two months. There are doctors treating Lyme under the table. There are doctors following the LLMDs in the US, but they can't draw attention to it or their licenses will be suspended. That's why we can't name doctors on the Facebook page. It's too dangerous for them.

The College can still go after them and they will. They went after Dr. B. They investigated and took his license I believe, and we all had to go to the US to continue our treatment, paying out of pocket tens of thousands of dollars to do so. Some people couldn't afford to go and they continued to get sicker. He was a HERO and saved countless patients' lives. He was careful not to say it was Lyme. Instead he said it's an infectious disease and I will treat it.

He saved my life and the lives of hundreds of others. Patients came for help from all over the province. He was our only hope at that time.

After 10 months of antibiotic treatment with him, I was walking, talking, driving, thinking, and so happy. He saved my life. I have had such an appreciation for every moment of every day. I was feeling so wonderful.

From 2008 on, when I discovered I had Lyme, I had no one to talk to as I was the only one in the region that I knew of who had it. I didn't have Facebook. I didn't have doctors who knew. I was alone and dealing with it alone.

People tell me "Well, don't you look great." They think they're giving you a compliment. They're not going to understand that for most patients this is extremely frustrating and insensitive but you're not going to change them. Most patients HATE when people tell them this but I try to take it as a compliment. I may not be able to control the illness on the inside, but I can try to make the outside look as well as possible. To me it means I'm winning against the disease if people tell me that.

I ask, would you say what you just said to a cancer patient? Lyme disease is just like cancer. Except that we have no medical support, no funding and no understanding. For years, I wanted people to know that I'm glad they say I look good on the outside, but try to understand that I'm rotting on the inside.

The local paper did an interview after my first time off of treatment when I thought I was cured and I started getting calls, including a call from a woman named Judy. It was the first time either of us had met anyone with Lyme. It was very emotional for both of us.

As my journey continued and I got sick again, twice more, and I found out that my children also had Lyme, I have gone through so many emotional highs and lows dealing with the terrible effects Lyme has not just on the individual but on their family. My entire family, especially my husband, was taxed to the limit—trying to help my kids, traveling to get treatment, paying for treatment, and keeping up with the normal, daily stress and activities of life.

I'm one of the very fortunate patients, in that my family and friends believed me, supported me and fought for my children and I. Everyone around my family is a positive light in our lives and without them I know that eventually, all three of us would have left this world one way or another.

Joan's Lyme Story

Here is a riveting Facebook message posted on November 27, 2015, by Lyme sufferer Joan Pifer in Ancaster, Ontario. Joan was eager to share her frustrations so that she could finally be heard—*by someone, somewhere*—and wanted her full name published. She eloquently and powerfully speaks for all Lyme sufferers in her frustration, helplessness, and desperation due to the lack of interest and acknowledgment by our medical system. This is her plea for more action, some action, any action on the government's part:

It has been a year now. A year. Since the government acknowledged the lack of treatment and incorrect testing on Lyme disease. All the articles, websites and Google searches, don't tell you even half of the debilitating symptoms or suffering. The details of how families are broken, jobs are lost, marriages broken, families split, and patients maimed for life, or even worse have passed…it does happen, a lot more than the general public thinks…I read in my group of people losing their lives due to this disease every month!!! How many must we lose before we matter?

All I know is I have an immense feeling of helplessness, my trust is gone, I no longer feel safe. I don't even know how to wrap my head around counting on the government while we wait around and deteriorate... It's a horrible feeling. It's unthinkable after you have felt this pain.

Not to be recognized, and no help from the government or the healthcare system for this disease. Infectious disease was no help either, they had their lines memorized well. Word for word, they all said the same thing, and they weren't helping, was very peculiar.

The other day I wrote about thoughtfulness. I try. I do try. To keep my head up, to appreciate life more, to make a difference in someone else's, and to be as helpful as I can. And to be honest, I guess I do this also, to pretend this isn't happening to me, to not let it break me.

But here I am, another night with insomnia, palpitations, numb limbs, aching bones, throbbing face, eyes in pain, pressure in brain, kidney pain, needles in my legs, feels like my ankles are sprained and vertebrae cracking.

How do you keep going on pretending that it isn't happening. I don't expect special treatment, I just dream of the same help anyone else gets here with a disease, I don't want to explain, and people don't believe me. I would love to go to a health facility and they teach me about my disease instead of vice versa, I would love to have help, and so would THOUSANDS of others.

Please, if any of you have any ideas on how to get the government on the fast track, please feel free to share. I also share this with you. If I had a disease that was recognized, that people were educated about, and received help and healthcare, believe me, I would be acting very differently, but imagine you were really sick, after years of being ignored, you finally found your own answer, then you rolled up your sleeves and accepted it, got ready for help, and treatment, there was no help or treatment. Just waiting...and more waiting. For the government to keep their word. Unfortunately, I think I'll be waiting a very long time...

If any one actually reads this, thank you for listening.[181]

Cody's Lyme Story

When I read Cody Glive's story on Facebook, my heart broke. I asked him if he'd be willing to share it. I know that since posting his story, healing has been a terrible roller coaster for him, as it is for all Lyme sufferers. Here is what Cody had to say:

Hello my name is Cody, thank you for welcoming me to the group. I am currently 27 years old but feel 67.

I used to be into hiking and outdoor activities and had plenty of energy. No one in my family has ever been sick or had any significant genetic conditions, except my grandmother had seasonal affective disorder in the fall but had proper medication.

Sometime in 2011 or 2012 I was hiking in an Ontario Park about 20 minutes from home, called the Long Sault Parkway which is a chain of small islands along the St. Lawrence River. I was making my own trails in tall grass and trees, when I got back to the car I noticed some bugs (only later would I find out what they are) on my clothing. I had heard about ticks and thought that only one in a billion could cause an infection known as Lyme, and that if I caught it, I'd probably know, and get treatment.

I brushed off the bugs and went home. That night when I was getting ready for bed I saw one of the ticks on the wall next to my bathroom mirror. I looked over myself and couldn't find any more evidence.

About two days later, I was at work and could feel a small lump on my back pressing against the chair. I started rubbing and feeling what felt like a skin tag in the very center of my back. Eventually I got hold of it and pulled it off, what I placed on the counter was somewhat alarming, it was a tick and it was still wiggling a little bit.

I thought to myself: "No one can get sick from a bug bite in Canada. What are the odds?" I discarded the bug and continued about my life.

About 2 years later, at the beginning of the fall, I noticed a lack of energy, a lack of being able to focus and think, and pain in the upper right of my ribcage. It persisted overnight and eventually I thought I was having a heart attack and visited the hospital, they did standard blood work (not for Lyme, as this was two years after the bite, Lyme wasn't even on my mind anymore).

They could not find anything wrong with me and sent me home. I sat up all night with back pain, brain fog, forgetting who I was, double vision, joint pain, and a huge amount of fear. Every time I fell asleep I'd jolt awake immediately in a panic as if I'd stopped breathing. I noticed over time more and more cherry angiomas forming on my body, my hairline, arms, torso, legs. (upwards of 15 or so currently)

I went to see several doctors, all of which "couldn't find anything wrong" with me. Finally, my mother told me about my grandmother and her slight seasonal depression she had and concluded that must be it and I should get medication. I didn't believe this was accurate but I needed to get my life back.

I started an antidepressant and it made little to no difference. I had major episodes of depersonalization, chronic fatigue, brain fog, and feeling of impending doom, rage, extreme emotions. Sleep medication worked, at least I could regulate my sleep.

Over the next year, it was like I was rebuilding myself mentally, but losing myself physically. I improved my diet significantly, but still kept losing muscle definition, losing strength, aging quickly and always black under my eyes. I gained weight and my body processed food very differently. I noticed this, friends and family also noticed this. I kept telling myself it would get better, it has to go away.

My vision deteriorated, I couldn't wake up for work. My limbs were always heavy and tired. If I had to do any physical activity, I would pour sweat and become tired, see stars in my vision and feel like I was going to faint. I read about heatstroke and it seemed very similar.

I had to plan my daily activities and leave spots for rest, I always had to have cold water and Gatorade to stay hydrated and it still only took the edge off of things.

Finally, at a car show on Labor Day weekend 2015, I collapsed. I was taken to hospital and during the drive started to rethink everything that had happened to me over the last two years: the decline. I thought about the tick bite and decided to really look into Lyme symptoms. I found a very detailed symptom list and realized I suffered from pretty much all of them.

I asked doctors to do a blood test for Lyme and they refused, I spoke to a nurse who said I would have to push to get tested, so I pushed and the doctor began to insult me and my general malaise. I asked him why he was so obtuse towards testing and he finally gave in "to make me happy." I thought my concerns were over and that hopefully I'd have an answer. I was told it would take several weeks to get results.

In the meantime, I wanted to research the illness I was so sure I had. I spoke to victims, people who had it for years and decades. I learned about Heath Canada and the government denying chronic Lyme exists and how doctors won't diagnose it or treat it in Canada. Other Lyme victims easily predicted my negative result with the Canadian test. In short; I learned about flawed testing.

I learned about proper testing, and how I'd have to go out of pocket for it, and now that I was barely functioning on 16 hours a week at work, I would have to figure something out. I spoke to a lot of people who had to put up their homes and max out their credit cards to get answers, to hope to get better. I was glad there were answers out there for them but I also became furious over the fact that I had never used (or abused) the OHIP health care system, but now that it came time to use it, it was letting me down at an incredible rate.

I tried to explain to close family how the illness works, how Health Canada and doctors deny it exists. How the numbers of people who have it are probably incredibly inaccurate and how many people are walking around sick, who are hospitalized with pain, heart issues, brain issues, paralysis. My family looked at me as if I was crazy. "Don't let it consume you." They didn't believe the Healthcare system would push back and not test. They considered the whole thing crazy. A conspiracy theory.

But when I spoke to people who had Lyme, and I described my life to them, and they described their life to me, it was all the same. I had finally found people who understood why I couldn't get out of bed. Why I couldn't go on a trip or go far from home.

I'm glad I found these people, I'm glad I found you [Facebook group Lyme: OHOH Canada]. It's been an incredible relief to know you're not alone in this illness, to know people are going through the exact same issues that keep my lights on at night. I am a warrior for proper testing, diagnosis and treatment of this illness and if I ever get better, I'll never forget this time in my life and I'll always be an advocate for anyone else with the same disease.

I want us all to get better, together, through life.[182]

A Mother Speaks Out

I met with Lisa, a Toronto mother, to hear her story about Lyme. It sounded frightfully like ours, complete with doctor mishaps, helplessness, no one listening or helping, and having to take matters into our own hands.

I am the mother of a 26-year-old boy who contracted Lyme Disease, some time in April or May of 2014.

During his initial emergency room visit in Woodbridge, I asked the attending emergency room nurse if it could be Lyme Disease and she asked me where I got my medical license because "No it was not Lyme because we don't have Lyme here in Ontario."

Suffice to say, almost a year to the day and following 30 emergency room visits in 26 days, numerous specialists and various tests that I demanded did we find a diagnostic specialist that immediately predicted what he believed to be the problem which IS in fact Lyme Disease. This physician said he would need to send the bloodwork out to 3 labs. 2 in the US and by law, 1 in Ontario but he already knew what the results would be. He said that the US would test positive for Lyme and that the Ontario lab will come back negative because of some kind of point monitoring system that we use. I have only recently become acquainted with this monitoring number system and it actually is used in a large array of tests for many diseases.

My son is in the entertainment business. It was through my reading of a People magazine article on Avril Lavigne that I knew in fact that my son had Lyme. All the same symptoms. All the same protocol from her Canadian doctors. All the same terminology and steering towards Anxiety and Depression. That was the most insulting part I think. That they actually almost had my son believing that he was going out of his mind and making up all the things that were wrong with him. That is what infuriated me the most. That they just didn't want to help this kid. Ugh! Don't get me started or I could be rambling all day.

There is something critically wrong with our healthcare system. Unfortunately, I had to find out the hard way. I had no idea about this point system we have until we got caught up in it.

My son went from being a vibrant, outgoing, six-day-a-week golfer and traveler to reclusive of his bedroom for 3 months with me bringing up food on a tray. He was almost convinced he had "anxiety" by our physicians and put on anti-depressants, which he had to wean himself off to being given antibiotics and reclaiming his life. There is something very, very wrong with what is happening in the province and perhaps country. He has been doing quite well for the past six months and had a minor recurrence of symptoms during this past week. As you know, there is no cure and remissions give false hope but at least we are being educated more and more after connecting with other people which is why I am reaching out to you today.[183]

Canadian Lyme Heroes—Rebels with Great Cause

In 1997, Apple created an award-winning ad campaign called "Think Different." The creative text written by Rob Siltanen went like this:

Here's to the crazy ones. The misfits. The rebels. The troublemakers. The round pegs in the square holes. The ones who see things differently. They're not fond of rules. And they have no respect for the status quo. You can quote them, disagree with them, glorify or vilify them. About the only thing you can't do is ignore them. Because they change things. They push the human race forward. And while some may see them as the crazy ones, we see genius. Because the people who are crazy enough to think they can change the world, are the ones who do.

This copy was a huge hit. Why? Because we love the underdog, the hero, the so-called "crazy ones" who break the rules in the name of justice. We love this copy because we relate to it. We love it because it hits a nerve. We love it because we know, without question, that it's the so-called crazy ones, the ones who go against the grain, the ones who have the courage to stand up to the powers that be, that push for change, who we root for and admire.

Think of David and Goliath, Nelson Mandela, Erin Brockovich, Norma Rae. Everyone loves an underdog. We can relate to this unlikely quintessential hero who has to work hard for his or her heroism. Fight hard for his or her cause. We long to support this archetypal character in movies, plays, literature, fables—and in real life.

The underdog allows us to root for the seemingly less powerful one, revel in a success story, feel something deeply, have our hearts and our minds captured by someone worthy of our attention and admiration.

While so many doctors are reluctant, even terrified, to speak out about chronic Lyme disease, there are some true heroes in the Canadian Lyme story.

Dr. Ernie Murakami of Hope, British Columbia, is one of these Canadian heroes. A rebel with just cause.

This passionate and highly compassionate eighty-four-year-old former MD and chronic Lyme activist is a voice of reason in the Canadian Lyme War. Murakami has been dedicated to understanding and healing chronic Lyme disease for much of his career.

Dr. Murakami is beloved because he is one of those round pegs in a square hole. Unlike the majority of doctors in this country, he is determined to help Lyme sufferers and to make sacrifices to do so. We admire him because he "gets it," because he is generous with time and knowledge, and because he cares.

This man has a big heart.

Throughout his medical career, having a degree in bacteriology and immunology, he directly treated more than 3,000 people with chronic Lyme disease, and another 6,000 indirectly. In 2008, after years of being investigated, bullied, and harassed by the College of Physicians and Surgeons of British Columbia, he relinquished his medical license.

He suffered at the hands of the College and it affected his health and well-being. Upon the insistence of his wife—who was worried about his health—he eventually decided to give up his license and find other ways to keep serving the Lyme community. But not without a good college try.

Today he stays in the Lyme world by teaching naturopaths in British Columbia how to treat chronic Lyme, by providing free information to medical doctors, and by focusing on his breakthrough research on cannabidiol (CBD)—a derivative of the hemp plant, which is an effective treatment for symptomatic control for Lyme and other chronic illnesses. He also makes himself accessible to support and direct Lyme sufferers by phone or by text when approached.

I had the pleasure of speaking with Dr. Murakami. Here's what he had to say:

The medical profession has been misdiagnosing Lyme disease for decades. In Canada, we have the highest M.S. cases in the world according to the MS International Society and we have the lowest Borrelia Burgdorferi cases in the world according to WHO (World Health Organization).

Germany has reported nearly one million cases of Lyme disease in one year recently as evidenced by the cases of Chronic Erythematous Migrans rash clinical diagnosis and laboratory tests. The temperature and environment is the same in Canada as in Germany but we barely come close to the reported number of cases. Canada reports that it has the lowest numbers of Lyme disease in the world by WHO and the highest number of Multiple Sclerosis cases in the world 240-340/100,000 population. No other country comes close to this figure. Germany's land size is 349,2233 square kilometers and Canada has 9,982,679 square kilometers or twenty eight times the land size and the rapid warming effect of the world is identical up to the Arctic circle in Canada and the European continent. It is long overdue that we demand an explanation and in my personal feeling a very obvious MISDIAGNOSIS by our medical profession.

The test results and interpretations of them that patients get from infectious disease doctors are seriously wrong because these doctors are uninformed, misinformed and closed-minded about chronic Lyme. In medical school, we are not taught about the Lyme spirochete and the survival forms which require specific prolonged therapy. Instead, the IDSA teaches members that thirty days is all that is needed to cure this disease at any stage.

The ELISA and Western Blot antibody tests are the same around the world. Our results in Canada indicate that there are very low numbers testing positive in Canada. This is not true.

And without question, the long-term use of antibiotics to treat chronic Lyme has more benefits than risks. I've seen what this disease can do to people when it's not treated long term. It can disable people for life.

Because there is not one doctor in Canada who can or will treat Lyme sufferers with antibiotics for more than the 28-day IDSA sanctioned protocol, we are being forced to tap into 'out of country' for Lyme treatment— primarily in the US. We are forcing patients to spend upwards of $50,000 for treatment.

Canadian doctors, like myself, who are vocal about treating chronic Lyme have been shut down. It's never stated directly. But they will harass you and bully you until you've had enough. They make you seem incompetent. That's what happened to me.

Murakami says doctors regularly phone him for advice about how to treat patients but don't want anyone to know that they're consulting with him for fear they will be investigated by their Colleges or peers. He continues,

My colleagues are all afraid that what happened to me will happen to them.

The only colleague of mine who stood by my side was Dr. Pat McGeer, Neurological Disease Researcher at UBC and because of his support, he no longer has a license. We have both suffered the same fate because we chose to help Lyme patients.

In my case, the College made me seem incompetent. I couldn't keep attending their mandated professional development lectures. In my career, I've gotten lots of letters of support and commendations. Yet they hired two doctors and sent them to my office—after 40 years of practice—to oversee my work. I ended up with hypertension, ulcers, mild strokes, bleeding bowels. My wife begged me to quit so I resigned, gave up my license.

I was condemned for making people better.

The medical world is petrified to diagnose or treat this disease because they will be investigated. It's tragic.

When it comes to chronic Lyme, there is pathological denial. I don't understand the resistance but I was a victim of it like all of the sufferers out there.

Murakami's passion is his research into the use of cannabidiol for the treatment of Lyme disease, as well as cancer, epilepsy, and other chronic illnesses. Says Murakami,

In the past 20 years, since my first case of this disease when the patients were telling me that when all the standard medications were not helping the severe symptoms of pain, arthritis, fatigue, depression (with suicidal ideation), mental fog with multi-organ failure, they resorted to smoking marijuana.

I was deathly against the use of pot and smoking but I was becoming more interested in the benefits mentally and physically and I directed them to use the cannabidiol

oil or paste since there were no psychoactive effects. Nabilone, a synthetic extract from marijuana, was used for my MS patients as a legal medication with a DIN number in 1985.

When Murakami learned that he, himself, had an asymptomatic brain tumor—discovered after hitting his head on a beam while playing hockey with his grandson—it led him to investigate the treatment of a brain malignancy.

It was then that he came across the use of cannabidiol in dissolving a glioma tumor. Says Murakami,

I thought this was an impossibility until I saw the MRI reports showing the absolute gradual resolution of the tumor in four months. Other anecdotal cases of cannabidiol treating chronic infections resistant to standard antibiotics convinced me that there was an antibiotic effect with cannabidiol. Patients who had used CBD for up to three years and were unable to continue due to the cost found their symptoms of Lyme disease did not return. CBD appears to also be effective treating other co-infections as well. This made me suspect a potential antibiotic effect on Lyme disease and co-infections.

Initial research with my colleague, Dr. Eva Sapi, has provided us with the positive evidence-based study we needed to continue with further testing on biofilm and eggs. The second-stage study is being conducted at a New Haven University and I am very grateful to all the donors who have made this possible through the Murakami Centre for Lyme, which is a charitable organization.

Dr. Murakami says there is good reason to feel that CBD and other compounds can have positive effects on the eradication of Lyme. "I can state with confidence that there was an increased spirochete, egg, and biofilm-killing effect with the increased concentrations of the cannabidiol in the test tube."

Cannabidiol can help reduce pain, spasms, headaches, brain fog, nausea, seizures, and all crippling symptoms most Lyme sufferers deal with. Many people will take opiate pain medication to deal with their pain, which can be ineffective, addictive, and can even end in overdose.

Initial treatment with antibiotics for Lyme disease can damage your gastrointestinal (GI) system as well as kill all the healthy bacteria in your system, leaving your body open to fungal and bacterial infections. Painkillers can also damage the lining of your GI tract.

Dr. Murakami's preliminary research suggests that hemp cannabidiol—which can be legally purchased at many of the same outlets as cannabis products—has multiple healing effects.

Par for the course, roughly fifty cannabis dispensaries in Vancouver, and about twelve cannabis producers on Vancouver Island, were notified of possible impending closures. Justin Trudeau, our Canadian prime minister, has promised decriminalization of these products. Dr. Murakami and thousands of Canadians hope that this law will be soon be enacted to relieve the suffering and anguish of so many. Anyone who doubts the medicinal benefits of THC, CBD, or CBD/THC should read the reports by Dr. Sanjay Gupta, MD, (neurosurgeon FRCP) Weed I, Weed II, Weed III.[184]

In addition to Dr. Murakami, other Canadian doctors have been harassed out of practice for treating Lyme patients. Dr. Ben Boucher of Port Hawkesbury, Nova Scotia, was apparently the only Lyme-literate doctor in all of Nova Scotia, and thanks to the powers that be, he is no longer in practice.

As posted on the CanLyme site,

> *Dr. Ben Boucher, in my opinion, is the most knowledge-able doctor in Canada in the field of Lyme and tick born diseases. He has empathy for his patients. [He's] what every doctor should strive to be like. But instead, some of these arrogant sociopaths who know nothing about Lyme, have driven him out of the business. What can we do now to get treatment?[185]*

Dr. Maureen McShane, LLMD, is *the* US Lyme doctor to most Canadians.

Her practice is "unusual" because she is a Canadian who resides in Montreal and travels to Plattsburgh, New York, each week to treat Lyme patients.

As she is not entitled to practice Lyme treatment in Canada, she crosses the border every Sunday to work in the US, where she is licensed, and crosses back to Montreal on Fridays to be with her family. Up to 80 percent of her practice is Canadian.

Having had chronic Lyme disease herself, she is passionate about helping others. Everyone I know who makes the trek to consult with her feels very supported and cared for.

"By the time they come to me, they're about one hundred percent sure they've got it, and when I listen to their stories, I know they have it," says McShane, who bases her patients' diagnoses primarily on clinical symptoms. She says many of her patients have visited dozens of doctors before seeking her out.[186]

While I have not had the chance to meet her myself, I feel indebted to her and the work she does to support, care for, and validate Canadian Lyme sufferers. She has saved the lives of many.

One of her patients told me she is incredibly open-minded; she will guide you where she has knowledge, and support you where she doesn't. She's extremely busy and not easy to get in to see, but once you're a patient of hers, I am told she always responds to emails with thoughtful ideas and direction.

Imagine how the thousands of sufferers in Lymeland Canada would fare if we could have many more LLMDs just like her proximally located to the people struggling. It would save so much heartache, time, money, and suffering.

Yet the Canadian government and medical powers don't seem all that interested in offering what works. They're far too busy defending something we don't quite understand rather than taking care of us.

A Canadian Anomaly

One morning, I had a pleasant surprise on Facebook.

I was responding to a post on LYME: OHOH CANADA (a closed group with 1,265 members) regarding the number of Lyme cases in Canada. I shared my understanding that our numbers are 10 percent of the US, or approximately 30,000 a year. And, more maddening, I noted there is not one doctor across the country who will recognize or treat this disease beyond the twenty-eight-day guidelines.

Lo and behold, a man named Ralph George Hawkins commented:

"You can't say not one doctor in this country will accept or treat Lyme."

Hmmmmmm. Who is this guy? I wondered. *An Internet troll? A government representative?* My curiosity was piqued.

Here's how our online conversation went:

Me: Name one that will or can please—without being annihilated by the College. I'd love to know. Beyond the 28-day guidelines, that is.

Hawkins: Me.

Hawkins: The guidelines are self-described as voluntary, and not intended to supersede the clinical judgment of the treating physician in any individual situation.

Me: You are an anomaly in Canada. Others who have attempted to treat beyond the 28-day guidelines have had their lives and livelihoods destroyed by the College.

Hawkins: Yes, that is true. I am proceeding in this regard within an academic clinic environment with institutional awareness and support. It is an innovation project. And, yes, I am anomalous. There are a few more MDs with intact reputations and licenses who provide prolonged antibiotic regimens. So you can't claim there are none. Your point that the status quo in Canada remains shameful is valid.

Me: Dr. Hawkins, can I please interview you for a more fully accurate story? I'd love to include your work with Lyme patients in my book.

Hawkins: Let me consider for a bit. I'm rather a recluse.

Dr. Hawkins emailed me and agreed to an interview. While trying to set something up, I looked at his ratings which seem to be very high. He does, in fact, practice medicine in Alberta, Canada, and his patients rave about his care. Nice to know! One doctor in Canada in our camp. Perhaps I stand corrected. Perhaps there are a few doctors here and there who stand by their Hippocratic oath and are willing and able somehow to do the right thing, regardless of the

College's strong-arming antics.

Another person commented on our thread:

There is the occasional doctor that follows the Hippocratic Oath and treats people, usually under the supervision of another doc, but there are very few of them and they're extremely hard to find. We would all like to think that clinical judgment would be used but many turn their heads when they hear the word Lyme. I have hope that with proper education, things will change.

Me on the same post, another day: Dr. Hawkins— your online reviews are outstanding. It's very heartening to know there is a doctor in Canada who can and will treat Lyme patients with understanding and skill. One who is still in practice and not shut down by the College. I'd love to have a conversation with you at your earliest convenience.

I reached out again. Hawkins went silent on me. I imagine he was self-protecting. I certainly can't blame him for doing so.

I tried one more time with this message,

Ralph—I keep reading your posts on Facebook and I really appreciate how empathic you are with Lyme sufferers. Who are you in the medical community, where do you practice, how is it that you are such an anomaly, do your colleagues know that you support those with chronic Lyme or are you helping people on the QT? I am very curious for obvious reasons. I would love to hear from you so that I can offer some hope to Canadians in my book Lyme Madness. *Thank you.*

He agreed to call me at the office that very morning. And what an amazing conversation it was.

Ralph George Hawkins is an MD, with a subspecialty in nephrology. He lives and works in Calgary. He is a gentleman and a scholar and an advocate of those suffering. He's truly one in a million.

Hawkins shared many insights and affirmed my understanding of how Lyme is being medically ignored in Canada and the US.

Saskatchewan born and bred, in the Tommy Douglas era of socialized medicine, Hawkins was raised with "a blue-collar mentality and a socialist political bent," he shared.

Getting down to brass tacks about this Lyme Madness, he explains:

Common beliefs are sometimes based on bad premises. It's simple. When roadblocks present themselves, you just need to revisit the premise.

When the common belief is that Lyme is an easy to eradicate, short-lived infection, and you see so much evidence to the contrary, then you know the premise is wrong. I take much of my inspiration and guidance from literature. Here I look to Hans Christian Anderson's "The Emperor's New Clothes" [a classic story of vanity, ego, and pride]. There are all sorts of parallels and insights with Lyme Disease. People are afraid to oppose the emperor for fear that they will look uneducated and foolish.

"And who is the emperor in this case?" I ask.

"The IDSA," of course, Hawkins answers firmly. "Led by a renowned rheumatologist, and co-author of the original report to the CDC describing Lyme as an arthritic condition back in the 1970s.

"What is he to do now other than to say 'Oooops, this is really a multisystem disease, not a narrowly defined arthritic one,'" says Hawkins with a heavily sardonic tone in his voice. "How can this rheumatologist—at the end of his long and distinguished career—admit to an error this large? It's too hard for the emperor to wear no clothes and look foolish. So you see, it isn't always money driving the false premise."

"And what about the CDC?" I ask.

The CDC is an American federal governmental body reporting ultimately through the Office of the Secretary of Health and Human Services, whose primary objectives include controlling costs. A cynic would say they don't want a chronic disease defined as an epidemic. That's a costly problem. And what's to stop them from defining the disease in such a narrow fashion that it becomes virtually impossible to diagnose, and then there's no need for a big budget.

It's easy. You define Lyme as so uncommon as to be almost nonexistent, and you don't have to support spending to deal with it. Government ethics are strictly utilitarian—sacrificing the (sick) few for the sake of the (healthy) many.

Hawkins has been treating Lyme patients since 2010, when his index patient [initial patient in the population of an epidemiological investigation, or more generally, the first case of a condition or syndrome] came into his office with all the hallmarks. Since then, he has been frustrated by the system, too.

Hawkins is a member of the clinical faculty of the University of Calgary, a site lead at a local hospital; he runs an outpatient practice and sees patients by referral. He said that it's common knowledge in his community that he is willing to see patients with chronic fatigue and symptoms of unexplained origin.

"There are two things I am NOT. I am not afraid. And I am not spoiling for a fight," he explained.

Hawkins also made it clear that he will NOT be bullied and he will NOT follow the herd. "How did that work for the Nazis? 'I just did what I was told,'" he retorts. "That won't work for me on Judgment Day. I just want to see people treated properly—humanely. I have a strong sense of social justice that is not being addressed here. Humanity is about caring for the individual that you've never met and are never going to meet. Doctors are supposed to be in the caring profession. Where is the care in our caring?"

Since speaking with Hawkins, I have since heard of a few other doctors in Canada who do treat Lyme. They are not easy to find. And they are cautious about using the term *chronic Lyme*. Lyme sufferers are protecting their doctors, careful not to give too much away, careful not to "out" them on Facebook. The common theme is that even when Canadian doctors are brave enough to treat chronic Lyme, they do so "in the closet." They are careful to say that they are treating the person, not Lyme, and they urge their patients to continue to see their US LLMDs because they are limited in what they are able to offer.

Perhaps there is a slight shift afoot. But it's not nearly enough for the people who are suffering without care.

A Breakthrough in Canadian Politics

As of October 2015, Canada has a new prime minister. One of the first policies that Prime Minister Justin Trudeau put in place was to take the muzzle off of scientists who, for the past decade—under Stephen Harper's government—have been forbidden to speak with the press without careful and strategic vetting by the higher-ups.

Scientists can now speak freely. Perhaps Trudeau understands how broken and corrupt science can be when important information is kept under wraps.

Mark Hume of *The Globe and Mail*, Canada's national newspaper, said,

> *It used to be that if you wanted to talk to a federal scientist ... you just called them up.*

> *And then Stephen Harper became Prime Minister and a dark curtain fell across Canadian science.*

> *Denied access to experts, reporters turned to those less informed or got what they could from published research papers, which are often so dense with data that they are difficult to unpack.*

> *That's why reporters want to talk to them, not to pry loose government secrets or embarrass Ottawa. Mr. Harper's government never understood that. The Conservatives wanted tight control on the message and didn't trust their own experts to be experts.*

> *That's all changed now. Mr. Trudeau has unmuzzled the scientists.*[187]

A Possible Breakthrough in the Medical System

In an open letter from Canadian physicians to Prime Minister Justin Trudeau, dated November 30, 2015, the authors state, "According to the World Health Organization, Climate change is the greatest threat to global health in the 21st Century."[188]

Among other ill effects caused by climate change, they mention that this threat includes "people affected by the emergence and spread of infectious diseases like Lyme disease, as climate change shifts the probability curve of a variety of illnesses, making them more common, and more severe."

Doctors recognizing the threat of Lyme disease—and, better still, taking action. Well, this is a first. Will wonders never cease?

The Lyme Conference Finally Takes Place

In April 2016, the announcement for the first-ever Canadian Lyme conference from Jim Wilson of CanLyme arrived in my inbox:

After many discussions and delays, the conference that is required under federal Bill C-442 will take place May 16th and 17th in Ottawa. We would like to have a public forum evening, preferably on Sunday May 15th, but the details will be decided by the planning committee for the conference. The conference is open to the public and medical professionals, and will be live-streamed online.

As most of you know, I am a co-chair for structuring the conference along with Dr. Gregory Taylor, Chief Public Health Officer, Public Health Agency of Canada, and Dr. Daniel Gregson, president of the Association of Medical

Microbiology and Infectious Disease Canada (AMMI).

This four years after the bill was introduced, and almost eighteen months after the bill was passed in the Senate.

And let's please remember that cochair Dr. Gregory Taylor, Chief Public Health Officer, said just a few years ago that it is *concerning* to see that the incidence of Lyme disease has risen from 128 cases in 2009 to 315 in 2012.

Concerning? Is that all you've got? Please, sir, check your numbers. Canada is far more likely numbering in the thousands, perhaps even tens of thousands, of chronic Lyme disease cases. Please, sir, have you not heard about the mass exodus of Canadians to the US—in a desperate effort to get extended antibiotic treatment?

Following the conference, Taylor thankfully told CBC, our national news station, "We think the numbers are much higher and it's alarming that the numbers are increasing continuously."

Taylor also said that he "expects the true number of cases is much higher since mild cases may clear on their own, or may never be reported to public health authorities, even though it's been nationally notifiable since 2009."[189]

Nationally notifiable? What on earth does that mean? Who are Canadians supposed to notify when there has been absolutely no one listening, forcing us to get a bill passed through the Senate and hold a national conference? As far as cases that clear on their own—just more of the same dogma and denial. There are no mild cases of Lyme. Yes, some cases are far more extreme and far more debilitating than others. But mild, I don't think so. This language has to change.

On a positive note, there were three significant bright lights at the conference—all of whom worked tirelessly to effect change and support the sufferers and all to whom we are grateful. Green Party leader Elizabeth May, responsible for getting Bill C-442 passed in the Senate, is continuing to lead the political charge. Jim Wilson, president of CanLyme, has worked fiercely on our behalf to create this conference and who for years has sat side by side with the many stakeholders to effect positive change. And Dr. Ralph George Hawkins, MD, clinical associate professor of medicine, University of Calgary, thoughtfully treats and supports the sufferers, and is a true anomaly within the medical community of this country.

Another beacon of hope at the conference came in the form of Lyme sufferers sharing their own personal stories—more than one hundred stories, representing decades of suffering, each carefully summarized in five minutes, no more, and heart-wrenchingly presented in person and via the web by the sufferers themselves, and in some cases their loved ones, out loud, for the world to hear. Fierce, riveting, real. Filled with courage, sadness, and outrage at a system that, for decades now, has denied each and every one of them proper medical support, forcing them to travel to the US for treatment and pay out of pocket at exorbitant costs, which many just cannot afford.

In stark contrast to the promise of so many voices finally heard and the potential for a glimmer of change was the obvious overhang of heavy, palpable darkness. Darkness in the form of information overload and emotional and physical suffering that felt simply overwhelming, difficult to sort through, with few solid answers. Darkness in the fact that we clearly have mountains to move in order to improve this unconscionable situation. Darkness in the form of subtle and not so subtle Lyme denial spouted by some of the IDSA and AMMI panelists, allowing us to hear it with our very own ears. Clear negation of the very nature and scope of this disease perpetuated for decades by those responsible for the slow and often nonexistent forward movement of medical testing, research, and treatment of a disease affecting millions worldwide.

There is no question that the conference was a watershed moment.

However, we need meaningful action—and we need it now. And so far, there is no noticeable or tangible progress seen or felt.

If a conference is the best that our politicians can do with so many people suffering and forced to cross the border for treatment at an outrageous financial, physical, and emotional cost to them, then all I can say once again is, "Oh, Canada—shame on you."

Prime Minister Trudeau—*I hope you're listening.*

9. LYME UPRISING

I'm late! … I'm late! For a very important date!
No time to say "Hello," goodbye! I'm late!

—THE WHITE RABBIT, *ALICE'S ADVENTURES IN WONDERLAND*

The Lyme movement is alive and well and fighting for the lives—and the quality of life—of millions worldwide. It is both an underground and aboveground lobbying group—looking to be seen, heard, and understood by the medical establishment, the politicians, and the insurers.

Advocacy work is never for the faint of heart. Look at how many have been fighting for so many years—from Polly Murray and Karen Forschner, to Kathleen Dickson and Beaux Reliosis, and so many others who continue to fight the good fight today.

We will NOT give up. We in Lymeland are determined to get our voices heard and effect change.

The Unequivocal Power of Facebook

Until recently, I didn't have much use for Facebook.

Then, suddenly, when I was faced with trying to understand this complex and overwhelming medical problem, Facebook became my savior. Because Facebook, in fact, is where Lyme sufferers congregate.

Slowly but surely, I connected with one Lyme Disease Facebook group at a time. One Lyme group member at a time.

I began listening—perhaps on the sidelines at first, and then with full participation. I scoped it all out. I read, observed, witnessed, queried, clarified, posted, shared, and bonded.

Before I knew it, I was a member of a growing number of Lyme Facebook groups, which have connected me to some of the most intelligent, passionate, kind, generous, and helpful human beings on this planet. And for that I am eternally grateful.

Not only have I met the most remarkable and courageous people online, but my membership in these groups has led me to new insights and ideas, new treatment protocols for my son, potential healers, fellow sufferers, caregivers, and loved ones alike.

Facebook has provided me with a growing Lyme community—new "friends" who have made this journey real, validating, less lonely, and slightly less terrifying. And many of whom have brought humor, wit, intelligence, reason, compassion, companionship, and understanding when it seemed impossible to find. I hope that *Lyme Madness* will do the same for them.

While chronic Lyme disease is being neglected and grossly undertreated by the medical community, we—the members of the chronic Lyme community—are not taking this lying down.

There is an online revolution happening. And it's happening on Facebook.

We are getting organized, we are getting informed, and becoming lay scientists, lay doctors, lay researchers, lay politicians. Why? Because we have no choice. Because we are not getting the attention and support that is needed. Because it's human nature to survive and to thrive and to fight when threatened.

We're fighting. We are fighting the establishment by supporting one another. Offering our knowledge and experiences and preferential treatments. We are sharing LLMDs' names—secretly—by private message because this information has to be kept hushed to protect our only supporters.

We are standing up to authority or government in this civil revolution. Facebook is a critical community for Lyme sufferers.

I don't think I could have written this book without the experiences I've had and people I've met down the rabbit hole of Lyme Facebook groups.

American author Herman Melville of *Moby Dick* fame said, "We cannot live only for ourselves. A thousand fibers connect us with our fellow men." This is the lesson this journey has taught me. We cannot do everything alone. We are meant to connect, to lean on one another. To share.

There are so many well-expressed ideas and opinions in these groups. I want the world to know that while we've been abandoned by the vast majority of the allopathic medical community, we are surviving through our own intelligence, strength, resilience—and by leaning on one another on social media.

Lyme is the tipping point for a sea change in medicine. There is a revolution happening. We are all part of it and we need our voices heard.

Michelle Thompson wanted to share her voice of gratitude, directed primarily toward her Facebook "friends" as well as her LLMD:

I have received endless help from this group and I wanted to update you all on my daughter. Sorry it's so long.

For some background, she got very ill in May. She had the gamut of Lyme symptoms, but I had no knowledge of the disease at all. I thought there was no way Lyme could make someone so sick. I was horribly mistaken. She ended up with a non-CDC positive Lyme test in August. Her ELISA test was positive and her blot showed 3 antibodies. I started learning, and our lives have been forever changed. Please let me say here, that if not for the care and support of all of you and a local Lymie from this group, I don't think we would have been able to do this. It has been life changing, truly.

Shortly after her test came back I was told I was crazy by infectious disease, and we had the door slammed in our face. Her pediatrician decided to treat with 28 days of Doxy after I had a breakdown in her office over my girl's failing health. During all of this I had an appointment scheduled for her with an LLMD in December.

Last Monday her Doxy cycle ended, and it happened to be a day her symptoms went into a tailspin. I brought my worries here and was told to call the LLMD, which I did. They got her in on Thursday.

That appointment was the breath of fresh air we had all been gasping for. She believed us, she cared about Riley, she was professional and understanding. She is aggressive and wants my baby well! It was everything we had been praying for!

She started treatment that day. We had a really rough weekend with some severe herxing, but yesterday my little girl came home from school happy and silly, she had no pain, she wasn't foggy, she got her assignments done in class and she had ENERGY! It was a miracle, truly. She is doing amazing, and she wouldn't be here without this group. Thank you!

Since my daughter's diagnosis, I have been concerned she got it congenitally. I have been ill for as long as I can remember, but I've never had an answer. My issues started in my kidneys and have just taken over my whole body. While we were in my daughter's appointment her doctor told me she thinks that the severity of Riley's case points to a congenital exposure, and she wants me to be tested.

So, it looks like I may be on this journey too, but I know that it will be ok with the support here. The thought of feeling human again one day is extremely exciting though, I have to admit. I see the LLMD in March.

Again, thank you all. You haven't seen the last of me here, as I plan to pay all you have done for my family forward. You ROCK!![190]

As a strong counterpoint to my trust and reliance on Facebook "friends," activist and Lyme blogger extraordinaire Beaux Reliosis claims:

The Internet is a terrible, scary place, full of truths, partial truths, misinformation, and flat-out lies—all indistinguishable from each other on their face. And speaking of face—we've got good old Facebook mucking it up, 24 hours a day, 8 days a week. I'd bet money that 99% of what you see on Facebook is false. What's a poor Lymie to do? How does one know where to get credible information about a disease that is the subject of the biggest medical fraud in the history of the world?

In the land of Facebook, many turn to "groups." There are groups that discuss treatment, groups for emotional support, groups for cousins of dogs whose hamster met a guy who got Lyme from a magical dragonfly. Frankly, these groups probably do more harm than good.

Granted, I probably wouldn't be where I am today, blogging about the science and the Cryme, if I hadn't crossed paths with certain people in certain groups. But I also had my share of run-ins with group administrators who were bent on protecting members emotionally. Yep, share a *real* fact (distinguishable by its proportional relationship to level of scariness), and get scolded, or worse—booted, for the egregious crime of intent to cause knowledge.[191]

I agree with Beaux, in part. We do have to be highly discerning about who we believe, what we read, with whom we share, with whom we connect, how to distinguish fact from fiction.

I learned this lesson the hard way when I inadvertently stepped on a land mine or two. It was then that I discovered that there truly is no bottom to this rabbit hole I've entered. I've come to see that Lymeland can be even darker, more terrifying, and more threatening than I ever understood, especially when those who are supposed to be one your side attack you for no apparent reason. When you live in Lymeland, you can easily get caught in the cross fire now and then.

Despite some head-shaking experiences of my own, Facebook Lyme groups and their thousands of members still remain a great resource.

I recently posted an image on my Lyme Madness Facebook page, which read: *Lyme gets "treated" more humanely on Facebook than in most doctors' offices.*

As of today, this post has reached more than 19,000 people with 180 shares. This message hit a sweet spot. This truth resonated far and wide.

Then I posted this: *Lyme sufferers are victimized in at least FIVE different ways: 1) by the disease itself 2) by doctors who turn their backs 3) by loved ones who roll their eyes and walk away 4) by insurers who refuse to provide coverage 5) by the CDC and IDSA who together say that chronic Lyme disease does not exist.* This post reached over 105,000 people with more than 1,000 shares.

The reach of these posts prompted me to message Jordan Banks, the managing director of Facebook Canada, as well as Sheryl Sandberg—the COO of Facebook and the author of *Lean In*. I wanted them to know this is an important story, a travesty affecting the lives of millions—one that lives and breathes on Facebook. I was hoping this "human interest" story, deeply affecting the lives of so many, would draw their attention. After all, it's attracting the attention of people who can make a difference, people who have some power and clout that we are so desperately needing.

I wanted them both to know that without Facebook, I

would not have been able to help my son get to where he is today. Without Facebook, I don't know that I would have been able to make sense of this madness. Without Facebook, I would not have had the resources, the wealth of information, and the personal encounters with so many brave and brilliant people who are making a difference, including the likes of Kathleen Dickson, Beaux Reliosis, Jerry Seidel, John Coughlin, Darrell A., Alison Childs, Donna Y. Jacobs, Kris Newby, The Better Health Guy, Jenna Luche-Thayer, Carl Tuttle, Bruce Alan Fries, Tick Chick, Dr. Ernie Murakami, Dr. Elena Monarch, Dr. Ralph George Hawkins, Dr. Kenneth B. Liegner, Dr. Robert Bransfield, Elizabeth May, Jim Wilson, Wendy Woodhall, Paula Jackson Jones, Mackay Rippey of Lyme Ninja Radio, Sarah and Aaron Sanchez of Lyme Voice Podcast, Robert Herriman of Outbreak News, and Tina J. Garcia—founder of Lyme Education Awareness Program (L.E.A.P) in Arizona.

Speaking of Garcia, she is a Lyme warrior, an activist extraordinaire, and a Lyme sufferer who I also "met" on Facebook. I would be remiss not to mention her advocacy work.

Garcia has been fighting the powers that be for years. Her greatest "weapon" in this war is her crystal-clear understanding of the falsehoods, unethical actions, and overall madness that ensues in the world of Lyme.

I urge you to read Garcia's letter entitled "Lyme Patients Angered Over New Vaccine," which you can find online. Her argument is sound, clear, and convincing, and it beautifully sums up all of the suffering and madness—ultimately emboldening each and every one of us in this crazy, topsy-turvy world of Lyme.

In her impassioned letter, Garcia says,

The horrible truth is the secret that is being kept from the public, a secret that the worldwide Lyme community already knows because we're living it—that Lyme disease is a very serious and complex infection, and a lot of money is being made through the manipulation of this disease through research funds, patents for test kits and vaccine development, resulting in the medical neglect of thousands, if not millions, of suffering people.

Chronic Lyme disease is a debilitating and torturous infection. Patients are bedridden, using walkers and wheelchairs, suffering relentless excruciating pain and inhumane denial of medical care. This is a shameful travesty that should shock our collective conscience and spur compassionate change.[192]

Mothers Fight Back

When it comes to Lyme activism, there is nothing like a mother—an outraged, brokenhearted, fearless mother who will do anything and everything to protect her child from this hideous, ravaging disease and from the medical community who has thrown her and her child under the bus. I've met so many powerful, fierce, intelligent, and resilient mothers who are now leading the charge in the decades-long battle of this disease.

As I was wrapping up this book and about to go to publication, I received a powerful and meaningful message from Dr. Kenneth B. Liegner, MD, of New York, who said, "Without the dedication of mothers, we would be absolutely nowhere with Lyme disease. It is MOTHERS, concerned about their families, their children, that has sparked ALL progress in this field!!!"

So here's to all the mothers who have made and will continue to make a difference. From Polly Murray, Karen Forschner, and Kathleen Dickson to Wendy Woodhall, Beaux Reliosis, Sue Burke Faber and so many others fighting for their kids, we collectively thank you, Dr. Liegner. Your words are a gift; your support and understanding so rare. And you are so right, Dr. Liegner. We are a force, we are a light in this darkness, and we will *not* give up the battle. Not until we see substantial change and solutions coming from government and medical communities worldwide.

Celebrity Lyme-Light

Chronic Lyme disease began to garner more attention when the likes of singer Avril Lavigne, model and actress Yolanda (Foster) Hadid, UK multibillionaire John Caudwell, and more recently Ally Hilfiger made the media aware of their own personal Lyme battles. The Lyme community is very grateful for their willingness to share their stories as they lend more credibility to the rest of us in Lymeland who feel stuck, unheard, and invalidated.

The most current celebrity Lyme story is that of Kris Kristofferson who, according to an article in *Rolling Stone* magazine, was suffering from debilitating memory issues, which doctors diagnosed as Alzheimer's or some other form of dementia. It turns out he has recently been tested for Lyme and, lo and behold, the test was positive. "He was taking all these medications for things he doesn't have, and they all have side effects," [his wife Lisa] says. "After he gave up his Alzheimer's and depression pills and went through three weeks of Lyme-disease treatment, Lisa was shocked. "All of a sudden he was back," she says. There are still bad days, but "some days he's perfectly normal and it's easy to forget that he is even battling anything."[193]

John Caudwell, with his massive fortune as the founder of the UK company Phones 4u—and a family that he recently discovered is ailing from chronic Lyme—has done a stellar job in pushing the political agenda forward and communicating with the Lyme community, all while focusing on getting his family back to a state of improved health. He is a *father* on a mission.

On September 27, 2015, in the British *Sunday Times*, the billionaire and founder of Phones 4u held back tears as he shared with the world how "his wealth could not protect him or his family from the ravages of [chronic Lyme disease], but he will not surrender."[194]

Caudwell, sixty-two, disclosed that several members of his family were exposed to and suffering from Lyme disease, including himself, his ex-wife, and three of his children. His son Rufus, twenty, has been the most affected. Rufus has reportedly been ill for ten years, bedridden and homebound for more than a decade. Until now, doctors and family believed that Rufus suffered from mental illness—a severe anxiety disorder, agoraphobia, health anxiety, and bouts of psychosis. Now they know that the root cause of the illness that has taken half of his life from him is chronic Lyme.

Caudwell is determined to make a difference. He is determined to restore his family's health—and to get the British government to listen and take action. I imagine he knows that money talks. And he has plenty of it. His business acumen and success over forty years must carry plenty of weight. So he is in negotiations, meetings, and ongoing discussions with government and medical officials to try to understand why this disease is so underdiagnosed and undertreated—in Britain and worldwide.

His questions are our questions. His confusion is our confusion. His outrage is our outrage. Facebook fans—and he has thousands—are depending on him to make a difference. He has the power that we don't. He has the voice that might be heard. We are hopeful he will be the catalyst we need to make traction.

We could use an almighty savior right about now. We are desperately in need of an agile and oh-so-accurate David to right the wrongs of the corrupt, slow, and half-blind Goliath—with a single slingshot between the eyes. Someone to right the wrongs of the greedy and betraying Judas.

Next to Caudwell, no public figure has had more media coverage of her struggle with chronic Lyme disease than Yolanda (Foster) Hadid, fifty-one, star of *The Real Housewives of Beverly Hills* and soon-to-be ex-wife of Canadian composer David Foster. She has been one of the highest-profile advocates and celebrity voices of this pandemic to date. (She has recently changed her surname to Hadid—the name of her first ex-husband and the father of her three children.)

There have been countless social media reports of Yolanda traveling far and wide for treatment.

In a highly charged, emotional speech at the Global Lyme Alliance Gala in New York City, Yolanda spoke about her suffering over the past four years. "I honestly don't have the proper words in my vocabulary to describe to you the darkness, the pain, and the unknown hell I've lived these past years," she said. "I actually did not live. I just existed in a jail of my own paralyzed brain. This disease has brought me to my knees. Many nights I wish to die. I pray that I will just wash away into heaven, where there will be no pain."

Yolanda has recently revealed that her children Bella and

Anwar Hadid have also been diagnosed with Lyme disease. She has also recently announced that she and her husband of four years, David Foster, are officially separating.[195]

I have never watched Yolanda's show, but my Facebook page blew up when her costar apparently accused her of faking her disease and declared that Yolanda is suffering from Munchausen's—a mental disorder in which a person pretends to be sick.[196]

I beg of her castmates to please get informed. I respectfully ask Bravo TV to stop using this show as a platform to misinform and do further harm. There is already enough misinformation, denial, and mockery about Lyme disease. The last thing the Lyme community needs is for you to perpetuate the long list of existing falsehoods. Would you ridicule an AIDS patient or a cancer victim?

Dr. Oz had Yolanda on his show to talk about her Lyme journey. She represented herself and Lyme well, candidly sharing with television viewers that she has been to eleven countries and has seen a hundred doctors over the years to deal with her illness. She reported that she has seen some incredibly dark days throughout her battle against Lyme disease, and that there had been some moments when she no longer wanted to live. Many nights her daughter Gigi (and her daughter Bella, too) drove her to the emergency room because the pain of the inflammation in her brain was too much for her to bear.

When it comes to media coverage of Lyme, the most accurate, in-depth, and powerful presentation on this subject to date recently aired on a Fox 5 News special report called "Lyme and Reason: The Cause and Consequence of Lyme Disease." The report featured such Lyme disease notables as singer and songwriter Dana Parish, renowned oncologist

Neil Spector, author Ally Hilfiger, Yale-trained Lyme specialist Dr. Steven Phillips, and twelve-year-old Lyme sufferer Julia Bruzzese who was literally touched by the Pope during his visit to NYC last year. This detailed report was driven by the TV station's vice president and general manager Lew Leone whose wife, Jennifer, has Lyme disease. The Lyme community is grateful to Lew Leone and journalist Teresa Priolo for the courage it took to tell the real story when most media merely scratch the surface.

Lyme Movement

Everywhere you look, the Lyme movement is happening and gathering momentum—protesting, petitioning, presenting, educating, informing, sharing, writing, drawing, quilting, creating, videoconferencing, YouTubing, Facebooking, speaking, and shouting out loud.

There is Josh Cutler who stormed a dinner party at the IDSA headquarters. Jessica Bernstein in the online mag called *Truthout* reported that Cutler—who was twenty-five when he watched his friend die of Lyme, and then got sick himself—could no longer tolerate the government's inaction as he watched millions suffer and the IDSA stand idly by.

As Bernstein tells us,

In May 2014, Josh led hundreds of irate Lyme sufferers in a massive protest in front of the IDSA headquarters, in a desperate attempt to change IDSA policies that prevent them from receiving care. In the tradition of ACT UP, the AIDS activist movement that sprouted up back in the 1980s when patients were dropping like flies and nobody cared, protesters took to the streets outside the IDSA building, demanding changes in diagnostic criteria and treatment protocols.

Sick patients descended on the place that became the office for the original dinner partiers, and conducted die-ins with protesters laying their bodies on the ground in order to block the entrance.[197]

Donna Y. Jacobs has a traveling art exhibit called *Drawing Out Loud*. Her art collection is quite something to behold. It's an eye-catching, heart-wrenching series of charcoal drawings and installations that represent her painful journey witnessing the suffering of her twenty-eight-year-old daughter, Bronwyn, who lives every day with the misery of Lyme. People stop cold when they see her work. They cry with Donna and share their Lyme experiences with her at each and every show.

There are Lyme walks, Lyme runs, Lyme books, Lyme art, Lyme cartoons, Lyme bracelets, Lyme necklaces, Lyme T-shirts, Lyme sweatshirts, and "Take a Bite Out of Lyme" challenges. Anything and everything that will grab the world's attention.

There are Lyme conferences and symposiums, Lyme support groups—both online and in person.

There are Lyme petitions, designed by Lyme sufferers, intended to get the CDC to change the status quo treatment protocols that are clearly not working.

There is "May We March For Lyme" at Lincoln Memorial in May to shine light on Lyme disease. May is also Lyme Disease Awareness Month.

The Mayday Project—a registered 501(c)(3) nonprofit organization founded by a group of volunteers who have all battled Lyme disease and coinfections—is now in its sixth year working to get Lyme disease recognized as a chronic, disabling illness. The project advocates for research and patient rights in the hope that there will one day be a cure. The group's most recent efforts to petition the CDC to "End Preferential Treatment of the IDSA Guidelines for Lyme Disease" accomplished its main purpose, which was to bring the misconduct to the attention of top officials at the CDC and the US Department of Health and Human Services (HHS) and force a response.

Despite the passion, drive, and best efforts of so many, the awareness, politics, and investment in chronic Lyme disease is slow moving—inching along decades later.

John Madigan, independent senator for Victoria, Australia, has "succeeded in establishing an inquiry into the incidence in Australia of a tick-borne disease that causes similar symptoms to Lyme disease."

Senator Madigan says: "The past few months have been a steep learning curve for me when it comes to Lyme disease. What has become clear over that time is there are thousands of Australians suffering debilitating symptoms who need answers. Hopefully this inquiry will put the issue on the radar nationally and bring us a step closer to providing those answers."[198]

Eighteen months after Canada Green Party leader Elizabeth May's private Member's bill C-422—the Federal Framework on Lyme Disease Act—was passed unanimously and became law, Canada finally took some action by holding a mandated conference to develop a federal framework on Lyme disease. On the heels of the Canadian Conference for Lyme Disease, two advocacy groups were formed—primarily out of the sheer frustration that not enough is being done to move the political agenda forward.

The Lyme Disease Society of Canada (LDSC), spearheaded by Elizabeth Rogers, was founded by several Lyme patients and their caregivers. Their aim is to educate and support both the public and frontline medical professionals in order to ensure that every Canadian understands the prevalence and very real, life-altering dangers of Lyme disease and the difficulties that patients face while trying to seek treatment.[199]

The other newly formed Canadian advocacy group is V.O.C.A.L.–Voices Of Canadians About Lyme–led by Donna MacPherson Lugar. V.O.C.A.L. is the first-ever annual Lyme awareness initiative, taking place in each province from coast to coast. On June 3, 2017, cross-Canada events will range from educational activities, fund-raisers, and marches to concerts, galas, and peaceful protests.[200]

On December 16, 2015, big news came from Silicon Valley. A local couple donated a $6.5 million grant to the Bay Area Lyme Foundation. This gift constitutes the largest private donation ever given to Lyme research. Generously gifted by the Steven & Alexandra Cohen Foundation, the money will support Bay Area Lyme's mission of using new scientific research and innovations to make Lyme disease easy to diagnose and simple to cure.

"I was shocked to learn how many people suffer from Lyme disease in silence, and how much we still need to do to raise awareness and help find a cure," says Alex Cohen, president of the Steven & Alexandra Cohen Foundation. "This gift is incredibly personal to me as I have experienced, first-hand, the chronic and debilitating side effects of this relatively unknown disease. We share Bay Area Lyme Foundation's desire to find a cure for Lyme disease and hope that this gift will help pave the way to that important work."[201]

And finally, a faint glimmer of hope shines through when I read about two more breakthroughs.

George Mason University has developed a urine test that detects the first stages of Lyme disease more accurately than the current testing available. According to an article in Science Daily, "After three years and 300 patients, researchers have proof that their early-detection urine test for Lyme disease works. In the case of Lyme disease, some patients may still have active cases but traditional tests don't register it, and these patients may not be receiving the additional round of treatment they need, authors say."[202]

The National Guideline Clearinghouse (US Department of Health and Human Services, Agency for Healthcare Research and Quality) has finally dropped the outdated and ineffective IDSA Lyme disease guidelines, and now only lists the ILADS guidelines. Until now, insurance companies have only covered the treatment plan of the outdated and IOM-incompliant IDSA Lyme disease guidelines. Hopefully, with this news, patients will be able to get doctors to prescribe antibiotics for more than the twenty-eight-day IDSA protocol and insurance companies will start to cover it.[203]

This is merely a sampling of the Lyme movement, actions, breakthroughs, and uprising taking place all around the world. Everyone's participation counts. Momentum is growing. We do have strength in numbers. Don't let appearances deceive. Lyme sufferers are WARRIORS. We will fight to the death. Sometimes at the cost of having to confront bullies and trolls who are determined to shut us up.

I am always asked, "What will it take for these Lyme Wars to end and for people to get access to the treatment they need and deserve? And when is this change going to happen?" The real answer is, "I don't know. Nobody does just yet." But what I do believe with certainty is that positive, substantive change will occur in one of two ways—or perhaps both.

First, by the continued daily actions of a critical mass putting pressure on the medical community and their political representatives.

Pressure means putting this disease on the radar of the majority of doctors who currently, for the most part, know next to nothing about this disease, who deny its very existence, and who undermine its severity. Deprogramming doctors from the party line "groupthink" is the first order of business—a change that would save months and years of suffering and heartache for so many, a change that would prevent a myriad of misdiagnoses and inadequate treatment, a change that would put an end to the prolonged suffering and daily medical invalidation. Next, or perhaps concurrent with this Herculean mandate, would be to make a viable, reliable, stable Lyme diagnostic test available everywhere and to everyone. Then there's finding and dispensing treatment that works—treatment that doctors are free to administer without having their licenses stripped and their practices closed.

Sigh! We have so much work to do. There's such an indescribable disconnect and detachment on the part of most doctors. How about this: Let's put them all in a room for an hour with thousands of Lyme sufferers—some screaming in pain for hours on end, others who look like mere shadows, skeletons of their former selves—and see how long doctors can continue to deny the suffering.

The second concurrent approach to change will happen as a result of the broad-sweeping actions of one or two whistleblowers—someone with a great deal of influence who has been personally affected by this hideous world of Lyme and isn't afraid to take on the political machinations, abuse of power, greed, and arrogance that lie before us.

And I suppose there is a third approach which most

of us have been forced to pursue. That is, to source out a myriad of diagnostic and treatment workarounds outside of conventional medicine which ultimately will render the majority of allopathic doctors unnecessary and ineffectual in this journey.

An uprising of enlightened sufferers, supporters, and whistleblowers will one day turn this tide—I witness it happening every day.

My hope is that sometime soon the Lyme Wars won't continue to require such a dramatic effort. I hope that soon we will gain the ear of the medical community whose ear we should have *always* had as a basic human right.

Doctors, politicians, world—are you listening? I hope so. It's only a matter of time before chronic Lyme disease affects you.

Toppling the Lyme Cabal

Every day I am asked: Why?

Why is chronic Lyme disease not recognized? Why is it not allowed to be treated? Why are doctors not taking it seriously? Why are so many people with Lyme not able to get medical care? Why don't doctors want to help people get well? Why don't they know more? Why do Canadians have to cross the border to the US to get an MD to take them seriously? Why in the US is there only a handful of LLMDs, many of whom have been annihilated by their licensing boards, associations and colleagues, despite the fact that they are the only ones actually helping Lyme sufferers?

If only I could answer these questions simply, confidently, and succinctly. If only it could all be easily and reasonably explained. If only after years of reading and listening and conversing and inquiring and deciphering and writing and speaking I was able to provide you with a clear and simple answer. If only I were an Erin Brockovich or a Michael Moore, someone willing and able to crack the code. If only I were a whistleblower or the Watergate "deep throat." I would love nothing more than to know exactly who is responsible for the untold suffering of millions worldwide.

I entered the Lyme world several years ago as a mother on a mission with only one goal in mind: to help my son get well. Little did I know that I would meet so many Lyme sufferers just like my son. And I could never have imagined that I was about to face such an ugly, dark, and cruel side of humanity within the politics of chronic Lyme.

I've read the documents. I've been privy to some of the most damning evidence. I desperately want nothing more than to see the Lyme cabal come toppling down and to know that justice has been done with regard to those responsible for this toxic mess.

Thankfully, there are people who are willing and able to get to the heart of these unconscionable acts. Some who are highly informed and courageous enough to blow the whistle and bring it all tumbling down.

There's Kathleen Dickson—the LYMErix whistleblower and former analytical chemist at Pfizer. On her website, ohioactionlyme.org, Dickson gives us her take on the who, what, when, where, why, and how chronic Lyme disease became an illness of outlandish proportions. She covers it all in great detail.

There's researcher and activist Carl Tuttle who has created a petition signed by 78,000 people worldwide, calling for a congressional investigation of the CDC, IDSA, the American Lyme Disease Foundation, and vaccine makers in order to uncover conflicts of interest, misinformation, and undue influences that are keeping people from getting diagnosed and treated for chronic Lyme.[204]

Bruce Fries, the founder of the Patient Centered Care Advocacy Group and a member of the Mayday Project advocacy group for Lyme patient rights, is a strong and powerful voice in these Lyme Wars. In one of his articles published in *Truthout*, Fries asks: "Why does the CDC, a public agency tasked with protecting the health of US taxpayers, promulgate the IDSA guidelines as policy, particularly when it can be demonstrated that the guidelines authors disallow, ignore, or reject a very large body of scientific evidence that contradicts their narrow view of this disease?"[205]

Another important advocate that I've had the pleasure of meeting is Jenna Luche-Thayer—a former senior adviser at the UN and other government agencies. Like Dickson and the others, Luche-Thayer herself has Lyme. It was misdiagnosed for fifteen years and almost disabled her; she has now been managing it for four.

What these two powerhouse advocates have in common is they both purport to be in possession of documentation that clearly points to the specific political players and their ugly deeds, the misappropriation of taxpayer money, violations of federal laws and codes of conduct, gross mismanagement, abuse of authority, and scientific falsehoods, among other things.

Luche-Thayer has never been a federal employee; however, she has worked on many federal programs and with a number of federal agencies. She was invited to be part of a Lyme Disease Science and Policy Challenges forum which took place in the congressional Rayburn Building in Washington, DC. Speakers included experts from the fields of microbiology, pathology, molecular medicine, integrative medicine, diagnostic testing, patient advocacy, and government oversight. This event was organized by the Patient Centered Care Advocacy Group and was hosted by the Lyme Action Network where she spoke about the need for congressional oversight of the CDC's Office of Infectious Diseases, National Center for Emerging and Zoonotic Infectious Diseases, Division of Vector-Borne Diseases, and the Bacterial Diseases Branch—all of which are responsible for federal policy and implementation regarding Lyme disease.

Luche-Thayer's analysis has been built upon her years of working with federal agencies where she witnessed and participated in ethics and inspector general investigations. She compares these situations to the CDC's highly irregular actions.

She is fearless, funny, brave, and in possession of well-documented sources pointing to those who have perpetrated these Lyme cover-ups, missteps, denial, and medical abandonment. She seems to know how and why the CDC and IDSA have been permitted to have so much political power around this disease, and why this madness regarding chronic Lyme and coinfections has been perpetuated and sustained for decades.

"This information is available," Luche-Thayer tells me. "I know where to look and what to look for because I have worked on so many different federal programs. And I have pages of well-documented answers—as to where, why, who, and how this Lyme agenda has been held in captivity. Other Lyme advocates have been very willing to share the documentation they have painstakingly amassed over many years...and this helps to show entrenched institutional patterns."

Why does the IDSA have so much power? I ask.

"The increasing threats of epidemics, pandemics, and

bioterrorism all combine to make infectious-disease specialists essential to concerns for national security. The IDSA is a big collaborator with Big Pharma, and Big Pharma outspends all the other lobbyists by hundreds of millions of dollars every year and have been rewriting the rules in their favor," says Luche-Thayer. "They're all enmeshed. The CDC. The IDSA. Big Pharma. Some higher-education institutions.

"This is how it all works," Luche-Thayer explains. "We can talk about the science forever. But until we dig out these truths and speak to how private economic interests are distorting our public institutions, the science won't help us.

"The promotion by the CDC of one private institution's Lyme guidelines is a clear appearance of preferential treatment. The name of this private institution is the Infectious Diseases Society of America (IDSA). The IDSA promotes the view that Lyme disease is easy to diagnose and simple to treat with a limited course of antibiotics... This appearance of preferential treatment for the IDSA by the CDC is further amplified by the following fact. *Out of all the diseases addressed by the CDC, it is only Lyme disease wherein the CDC promotes one private institution's medical guidelines.* This is a strikingly unique and highly unusual situation," says Luche-Thayer.[206]

According to Luche-Thayer:

Since 2001, the CDC has disregarded congressional legislation to do something about Lyme; they have ignored congressional directives. The CDC is enmeshed with the IDSA and it is the IDSA's financial interests that are setting the Lyme guidelines and programs. The IDSA shares the same economic interests as Big Pharma—development of vaccines, drugs, therapies, and diagnostic tools for public health medical emergencies—that's a given. The IDSA members sit on the board of almost every major institution that does research. Funding for the Department of Health and Human Services represents one of four tax payers' dollars. The federal government is an annual big funder of IDSA and Big Pharma products, such as CDC's vaccine programs.

"Big Pharma's profit motives do not serve public health very well. What does or doesn't get done is driven by greed and economic interest; when it does get done you have a 'happy' coincidence," Luche-Thayer explains. "The NIH, two major universities, and the IDSA are directly implicated in the misappropriation of six federal grants. Monies from these grants were used to:

- *discredit the Lyme community and its advocates;*
- *invalidate their experience of the disease;*
- *marginalize the Lyme community and its advocates from the decision-makers that determine access to care and insurance coverage of Lyme;*
- *undermine their access to discourse and engagement with scientific and medical communities; and*
- *deny their full rights as citizens to engage as stakeholders with government officials on topics of their deep and valid concern.*

"The CDC appears to allow IDSA's financial interests regarding Lyme to overwhelm CDC's core mandate to protect the public health. A number of the directors and officials responsible for the CDC Lyme policy and programs are themselves members of the IDSA. They appear too enmeshed and personally vested in the IDSA to: (1) be

able to correct the balance of power; and (2) make Lyme policy and programs that represent the best science and are patient-centered. This dysfunctional enmeshment has been heavily documented and is on public record. State and federal government and legislators have been repeatedly apprised of this escalating situation that continues unabated. Despite corrective efforts, such as appropriations committee language and state laws, the situation has not improved. With regards to Lyme, the CDC has broken the public trust and systematically marginalized Lyme patients. For all these reasons, formal oversight of the CDC is required.

"This array of behaviors and affiliations by the CDC-touted Lyme experts is disconcerting. Formal ethics complaints to the CDC regarding preferential treatment for the IDSA have been met with silence. The over seven hundred peer-reviewed and published studies indicating and/or proving persistent Borrelia infection gather dust on CDC shelves. Patient and medical expert testimony and documentation regarding the improved health of patients from a variety of non-IDSA protocols remain ignored. The CDC appears to be insensitive to and dismissive of the Lyme community.[207]

"I have to wonder why the IDSA is talking about Lyme training on their website for new recruits, spending time, money, resources, shaping law and policy on a disease that they say is not all that significant. If it were really that 'difficult to catch, easy to diagnose, and easy to treat,' you wouldn't be spending so much time and resources training new members. What they do and say on their website doesn't match up with what they say to patients and the public at large.

"I am compelled to dive deep and unpack this Lyme travesty."

To all the advocates and whistleblowers of chronic Lyme, we thank you. We trust that with your help the truth will reveal itself. Hopefully soon.

CONCLUSION
STILL BATTLING, BUT HOPEFUL

When I get home I shall write a book about this place...
If I ever do get home.

—ALICE'S ADVENTURES IN WONDERLAND

I was fortunate enough to write the first draft of this book on a writing retreat in Bali, something I signed up for on a complete whim. I actually felt driven by something much larger than myself. There was no other way to explain my impulsivity.

It was April and I had just returned home from a special trip with my daughter. I had no intention of traveling again. Yet there it was—on my Facebook newsfeed—an invitation asking ME to come to Bali to write that book I'd always wanted to write.

I knew I had to go.

I spent the next two hours filling out the application. *What am I doing?* My inner voice kept disrupting the flow. *I'm going,* something much more powerful inside of me replied.

As I completed the application process, I thought, *But what about Matt? Will I be able to go by November? Will he be okay? Can I be that far away?*

I had to write this book. I had to lighten my own load. I had to write from my own truth. I had to heal my despair and that of others. I had to move all that I'd read for months on end from head to paper. I had to make sense of the *madness* of these past few years. I had to try to explain the political underpinnings of this disease. I had to be a voice and a platform for those who needed to be heard.

I thought about these powerful words by writer Sarah Manguso:

> *The purpose of being a serious writer is not to express oneself, and it is not to make something beautiful... The purpose of being a serious writer is to keep people from despair.*

As soon as I signed up for this retreat, Matt began to have a rough time again.

Inch by inch, hour by hour, day by day, we never knew how he was going to be. His progress was rarely linear—there were lots of ups and downs. New symptoms appeared when old ones let up, and old ones returned and became acute. Sleep was hard to come by. Every hour, every day, brought something new—usually something worrisome. There was little time to breathe.

I don't know how Matt continued to work. The mother in me wanted him to come home. But, of course, he had a life in NYC. Coming home to Toronto would mean that life had stopped for him. He kept repeating, "I'd rather be sick with a job than sick without one."

He needed to have some normalcy. He needed to stay with Shayna, in their apartment together in NYC. I knew this was true. But it was hard to be so far away and not be able to see him, and help him.

It killed me—every day. He would reach out with texts when he wasn't feeling well. I inquired daily, trying not to crowd, wanting to honor his space, but I was always worried.

The days and times when his voice sounded strong were all that I longed for.

I listened to the lyrics of songwriter Anthony Rapp's "Carry Me Home" over and over and over for months. The song is about a grown son who knows that his mother wants nothing more than to carry him home so that she can love and protect him from his struggles in life.

I listened to it again and again...

Yes—I'd love nothing more than to carry him home.

A Relapse

I love the line from the film *The Best Exotic Marigold Hotel*—the one where Sonny, the main character, says, "Everything will be all right in the end...If it's not all right, then it's not yet the end." Or was it John Lennon who first said this? I'm not sure. But in any case, it is both circular thinking and divinely guided all at once. It's clear, optimistic, and hopeful.

Six months of oral antibiotics got Matt to a better place than the months before his diagnosis. From June to December 2014, he was on a combination of several oral meds—administered by "pulse dosing," as we say in Lymeland.

His second test from Advanced Labs showed he still had spirochetes in his blood. So with his LLMD's guidance,

Matt decided to go for broke and try the most aggressive treatment: IV antibiotics.

This meant having a Hickman line—a silicone intravenous line surgically attached to his chest, and inserted into a large vein near his heart—giving the poison a more direct line to his brain and his nervous system.

I hated that Hickman line. I hated that Matt had to feel like a hospital patient twice a day, every day, feeding his body with antibiotics directly through his veins. I hated that he had to keep the tube immaculately clean at all times, reminding him of the potential for serious infection. I was relieved to know that a nurse came to his apartment once a week to check on his line.

When he was home visiting for a weekend, I watched him set up his Lyme patient ward—creating a makeshift IV stand, hanging his line on a wire hanger attached to my living room painting, high above his head so that the medicine would drip freely through his line and through his bloodstream.

Matt has always been organized, meticulous, fastidious. So I knew he was taking great care. But this IV method of delivery felt so over the top. Did he really need this? Was it doing any good?

I worry. I worry about him having so much medication in his system. I worry because he looks pale and unhealthy. I worry when I see the constant look of intensity and lackluster in his face. I worry that this will never end.

Last June, he went to Prague with Shayna for a much-needed holiday. By the end of their ten-day respite, he relapsed so far from home. Severe diarrhea, unable to leave the hotel room and not sure how he was going to make it home. He called his doctors in NYC. They prescribed an antibiotic that couldn't be filled at the pharmacy there. He called a local doctor (a Mrs. Doubtfire doppelgänger, I'm told) whose remedy was to aggressively boss them around to fetch some sugar, salt, and water. Apparently, this doctor went to med school to dispense this sage advice.

Any sudden illness—on vacation or not—is upsetting, but usually quite manageable. When you have chronic Lyme, any setback—especially far from home—terrifies you because you don't know what's triggering it. You feel like you don't have any control, and you don't know when, how, or if this health roller coaster will ever subside.

I wondered and worried. And I was weary along with him.

Is this a Lyme setback, a herx, a new opportunistic infection, food poisoning? We had no way of knowing.

Over the past three years, Matt and I have done this dance. A dance between treatment protocols where I look for windows of opportunity so not to overwhelm him, but to suggest, advise, and provide new ideas. I'm always searching, asking Matt to put new findings in his back pocket.

There's a new research study that says that Claritin—an over-the-counter allergy medicine—can treat Lyme. We try that. There's the BioMat that I discover from Mindy Haber, another Lyme mom, who wrote the book *Lyme Rage*. It emits far-infrared rays and negative ions to relieve pain and boost the immune system. Matt agrees to try this too. He's open to everything at this point.

I don't want to cause him to stop believing in his antibiotic treatments, but I'm hyperaware that we need to plan ahead for the time when antibiotics are no longer appropriate, no longer serving him, no longer effective, or too much of a toxic overload.

Following his relapse, Matt continued to have a rough summer. He went to work with a fever. Took more antibiotics—Cipro this time, which has an FDA black-box warning for permanent peripheral neuropathy, severe tendon damage and actual tendon ruptures, and acute liver toxicity. I only learned this after he took it. Great, more poison in his already compromised system. Where does it all lead?

One day this past summer, Matt got a call from his Lyme doctor telling him his liver enzymes were too high. He suggested that he see a specialist.

Matt got in to see a hepatologist the very next day. The doctor took all kinds of blood tests and sent him away until the results came in. As potentially distressing as it sounded, I quickly learned that hepatitis is an infection of the liver, and there are all kinds of causes and three different types—A, B, and C—both chronic and acute. We believed that Matt had the treatable kind—acute, not chronic—but it presented us with yet another health issue to worry about.

I desperately wanted that Hickman line out and to have him off the IV antibiotics—and off *all* antibiotics, for that matter. I was convinced that several months of antibiotics in his system was one reason his liver was so compromised. His body was saying, *Enough! Stop giving me toxins. I can't take it.*

I wanted him off these drugs, but I tried not to push. Matt knew how I felt. He can read me well—I'm not much of a poker player. My face, my voice, and my body language say it all. I have to wait patiently for him to be ready. He's a smart and responsible guy. He'll do it when he thinks it's time, I tell myself.

In the end, it was his pharmacist who called him and told him it was time to get the Hickman line out. That is was risky to keep it in for so long if he wasn't continuing to take the antibiotics. That he could always have it reinserted if need be.

I hope that is never the case.

A "Guide" Named Darrell and Then Dr. D.

So with antibiotics no longer being a viable protocol, Matt needed something else to work with. He could not stop treating. If you stop treating, this disease wins.

Serendipity struck. I met Darrell A.

Darrell, who I met on Facebook, lives in the US and claims to have healed himself, his family, and thousands of others using the Rife machine.

Huh? Is this possible? Is this not too good to be true?

With great skepticism, I spoke to Darrell on the phone. He is smart. Passionate. Quick-minded. A man of faith.

He truly believes his mission in life is to help others heal from this disease. He sees it as his calling because—at the very moment he was about to put a gun to his head to end his life due to years of excruciating, debilitating pain and no relief in sight—he experienced the presence of a higher power showing him a way to heal.

Darrell's personal Lyme recovery seemed compelling, for sure. But still too good to be true. If this is *the* answer, then why doesn't everyone in Lymeland use a Rife machine?

Matt and I knew about Rife from the start—it wasn't a new idea to us. In fact, it was one of the first treatment protocols we had read about months before. Matt had asked Dr. R. what he thought about it. He was supportive of it, but didn't know enough to be able to guide him.

So here appeared Darrell—out of nowhere. And I was game to learn more.

Darrell emailed me about fifty PubMed, evidence-based, peer-reviewed journals about Lyme. He had clearly done his homework. He could wax poetic about this disease in a way I had never heard anyone do before. He understood the bigger picture, the corruption, the medical cover-up. He was far more self-educated than I was, as he had been dealing with chronic Lyme for more than fifteen years.

He says he has healed himself, his entire family, and over a thousand more people with his Rife protocol. It now seems that Matt just might heal because of the kindness of a stranger named Darrell. I will personally throw him a parade if Matt gets good results.

Is this all just magical, wishful, fanciful thinking? Perhaps. Nevertheless, for now, Matt and I are choosing to believe. There is a lot of power in that—all in itself.

Darrell's Lyme Story

Here are some excerpts from Darrell's story—in the form of a letter he wrote to me and happily agreed to share:

Dear Lori,

Thank you for reaching out to me via Facebook. I sincerely believe I can help guide your son to beat this terrible disease once and for all!

I tried just about everything to eliminate the devastating effects that Lyme Disease (LD) was doing to me after having it for many years, even possibly being born with it, however the last 2 years were absolutely shattering. I am very thankful for my Lyme Literate Medical Doctor (LLMD) because other doctors thought I had MS or Lupus since they have such similar symptoms.

My LLMD and I still think I was infected by a mosquito because after being bitten it looked really infected. I was put on 3 types of oral ABX for many months and then I even had an IV PICC line with several different ABX for 5 months; I was only getting worse. Then I treated with 35% hydrogen peroxide chelation mixed with a Vitamin "cocktail" performed by a MD three times a week for 6 months.

I was still very sick. I then purchased a hyper-thermic chamber (steam sauna) and a medical grade ozone machine and I did two treatments per day for well over a year. I also did rectal insufflation treatments once each day.

The first 4 months I broke out in oozing and bloody boils from under my chin to the top of my feet. Some of my symptoms were being relieved however most of them were still debilitating and destroying me.

My LD symptoms were severe migraine headaches (constant for 2 years), joint pain, dizziness, balance issues, confusion, memory loss (short term and mid-term), hypothyroidism (Hashimoto's disease), ocular blurriness, rash and boils all over my body, severe itching (under the skin crawling), severe stomach cramps, restlessness, mental fogginess & confusion, constant fatigue (sleeping up to 20 hours per day), hiatal hernia/esophageal vasospasms, acid reflux, uncontrollable twitching, drooping eyelid, systemic candida, heart pain & palpitations (docs initially thought I had a heart attack), facial/oral facial/dental pain, jaw pain, difficulty talking in sentences & slurred speech, swollen & painful lymph glands, shortness of breath, suicidal tendencies, hypersensitivity to sound, ringing and pain in the ears (tinnitus & Ménière's disease), thrush, difficulty swallowing, metallic taste, carpel tunnel syndrome, panic attacks and anxiety. My LLMD believed I had many of the 300+ co-infections of LD and it was a brutal struggle for survival.

I eventually spent north of $300,000 trying to get better but to no avail.

LD almost killed me!

When I was at my lowest point, I found a flicker of hope. I talked to a complete stranger, my guardian angel, and he guided me to find a Rife Frequency instrument. It destroys the late stage LD bacteria and it has been scientifically proven on all other bad bacteria and viruses in the body without hurting any good cells of your body. It can only eliminate the bad bacteria and viruses. A similar form of it was originally designed, manufactured and used to treat TB and cancer in the 1930s. I used it regularly for less than 180 days and finally got completely healed! My LLMD friend and his family were all healed as well as my entire family. He later tried using it in his practice and was threatened.

I have been completely healed now for over 15 years. I finally beat the LD before it totally wiped me out. Now for many years I have been helping people to get well for no charge because someone reached out and helped me. It has become my passion to help others. Since I am fully recovered, in the last 15 years I have been fortunate enough to help over a thousand people get completely well and become symptom-free.

It is so sad that doctors are only allowed by their governing bodies to practice inside their box. They are not allowed to venture outside for solutions because they are criticized, fined or their license to practice is revoked.

We can step out of the box and own and use the machine on ourselves and family members. Furthermore, the machine is extremely safe because no good cells can be harmed from the frequency range of the machine, because bad cells and good cells have completely different frequency ranges to be destroyed.

I was desperate to get well and I used these machines to finally conquer the LD giant and I am confident it will help you too.

I read Darrell's story—in its entirety. Not once, not twice. But a third and then a fourth time. I looked for holes. For reasons that this was ridiculous. Impossible. I listened carefully.

As much as I had a hard time believing his story, he possessed a great deal of knowledge and he made a lot of sense. I wanted to trust him. It felt like the real deal. What on earth were we doing being guided and healed by Darrell—a non-medical professional whom we'd never met? Why weren't doctors helping us find solutions, thereby forcing us to rely on strangers without medical credentials?

Sometimes our non-linear thinking kicks in when we need it most. Our ability to suspend rational thinking, to take a leap of faith, to trust and believe in something bigger, perhaps a force we can't explain.

I do so—with great skepticism and high levels of trepidation. But sometimes all you've got is to trust the seemingly impossible—even when others are rolling their eyes at you.

I talked to Matt about Darrell. He was ready to try something new. He recognized he could no longer rely on traditional, conventional, Big Pharma protocols. He was willing to speak to Darrell—with an open mind.

We bought the Rife machine that same week. And he's been using it ever since. With Darrell's self-created frequency protocol and his most generous personal guidance.

Darrell has promised—often and consistently—that he can get Matt well using the Rife machine daily, ramping up the frequencies in a slow and studied manner.

Several months in, Matt has had yet another relapse and still suffers from a myriad of symptoms, including brain fog and a leaky gut, which are some of the toughest symptoms to heal.

When Matt asked one of his Lyme docs—an NYC MD who specializes in tough cases of chronic Lyme and its coinfections—what she thought about using the Rife machine, she told him she had just come back from a conference where the theme was energy medicine as the guiding treatment force. Energy medicine including Rife, bioresonance, low-level laser, Reiki, and many other protocols, are all being used with some measure of success in eradicating this stubborn disease. Or putting it into remission at the very least.

In addition to the Rife machine, Matt has also tried CBD, which is soundly researched and generously guided by Dr. M., whose expertise has given us and thousands of others that extra boost of confidence we're looking for.

Cleaning Up

In September, Matt had a long-standing appointment with a Toronto Lyme-literate naturopath, Dr. D. I made the appointment for him several months earlier because I had heard this doctor had a very unique and advanced practice. He trained in Germany where they are far more up to date on frequency technology and state-of-the-art protocols.

The appointment with Dr. D. was overwhelming to say the least. He tested his immune system. He looked at his blood sample through a dark field microscope. He found that Matt's immune system was the equivalent of an eighty-year-old's. That was devastating to hear and to process.

He found mold, parasites, and a leaky gut in Matt's cellular environment. He explained that we are bacteria having a human experience—that we are composed of one hundred times more bacterial DNA than human DNA, as evidenced by Matt's blood sample.

It all had to be *cleaned up* with a new supplement protocol, filtered water system, filtered air system, and an even more refined diet.

"We have to change the terrain first, then go after the infection," Dr. D. explained. "I don't see biofilm, but Matt's kidneys and liver are working too hard and his immune system is badly compromised. This infection is stealth and will do anything and feed on everything to stay alive. We want to change the cellular environment [that is, the space between the cells] to give the spirochetes fewer places to attach themselves, to hide and stay alive. Let's take a step back, bring down the toxic load, and then go after the infection again."

The appointment felt disheartening, a bit of a setback. But the information we received and this new approach were really important. And very much in keeping with everything I'd read about the Lyme journey. Once you've treated the most acute symptoms, the next steps are to clean up the cellular environment, boost the immune system, then—when Matt's system is strong enough—go in for the kill with heavy-duty antibiotics to eradicate all leftover parasitic invaders in a head-on, military-like fashion.

We're scheduled to see Dr. D. again. His waiting list for new patients is now twelve months long. He is very knowledgeable, kind and respectful. And we feel lucky to have him on our team.

And thanks to another far-reaching, deep-thinking,

innovative doctor—Dr. K. in Toronto—Matt has also tried using a high-grade, low-level laser for healing, with specific protocols programmed specifically for his symptomatology, including a leaky gut and brain fog.

Make no mistake. Healing from Lyme is a complex, multilayered, do-it-yourself guessing game as to what is causing the symptoms and how best to address them. And while Matt has some very good doctors on board, the moment-to-moment, hour-by-hour shift in his health requires us to continue to be our own sleuths, researchers, doctors, diagnosticians. Matt and I are constantly searching for new ideas as his various symptoms wax and wane.

Without question, this process is expensive and draining, as it requires throwing all kinds of things against the wall to see what may or may not stick. If the medical system would just do its job, perhaps this journey could be a little less do-it-yourself with a lot more certainty.

The Cause of Lyme Turned Upside Down

Are you ready for a final piece of Alice-in-Wonderland-style madness? Where I now begin to question whether this never-ending journey down this never-ending rabbit hole to the darkest recesses of the earth has been real, or just a very bad dream?

Whether all of this reading, researching, interviewing, learning, gathering information, recognizing misinformation, and weighing opinions and theories about chronic Lyme disease is nothing but a misbegotten journey or an incomprehensible nightmare of sorts.

Where nothing seems true and everything feels false.

Where the medical system is nothing more than a bunch of anthropomorphic animals (the Mad Hatter, the March

Hare, the Cheshire Cat), governed and oppressed by a monarchy of playing cards.

I don't know how else to explain this final piece that confirms what very, very few have said and known to be true all along. That all that we understand to be chronic Lyme has been nothing but a pack of lies and misinformation fed to the suffering Lyme community.

According to many, illusion, delusion, distraction, greed, profit, laziness, herd mentality, gaslighting, sociopathy, and a broken medical system's psyche have caused the medical world to lie, deflect, and simply not care—causing millions to suffer.

As Lewis Carroll said, "Madness is a fact of life in Wonderland. No matter where you go, everyone there is crazy. This ubiquitous madness seems to make everyone equivalent in some way—the Hatter is exchangeable with the Hare because they're both mad."

I purchased the book *Medical Medium: Secrets Behind Chronic and Mystery Illness and How to Finally Heal*, by medical medium Anthony William. This much-anticipated book provides an entirely new perspective on what I've been researching for so many months—with mind-blowing, astonishing, alarming insights.

The book arrived on the heels of finishing my first draft. After reading it, I thought, *Well, isn't this the perfect cliffhanger to the madness that is Lyme?*

I turned to the chapter on Lyme disease, and the first thing I read was,

*Truth is, **Lyme disease isn't the result of ticks**, parasites, or bacteria. **Lyme disease is actually viral**—not bacterial or parasitical. When medical communities finally awaken to this fact, there will be hope for Lyme patients.*[208]

The bacteria—*Borrelia burgdorferi*—has nothing at all to do with Lyme! William goes on to say,

The true cause of what's being called Lyme disease varies in each individual. People who have different varieties of Epstein-Barr can have Lyme symptoms, as can people who have HHV-6 and its various strains. People who carry any of the different strains of shingles can exhibit Lyme symptoms, with the non-rashing varieties causing the most severe cases, including symptoms such as brain inflammation and other central nervous system weaknesses. It's the same for any number of viruses.[209]

When you contract Lyme, William tells us, the herpes-family virus that was dormant inside of you has now been triggered by any one of a number of twenty-one things that can weaken your immune system. These triggers include mercury in any form (read *flu vaccine*), mold, stress, insomnia, and tick bites, which he lists as number twenty-one—last on his list of triggers.

He says that tick bites are responsible for *triggering*, not causing, Lyme, and that this is the case in only 0.5 percent of sufferers.

The triggers of the dormant herpes-like virus manifest a whole host of unexplained symptoms, including fever, headaches, joint pain, muscle pain, fatigue, neck pain, burning nerve pain, heart palpitations, and almost any neurological symptom.

To summarize William's theory, the causes of Lyme disease are herpes-like viruses that were once dormant and have now presented in a constellation of chronic neurological symptoms that have been dubbed Lyme disease.

After reading William's chapter on Lyme, my head spun. No one in my world wants to hear it. "She's listening to a medium now—uh-huh! She's officially lost it!" read their forlorn expressions and the pitying tone in their voices.

"Why do you think I wrote a book, people?" I mutter under my breath. "Do you think I've been spending all of these hours poring over the research because this subject is simple? Because doctors have all the answers—or any answers, for that matter? Because sufferers are all "mad," and I voluntarily decided to join them in this crazy world called Lymeland?"

No. I'm still caught in the muck and mire of this dark, nonsensical, certifiable, psychotic, unending rabbit hole *because* my son is sick and and I'm compelled to understand. And we are all forced to figure out this madness for ourselves.

Despite what others choose to think, I believe that William's theory makes sense and is a closer fit to our experience than any others I've heard along the way, except for that of our current LLND. I am going to give a copy of this book to him at Matt's next visit. I'd love to know what he thinks.

For years, I have admired medical intuitives like Caroline Myss. Her work, in conjunction with Harvard-trained neurosurgeon Dr. C. Norman Shealy, allows Myss to understand complex medical issues in a way that most doctors don't—using her highly attuned intuitive skills. Imagine if we could find doctors who were adept at combining these two critical types of intelligence, medical and intuitive. How medicine would thrive again.

William's theories pose some important questions: *Is chronic Lyme primarily bacterial? Is it viral? Or both?*

The Mayo Clinic says,

Many human illnesses are caused by infection with either bacteria or viruses. Most bacterial diseases can be treated with antibiotics, although antibiotic-resistant strains are starting to emerge. Viruses pose a challenge to the body's immune system because they hide inside cells.

In some cases, it may be difficult to determine whether a bacterium or a virus is causing your symptoms. Many ailments—such as pneumonia, meningitis and diarrhea—can be caused by either type of microbe.[210]

Many will argue that Lyme is a bacterial illness and that it is confirmed because they got their lives back by using long-term courses of antibiotics.

We also know—without question—that Lyme can put tremendous stress on your immune system, rendering you sensitive to chemicals and mold and all kinds of toxins. And if your immune system is stressed, dormant viruses can be reactivated with Lyme disease.

My experience—and that of so many others—informs us that chronic Lyme disease is a toxic stew, a holy mess of things that, apart from spirochetes, can and often does include parasites, mold, fungi, cell-wall deficiencies, biofilm, chemical and toxic overload, a leaky gut, immunosuppression, OspA I'm told as well as a relapsing fever. And, without question, Lyme disease can include a viral component whereby dormant viruses like EBV become activated and wreak havoc on your immune system.

So...is Lyme disease bacterially or virally driven?

Perhaps both.

William's views closely align with this and with everything we've experienced on Matt's journey. For some time now, I've been convinced that his illness was triggered by a flu shot, *not a tick bite*. And Matt did have a short bout of EBV (that is, mononucleosis) as a teenager, so this also fits with his medical history.

With hindsight, and with William's affirming theories, it's beginning to make more sense.

Let me assure you that I do recognize I am now listening intently to a medical medium—one who gets his wisdom from spirit, a higher power, an otherworldly place. I realize that many of you will furrow your brow, shake your head, and wonder whether *I* have now turned mad.

The answer is yes. I am mad. Mad enough to remain in this rabbit hole until I get answers that make sense and confirm what certain wise ones have been saying all along. And other than our current doctor, who seems to "get it" more than most, I have not heard any other medical professional put any of this together for us, or help us to make sense of it all.

And what, by the way, is *"madness"* but a natural by-product of our overriding confusion as we are forced to seek out and reconcile multiple irreconcilable messages—— in a desperate attempt to make sense of it all.

I am gobsmacked by William's book. It turns all conventional wisdom on its head. At the same time, it confirms what very few—only the Yodas of the Lyme world who I can count on one hand—have been saying all along.

More information, new ideas, require further understanding of some of the missing pieces. I want to understand the role of B cells in Lyme (something Kathleen Dickson speaks of). For this, I take a cursory glance at the work of Nicole Baumgarth, Professor of Pathology, Microbiology & Immunology, Center for Comparative Medicine, School of

Veterinary Medicine, University of California, Davis, CA. Dr. Baumgarth studies the regulation of immune responses to infections and focuses on T cell interactions with B cells and how these cells become unable to promote the production of anti-Borrelia antibodies.

And then I briefly take a look at the work of Dr. Armin Alaedini, Assistant Professor, Department of Medicine at Columbia University Medical Center, NY, whose research has focused on the gut-immune-brain connection in chronic Lyme disease and the role that it plays.

Then came this! An article written by John P. Thomas of *Health Impact News*. In this piece, "Vaccines and Retroviruses: A Whistleblower Reveals What the Government is Hiding," Thomas reports that,

> *Data suggests that 6% of the US population is harboring a retrovirus in their bodies that can develop into an acquired immune deficiency. This is not the well-known AIDS caused by HIV, but Acquired Immune Deficiency Syndrome (AIDS) associated with other retroviruses. These non-HIV retroviruses were unintentionally introduced into humans over the past 75 years.*

According to Thomas, twenty million Americans are likely infected with retroviruses, although not everyone will end up being chronically ill.

> *Retrovirus exposure intensified in the 1970s as new vaccines and pharmaceutical products were developed. These retroviruses and related infectious agents are now associated with dozens of modern chronic illnesses—perhaps nearly all of them. In these diseases, infection*

leads to inflammation—and unresolved inflammation can lead to chronic disease.

Even though 20 million Americans are likely to be infected, not everyone will develop serious illness. Retroviruses in the human body are like sleeping giants. They are quiet until they are activated in immune deficient people.

*Once activated, they create diseases such as Myalgic Encephalomyelitis, also called Chronic Fatigue Syndrome (ME/CFS), **Chronic Lyme Disease**, Chronic Lympho-cytic Leukemia, autism spectrum disorder (ASD), numer-ous cancers, and a wide range of other autoimmune, neu-roimmune, and central nervous system diseases.*[211]

Thomas's main source is Judy A. Mikovits, PhD, who was fired as a research director, locked out of her lab, and put in jail for stealing her own notebooks that contained confidential names and addresses of every patient in her gammaretrovirus research studies.

Mikovits's book, *Plague: One Scientist's Intrepid Search for the Truth about Human Retroviruses and Chronic Fatigue Syndrome (ME/CFS), Autism, and Other Diseases,* has many of the answers that may bring this search to an end.

As a side note, I recall seeing a copy of this very book on Matt's LLND's desk at our last visit.

Mikovits was put in jail and her career was decimated because,

She spoke the truth about the fraudulent use of govern-ment research money, the marketing of inaccurate ret-rovirus tests, Medicare fraud, the contaminated blood

supply, and the harm that is associated with vaccines and their schedule of administration. Her research showed how retroviruses are linked to the plague of modern illnesses that are bankrupting the U.S. healthcare system.[212]

This sounds all too familiar. Mikovits's story reminds me of another whistleblower I've referred to multiple times.

Back to Kathleen Dickson—One Last Time

I made one last-ditch effort to contact Kathleen to be sure I've got it right before I go to print. If we can figure out how we got here, then maybe we can figure out how to get out of this insane rabbit hole. *Isn't that the point of all this, after all?*

I join her message group. I keep listening and learning. Still not sure I've fully got it. Then I begin to get messages from some of her cohorts—members of the Dickson School of Lyme, or as they are more formally known, the Society for Advancement of Scientific Hermeneutics (SASH). The members of this medical abuse victims' rights group have been working together for years, trying to get the US Department of Justice (USDOJ) to hear their pleas. As chronically ill and disabled activists, they want the USDOJ to know that medical abuse has been inflicted upon them—how, when, why, and by whom.

So please, I ask Kathleen—one last time...

"What is the disease we know as Lyme?"

"The disease is the cryme," Kathleen Dickson lobs back a riddle, wrapped in a mystery, inside an enigma-style explanation.

"The vaccine caused the very same systemic neurologic disease we know as chronic neurologic Lyme. That was why they excluded it from the case definition claiming there was 'no such thing as the disease created by injecting people with a fungal antigen.'

"Both the disease—transmitted in a myriad of ways including tick bites and human interactions—AND the cryme which is the vaccine we knew as LYMErix deliver a fungal toxin that causes a slow septic shock outcome. A non-HIV/AIDS-like post-sepsis illness that reactivates a dormant virus like EBV and leaves sufferers with a relapsing fever illness. Borreliosis means relapsing fever," says Dickson.

And here's what I've been trying to understand for a very long time. It's all got to do with something called OspA—outer surface protein antigen—which Kathleen always underscores when speaking about chronic Lyme.

Please remember this term. It's taken me a long time to understand how this fits in. OspA is the key word we all need to understand. It is apparently the *epicenter* of this hell we know as chronic Lyme disease. And, in fact, OspA may be a more fitting name for the disease itself—chronic OspA, rather than chronic Lyme.

OspA (the outer surface protein antigen on the spirochete, a.k.a. Borrelia) is transmitted in a least two ways—by two specific "dirty needles": the tick (mosquito, flea, spider, mite, etc.) and LYMErix. This protein antigen is what creates the fungal synergy awakening dormant viruses like EBV in humans.

"Spirochetes 'stealth bomb' your immune system by shedding toxic fungal antigens (OspA). The bacteria become stealth, and your immune system stops producing antibodies," says Dickson. But it seems that no one else is talking about OspA disease.

"OspA is Lyme. This is what the disease is all about.

"Once you understand the biological mechanisms by

which Lyme sufferers are sick, then the question becomes, 'Who scammed us and why?'" explains Dickson. "The answer is simple. It's CDC officers who own most of the patents. They found OspA caused the same disease as chronic Lyme (EBV, mainly) so they deleted that definition from the case definition at Dearborn."

Why did it have to take so many months of racking my brain to understand this? So many pieces of this puzzle. All scattered about for someone to assemble. I'm doing my best.

I continue to ask questions of Kathleen. Where does the OspA come from? She tells me it comes via a bacteriophage, perhaps from mycoplasma—and so on and so forth. My feeble brain can only absorb so much.

Yet there is one more scientific piece that needs to be addressed vis-a-vis this medical nightmare we know as chronic Lyme. That is, EBV mutated B cells ——one of the most central outcomes of this disease, leading to chronic fatigue, cytokine storms, relapsing fever, and immunosuppression. According to Dickson, if there is a so-called 'cure' for chronic Lyme at this time, the only thing that may possibly provide any chance of recovery or at best remission is a drug called Rituximab, which is primarily used for cancers like Non-Hodgkin's Lymphoma, and which has been shown to have a high 'cure' rate for cancer patients with chronic fatigue syndrome.

I won't begin to pretend that I understand this fully. I've done my best. But I would be remiss if I didn't make reference to the importance of T-cells, EBV mutated B cells, blebs and the like. We all have a lot to learn still. A great deal to study. A lot more to understand and research.

Kathleen Dickson. I thank you for your dogged pursuit of the scientific truth.

I've come to comprehend these scientific facts to the best of my ability—in my own time. We've all had to explore this rabbit hole for ourselves. Talk to many experts, write blogs, write books, chat on Facebook, experience heartache, read a copious number of research articles till our heads hurt—just to arrive at the conclusions you discovered long ago.

You, I now see, are the reigning queen in this mad, mad world of chronic Lyme disease.

I hope the world hears you—loud and clear!

Now I will conclude with my own definition of Lyme disease, in the clearest language possible, based on everything I've learned to this point. Many thanks to Kathleen Dickson and Beaux Reliosis, as well as Anthony William, Judy Mikovits and many others for this hard-won grasp on a disease that is so highly complex. And while this disease is still not entirely understood, continuing to decode the mechanisms by which it is transmitted, persists and destroys our health is of course necessary before any fully effective treatment solutions can be found:

Chronic Lyme disease (which is often seronegative) is a disabling, complex, multisystem, post sepsis illness of immunosuppression likened to a B-cell AIDS.

Borreliae, the causative organisms, damage essential lymph node structure while B cells mutated by Epstein-Barr virus (EBV) become non-functional and are unable to undergo programmed cell death.

Outcomes include multiple infections of the central nervous system, including reactivated herpesviruses, and systemic opportunistic infections—bacterial, viral, fungal, and parasitic.

OspA—a fungal-type toxin and one of the major antigens of Borrelia burgdorferi—is the main detonator, causing a septic response, immune system damage and chronic illness. This antigen can be transmitted in a number of ways ... including ticks.

Chronic Lyme disease (or OspA) is known as the New Great Imitator (or detonator) mimicking hundreds of other conditions primarily due to the reactivation of the latent herpesviruses.

Oh how I miss those earlier days when I thought chronic Lyme disease was simply about ticks.

The Gut—A Missing Link

I was visiting my son in NYC. He had just had another three-month relapse and we were working hard to help him get back to a more stable place. For a few months, he had been struggling with an even more pronounced "leaky gut," which for a while now we believed was the primary cause of his continual brain fog, achiness, chronic fatigue, and other flu-like symptoms. Of course, every relapse sets me into panic while he remains calm and steady.

Why can't he get better? Why does he keep taking multiple steps back? Is the bacteria still active in his system? What is going on in his body that is not allowing him to secure a steadier course of recovery? A highly compromised immune system, no doubt.

Upon several recommendations, Matt ordered the book

Eat Dirt: Why Leaky Gut May Be the Root Cause of Your Health Problems and 5 Surprising Steps to Cure It by Dr. Josh Axe, a chiropractor and naturopath. In this ground-breaking work, Dr. Axe explains that 70 percent of our immune system is located in the gut. When the gut is compromised or permeable due to a number of factors, including an imbalance of good and bad bacteria, environmental toxins, inflammatory foods, and overmedicating, our immune system becomes compromised and so does our general health. When you have a leaky gut, which Matt's LLND diagnosed, a number of factors can lead to a breakdown of the intestinal wall, allowing food, bacteria, and toxins to seep into the bloodstream. This is what Dr. D. was trying to tell us many months ago. Dr. Axe's book has helped Matt understand this in more detail.

So how does a leaky gut relate to Lyme?

When Matt read *Eat Dirt*, a lightbulb went on for him. No, make that a floodlight.

After searching, reading, guessing, analyzing, and consulting so many healers and practitioners about his health for almost four years, thanks to the work of Dr. Axe, Matt now has a new theory about chronic Lyme disease—a theory that says that the rest of us in Lymeland may have it all backward. Matt now believes that everything we have read and understood about chronic Lyme disease to date may actually be *the tail wagging the dog.*

Matt conjectured: What if his illness all began because of a leaky gut that he may have always had? What if his leaky gut, which once kept the *Bb* bacteria in check, somehow became compromised, allowing all of these antigens to enter his system, which ultimately wreaked havoc?

This, by the way, doesn't change the theory of OspA as

the immune system detonator with chronic Lyme. It doesn't change the theory of *Bb* bacteria as a destructive pathogen. It merely speaks to the potential passageway that *Bb* and OspA, and perhaps the once-dormant EB virus, may have had to Matt's being—his brain, his nervous system, his liver, his cellular environment—making this thing we call Lyme a systemic and chronic disease.

"Why," he wondered aloud, "do so many people carry the *Bb* bacteria and they don't all necessarily become chronically ill?

"Why is it said that we are bacteria living a human experience, that our bodies are host to millions of microbes, rendering our microbiome an influential driver, unique to each and every one of us?

"With regard to the *Bb* bacteria and its transmission of OspA, why is it that only 20 percent of people see the tick that bites them, and the other 80 percent are sick without clear evidence of causation?

"Why is it that there is a 'whack-a-mole' approach to the treatment of this disease we know as chronic Lyme and no one—not even LLMDs—are looking at it from a 10,000-foot view, but rather playing guessing games, and treating isolated symptoms only?

"What if we flipped the current paradigm—that is, killing the bacteria as the first-line treatment response—to healing the gut instead?" Matt wondered. "What if a leaky gut is the missing link, the primary reason as to why Lyme is the New Great Imitator, mimicking 350-plus medical conditions of an autoimmune and immunosuppressive nature? What if a leaky gut is the key to unlocking all these conditions and more?"

Matt explained, "Mostly, I think it is important to understand that Lyme is not necessarily the great imitator, but rather all these diseases with overlapping symptoms perhaps come from the same place—a leaky gut."

He reminded me: "Remember how Dr. D.'s testing showed my immune system was working hard but inefficiently? This also corroborates my theory that things are entering my system through my gut that shouldn't be there (i.e., food, toxins, pathogens) and they are giving my immune system too much work to do, causing it to be inefficient and attacking everything almost indiscriminately, not just the dangerous pathogens, and thereby causing systemic inflammation."

Now, after all that he's experienced, all the reading we've done, all the people we've consulted with and all the guesswork that has been and continues to be required of him, Matt believes he has found a missing puzzle piece that may allow him to take a giant step toward recovery from this disease. He now firmly believes that recovery for him—and perhaps all Lyme sufferers—starts and ends with the gut. He now knows with certainty that the gut is the gatekeeper to pathogens and toxins, and when it's leaky, these pathogens and toxins, including Borrelia and OspA, wreak havoc on his immune system. He now gets that the gut is the protector of his overall health, and if his gut is not strong, then all kinds of bacteria, including Borrelia, can lead to a multisystem, immunosuppressive, post sepsis, AIDS-like illness we know as chronic Lyme.

Matt may have been bitten by a tick, or not. Or he may have carried Borrelia since birth. We simply don't know. What is clear, however, is that his gut is leaky, his gut has clouded his cellular terrain (which we witnessed with our very own eyes under a dark field microscope), and that his leaky gut has compromised his immune system and is keeping him chronically ill. What Matt now believes is that until his gut is healed, he won't fully recover. And that no amount of antibiotics designed to kill the bacteria will heal his gut—but, in fact, will only damage it further.

It leaves us puzzled still. How is it that so many attest that their recovery is due to the use of long-term antibiotics? Why is it that Matt's system couldn't tolerate this protocol beyond his initial six-month acute phase? Why is it that his lingering symptoms all seem to be gut-related? How did he fall into an acute phase of illness one week after having a flu shot? How exactly did the flu shot tip the scales on his gut, opening the floodgates to the bacteria in his system and further destroying his already compromised immune system?

It might have eliminated some of the madness for us if just one of the forty-plus and counting medical professionals that Matt has seen over the past four years could have put the full picture together for us—helping us to understand the significance of this missing puzzle piece. But alas, no one we've come across has even made mention of the gut, save for his LLND whose practice is so full that Matt can only get to see him once every four months. This doctor has been the closest by a long shot in recognizing this issue and treating accordingly. And for that we are grateful. So, along with his guidance, Matt will keep attending to his leaky gut in the hopes that this will take him where he needs to go for a full recovery.

What I Know for Sure

Here's the one and only thing that I know for sure: healing chronic Lyme disease will *never* take place within the narrow confines of allopathic medicine.

So whether you use a Rife machine, a low-level laser,

ozone therapy, IV light therapy, CBD, bioresonance, infra-red saunas, GcMAF, supplements that resonate, and a very clean diet, or whether you decide to try the latest and great-est invention that comes along tomorrow, you have a far bet-ter chance of getting closer to recovery than waiting for Big Pharma to rescue you. *That's never going to happen.*

So I know that Matt has to keep trying new things that just might make him feel better, and years of antibiotics is NOT the answer for him, as it is not the answer for many. Yes, this approach is expensive, challenging, and not a straight line. Yes, we have to beware of charlatans who take advantage of the sick and infirm. And yes, it can be extremely frustrating, discouraging, disheartening.

But if we don't keep trying new things, then hope will die. And I, for one, am not prepared to give up hope—ever.

The Heart Speaks

My heart has taken a beating—so many times and for so many reasons in my life.

My father's death thirty-plus years ago. Financial ups and downs. My mother's death from Alzheimer's (*or was it Lyme?*) just last December.

With Matt's illness, my heart broke into a thousand tiny pieces, in a way that I last felt at age twenty-five when my father was sick and dying. In both of these life crises, it felt like the ground was pulled out from under me, that my energy and life force was sucked dry, and that my heart would never be whole again.

But the truth is that when our heart breaks, it can be the gateway—painful though it might be—to heart opening, heart strengthening, heart resilience, heart connections, and a deeper, heart-driven life.

It's not easy to remember all of this when our life is crumbling and our heart is being shattered. In those moments, we only see a dark, negative, scary abyss of emptiness. We think we can't go on—but we do. We don't see possibilities—but they're there. And when we get to the other side of brokenness, we emerge a stronger, better, more whole, more integrated, more congruent, and empathic being.

I have learned to embrace my broken heart. It's what guides me, connects me, allows the light to shine through. It's the very thing that allows me to deeply touch others and let others deeply touch me.

My heartbreak was validated by Ketut, a Balinese medicine man whom I had the good fortune of meeting on my writing retreat. This ninety-year-old man with dark, weathered skin, bright blue eyes, and a luminous white smile offered an experience to behold. It was my very own 'Eat, Pray, Love" moment.

His office (an open-air deck adorned with statues of the Hindu gods) opens to patients at 8:00 a.m. Tourists and locals line up to see him. He takes each person, one at a time, and for 300,000 rupiahs—the equivalent of twenty American dollars (which we later learned he will use for his great-grandchildren's education)—he offers ten minutes of his undivided attention. He begins the session by putting his hands on the crown of your head, your neck, and your sinuses—trying to determine the lay of the land.

Then he motioned for me to lie down on a mat, asked me how old I was, and proceeded to tell me that I have recently had a very stressful, traumatic time. He said that while I am getting better, my heart has been covered with a lot of scars. "A lot of scars," he repeats.

This sounds like a cookie-cutter diagnosis—one that

could apply to anyone. Who, after all, doesn't have heartbreak in their lives? But after consulting with my friends who joined me on this excursion, his diagnosis and treatment was very particular to each one of us. His was not a one-size-fits-all approach.

Using a hard, plastic stick, Ketut then proceeded to poke my toes—starting with the smallest one. When he got to my middle toe, the pain was so severe, I winced and pulled away. He poked at it again. Again, I winced and pulled away.

"That is your heart," he said, pointing to my middle toe—the toe that made me want to go through the roof when he poked at it.

"Very scarred. Very scarred. You have a lot of stress and trauma in your life. You worry a lot. Your heart is scarred. Many scars. We must get rid of the scars."

He stood over me, moving his arms, chanting and pulling my energy to him and waving the energy away. He sat down again, tested the same toe with his medicine-man stick, and, lo and behold, there was no pain. He used the same stick to draw an X across my heart three times, then he said, "There—you have no more scars. Your heart is new. Empty. Clear. You must stop worrying."

He took a long, hard look at the necklace I was wearing—a medallion-shaped pendant with the word *love* inside—and, holding it between his fingers, he finished our session by saying, "There, that's all that you put in your heart now. No more worries. Just love."

The session was over. I felt light and free.

My greatest lesson going forward is to remember to find some kind of balance in heartbreak and uncertainty. To remember there is always light, even in the darkness.

The magic of life lies in the ebb and flow of ambiguity,

how we handle the "not knowing." The magic lies in how gracefully we bend and twist with the forces, rather than our programmed response to push and resist.

Grace under pressure has never been my thing. I am learning, though. And I am getting better at it.

By writing this book, I've rediscovered the power of channeling my angst and heartbreak into something positive that will both contain and share my emotions. Something that allows me to connect with others who are also suffering, while helping and serving them along the way.

Expressive writing—journaling, poetry, prose—has tremendous benefits for one's mood, health, and well-being. The power of writing—and then rewriting—your personal story has great therapeutic effects, as we change our narrative from one of a victim stance to a hero's journey. Writing down your worries allows you to have a container for them so you don't have to lug them around all the time. It takes a load off.

Practicing gratitude is also powerful. The word *gratitude* comes from the Latin *gratia*, which means graciousness, grace, or gratefulness. The practice of gratitude is known to be able to increase our happiness quotient by forty percent. Gratitude is a powerful tool, but difficult to practice when we're suffering. It may sound simple, but it's not easy. Nothing worthwhile ever is.

To exercise our "gratitude muscle," we have to get into the habit of writing down things we're grateful for every single day. It can be one thing. It can be ten. But it needs to be a dedicated practice to keep our perspective fresh, positive, and buoyant.

Meditation is another practice that we need to dedicate ourselves to—in good times and in bad. The daily practice of meditation—whether we do it for five minutes or fifty—reminds us to breathe. It reminds us to be connected to our heart and to keep it open. It reminds us that we're not alone. It reminds us that there is a force bigger than we are—a force that will guide us through. Meditation can help us with all kinds of mental and physical disease and discomfort. It may create discomfort at first. But that will all dissipate while the benefits of regulating our moods and providing a vacation for our thoughts will become clear. As Deepak Chopra tells us, "Meditation is not a way of making your mind quiet. It is a way of entering into the quiet that is already there—buried under the 50,000 thoughts the average person thinks every day."

Moving our bodies is also a critical life lesson in our stuck times. Our natural inclination is to freeze, stay very still, and perhaps the nightmare will end. But we have to fight that instinct and push ourselves to walk, do yoga, Pilates, cycle, hike, swim. Whatever you do to move your body will help your energy to get unstuck and will help your mind to stop perseverating.

Above all, we have to remember to get out of our own way—by getting out of our heads, listening to the wisdom of our heart center, laughing often and freely, celebrating small moments, connecting with loved ones, and trusting that good things will come.

We have to continually look for ways to shift our own thought paradigms in order to heal from deep inside. Answers are clearly not going to come from outside of ourselves——from the people and places we once depended on.

As David R. Hawkins, an internationally renowned psychiatrist, consciousness researcher, spiritual lecturer, and mystic wrote in *Power vs. Force*, "In every studied case of recovery from hopeless and untreatable disease, there has been a major shift in consciousness, so that the attractor patterns that resulted in the pathologic process no longer dominated."

There is no simple blueprint to put this concept into action. A major shift in consciousness takes a great deal of time, focus, and effort. But it is doable, and we must all keep searching for ways to get there.

Ultimately, what I know for sure, is that we cannot really cure anyone of their pain and suffering. We can only help carry them through it. Which I certainly hope will be enough as I continue to stand by Matt's side.

My Hopes and Dreams—If I So Dare

What hasn't fully killed me in this lifetime has made me stronger. More resilient. Wiser. What choice have I had?

With each and every challenge, I grow and stretch in ways that are uncomfortable, in ways that I never imagined, in ways that really matter—building heart, courage and resilience.

It takes tremendous heartbreak—over and over again—to emerge a different soul. Like the phoenix rising from the ashes, I have done this more times than I care to count.

With each and every crisis, I have emerged more open-hearted, more flexible, and much less fussed about the small stuff, for the most part. Not in a saintly kind of way. And not without a great deal of pain and suffering. But in a more evolved, core strength, grounded kind of way.

As Kahlil Gibran, the Lebanese-American artist and poet said, "Out of suffering have emerged the strongest souls; the most massive characters are seared with scars."

In one of my very favorite books, *Survival Lessons*, writer Alice Hoffman says, "In many ways, I wrote *Survival Lessons* to remind me of the beauty of life, something's that all too easy to overlook during the crisis of illness or loss."

The purpose of writing this book has been to heal my own heart during this crisis, and, in doing so, to help you heal yours, I hope.

After four-plus years of Matt's health journey, during the brief moments when his health seems to improve, I feel like we might be ready to move along. To let go a bit. To trust that this crisis will one day pass. That he will recover—and so will I.

I'm slowly regaining my faith in Matt's future, and I'm once again seeing and believing in the full and exceptional life that lies ahead for him.

This journey has stripped us all of so much: Faith. Hope. Time. Opportunities. Dreams.

My relationships have suffered. As has my own health and well-being. It's been a single-focused period where the rest of the world has necessarily faded away. Where my world has been nothing but Lyme, Lyme, and more Lyme.

Suffering—especially chronic suffering—can be an enormous burden. We are sometimes forced to live a smaller, more insular life. A more internal, isolated experience, trapped in a parallel universe where it often feels like us versus the rest of the world.

We are forced to live in a constant state of vulnerability, made to examine and reexamine the meaning of our life, often recoiling from and resenting what once seemed normal and easy and pure. What we once took so easily for granted.

Suffering often forces us to be hyperfocused on the small things. The little things we can control. The simple things that allow us to breathe. That may give us just a brief moment of pleasure.

Of course, we all respond to suffering in our own idiosyncratic way. I marvel at the strength and resilience that my son has mustered in his suffering, as well as the courage of so many others that I've met along the way.

I was recently introduced to the concept of "sisu," a word used to describe the Finnish spirit of endurance, tenacity, resilience, and perseverance. Urban Dictionary explains, "It doesn't take sisu to go to the North Pole; it takes sisu to stand at the door when the bear is on the other side." Sisu requires us to confront our challenges head-on, every day, despite the obstacles before us, taking small—sometimes large—meaningful actions, while standing in the face of heartache and fear. Matt and I have clearly practiced sisu for years now. We just didn't know that it had such a poetic name. And we will continue to practice sisu together until he recovers his health—and beyond. It's all we know to do.

I want to believe that it's time. Time to move out of the suffering and begin to trust that Matt is on a positive healing path. I want to put an end to my chronic worrying. To depart from Lymeland for a bit, get out of this insane rabbit hole, and move into not Alice's but some other glorious Wonderland—where, during my month in Bali, for a very short while, I felt like I had landed.

While in Bali, I was so grateful to be there. It's a magical, spiritual place, perfectly appointed across continents, so far from home.

Bali means "mighty warrior." That's Matt. That's me. That's all of you Lyme sufferers and loved ones.

There was no doubt that I had come to the right place.

Bali is a place where the ocean cradles the sun. A place where the sky illuminates with colors so saturated and rich that they appear otherworldly. A place where there is great reverence, unspeakable beauty, humility, and grace. A place where the heart sings.

Bali is the island of gods—and I could feel it at work in everything I encountered. Vibrations that elevate. Volcanoes that erupt. Geckos that "gecko" all night long. Plumeria that lovingly dust the pavement. Prayer beads and offerings that lay at your feet in pure abundance.

I hope that my book helps you find your own healing path—whatever that might be.

I pray that together we continue to work diligently so that each and every one of you will receive the medical support, the recognition, the understanding, the validation, the heart, the soul, the caring, the empathy that you so deserve.

Above all, I pray for a way for everyone to get well while keeping our hearts wide open, our wits about us, and our souls eternally grateful for the support we have shown one another.

I am grateful for each and every one of you. I'm in awe of your unending courage and your warrior spirit.

Ubuntu. Namaste. I see you, I honor you, and I reflect back the divinity in you.

Together, let's find our way out of this crazy, mad rabbit hole—healthy, whole, renewed.

POSTSCRIPT
STORIES OF SUFFERING, RESILIENCE, AND HEALING

"I can't go back to yesterday because I was a different person then."

—ALICE'S ADVENTURES IN WONDERLAND

This section is heartfully, tearfully, lovingly devoted to all chronic Lyme sufferers far and wide. A section to satisfy the most basic of human needs—the need to have our stories known.

Here I share with you twelve chronic Lyme stories. These stories, written with great courage and the need to be heard, are about pain and suffering, fear and anger, confusion and madness, frustration and hopelessness, resilience and hope. Above all, these stories are about lessons in faith, perseverance, and survival.

I am grateful to those who have agreed to share their stories here with you in Lyme Madness. There are so many more personal Lyme journeys that I would have included if I'd had the space. Just know that I appreciate everyone's contribution, your willingness to put your hearts and vulnerabilities on the page, your openness to tell your Lyme stories in alarming detail.

I know that each and every one of your stories will resonate with millions worldwide. You, after all, are *the* voice of chronic Lyme disease, the voice of the infirm and downtrodden who will one day find truth and healing on this mad, mad journey called chronic Lyme.

Our stories—written, expressed aloud, and truly heard—connect us, bond us, comfort us, help us to feel less isolated, less alone. Let's keep sharing our stories as we work together to create change.

The Better Health Guy's Lyme Story

From Wrecked to Recovered by Scott Forsgren
Imagine a life where you seemingly have it all. Imagine wanting for nothing more, except for the continuance of your already blessed life. Actually, I never really wished for that as I always took it for granted.

Now imagine that almost overnight it is taken away. This is how it happened to me. It all began with what seemed like a viral infection, and in just a few short days had become a major illness which continued to baffle the best medicine had to offer for days, weeks, months, and even years. My life was forever changed.

Imagine the fear one feels when presented with the unknown. Imagine the isolation and the desperation that one might experience when being confronted with a serious, unknown illness that, at the time, felt as though it literally could have taken my life. Unfortunately, it does not take imagination to understand what this might feel like; for this had become what was left of me.

Imagine a constant burning sensation throughout your entire body that is at times almost unbearable. My body burned like someone had poured acid on it. Beyond the physical pain, there was the emotional pain, which was generated by the uncertainty of what had become my existence.

Imagine having a fever that lasts for over a year, all the while having doctors and others trying to convince you that it might be "normal." In your heart, you know that this is far from normal, but you find it impossible to convince anyone that it is a sign of something gone seriously awry.

Imagine that you no longer have to imagine what it is like to feel sick day in and day out. Suddenly, it becomes you. You become it. Nothing else matters except the quest to return to your previous life. In fact, this was a new life filled with fear as well as physical and emotional pain unlike anything I had experienced in the past.

I remember it all so vividly from head to toe. Odd tingling sensations ran through my body. My vision was blurred more often than not. My ears were full of pressure and popped with every swallow.

Walking was a challenge due to the weak muscles in my legs. For several months, I could barely walk at all. Of course, that fueled my fears that I had a serious neurological disease. Simpler physical acts were also surprisingly difficult. Sitting in a chair proved challenging as my balance was off. I constantly felt as though I was falling to one side. No matter how much I propped myself up, the falling feeling never went away.

I always felt as though I was going to roll off the bed and land on the floor.

Every muscle in my body was sore and every joint even sorer. I cannot count the nights that I cried myself to sleep due to the intense pain. It seemed to get worse as time went on, and I knew that the illness was progressing and the need for answers grew stronger and stronger each day. I would stare at my hands and feet, feel the pain, and wonder what it was that was causing it. It was undoubtedly the biggest mystery I would be faced with in my life, and I set my sights on solving it.

I had muscle twitches throughout my body. Eventually, almost every muscle in my body would at one time or another have these annoying little reminders that something was wrong.

My stomach was an entire set of problems and symptoms in and of itself. It hurt all the time. There was an intense burning that never seemed to end. If there was a list of GI symptoms that one could have, I certainly had almost all of them.

Imagine a motor-like, tapping sensation felt continuously in your arms, legs, and feet. Twenty-four hours a day, I felt this constant tapping sensation. Imagine that every doctor to whom you described this sensation looked at you with a blank stare as if to say they had no idea what was causing the problem; or if the problem was even real.

Imagine the day that you open a book which describes a "motor-like" sensation as a symptom of something called "Chronic Fatigue Syndrome." Imagine you search the Internet to find information on CFS which states that, "The illness varies greatly in its duration. A few recover after a year or two. More often, those who recover are more likely to do so from 3 to 6 years after onset. Others may recover after a decade or more. Yet for some, the illness seems to simply persist." Great, so now I had a disease which had no known cause or origin, no known cure, and even worse, it could last for decades. Oh, the fear and desperation that I felt, and yet, I could think of nothing more than to continue the quest to research and figure out how to get myself out of this situation. I was certainly not giving up!

Imagine that one day you find out that the cause of your unexplained illness is actually "Lyme Disease" and all of its not-so-delicious trimmings. Imagine you find a doctor that specializes in your particular illness and becomes your biggest mentor and influence as you now have something tangible to work with. Imagine that you work hard over the next several years to make a comeback. It takes work, hard work. You struggle. You sacrifice. You listen, not only to your doctors, but to your own body and your inner-wisdom.

After eight years of being seriously ill, I found Dr. Dietrich Klinghardt, MD, PhD in Seattle, Washington, to whom today I express infinite gratitude for having changed my life in so many ways. It was his "Klinghardt Axiom" that became the blueprint for my recovery. It was the understanding that getting well is about much more than killing infections and that the infections themselves are often not always even the most important thing to address. It was learning about toxicity and how toxins are a significant factor in why we become ill *in the first place. All of this occurs within the backdrop of emotional conflicts and traumas that we have experienced within our lifetime. The axiom is about the inter-relationship between emotions, toxins, and infections and how we must focus on all of these simultaneously to truly regain health and wellness.*

When I first started down my Lyme recovery journey, I was certain that infections were the most important thing to address and that I could kill my way back to health. Then, I began to understand that toxicity was an important consideration. I put the emotional contributors last on the list at the time; even though I knew I could certainly benefit from some work in this realm. Today, I see things exactly the opposite. Getting one's emotional health in order is a top priority. Feeling we deserve to be well and remediating any false beliefs is critical. Detoxification became a major area of focus, and as time progressed, infections became less and less of a consideration. I ultimately went from viewing infections, toxins, and emotions as my priorities to an understanding that it was really emotions, toxins, and then infections.

Dr. Klinghardt pushed me to think outside of normally accepted ideas. I had to consider a number of new concepts such as how living in an environment with toxic mold impacts health, how parasites affect us, how electromagnetic fields add further stress to our already weakened bodies, the impact of diet on inflammation and immune health, and how other factors such as underlying dental issues contribute to the imbalances that we perceive as illness. The next several years became a process of removing stressful items while adding numerous health-promoting ones to shift the balance back to my favor. It was not easy, but it was so worth it.

Imagine that little by little you improve. It takes time. In fact, at times, the improvement seems so slow that you almost don't notice that you are still improving, but you are. Imagine that one day, you don't think of yourself as having an illness anymore.

Imagine that you learn so much from the struggle and gain so many unexpected gifts along the way that you never again look at life in the same way. Imagine that life is good and you feel at peace...at last you feel peace. Imagine, you are well.

Now, this was at one time hard for me to imagine, but fortunately, it did not take imagination because this became my reality. In my wildest imagination, I could not have believed that I would ever have gotten back to the place that I am today; I have literally gone from wrecked to recovered. I am truly blessed and forever grateful. Hope abounds...

Scott Forsgren is a blogger, health writer, advocate, and coach. He is the editor and founder of BetterHealthGuy. com, where he shares his nineteen-year journey through the world of Lyme disease and the myriad of factors that it often entails. He has been interviewed on Lyme Ninja Radio, Lyme Less Live More, Essential Medcast, and Beyond Wellness Radio. He has been fortunate to have written for publications such as *Townsend Letter, Public Health Alert, Explore,* and others. He serves on the board of directors of LymeLight Foundation, which provides treatment grants to children and young adults dealing with Lyme disease. Today, Scott is grateful for his current state of health and all that he has learned on this life-changing journey.

Dietrich Klinghardt, MD, PhD, is founder and medical director of Sophia Health Institute in Woodinville, Washington, where he treats patients with complex chronic illnesses. More information on his clinical practice can be found at www.sophiahi.com. To learn more about his work, Klinghardt Institute can be found at www.klinghardtinstitute.com. Scott is eternally grateful to Dr. Klinghardt for having touched his life and the lives of so many through his unique approaches to healing.

Source: The "Klinghardt Axiom" was discussed in a previous article entitled "Microbes, Toxins, Unresolved Emotional Conflicts: A Unifying Theory," which can be found at www.betterhealthguy.com/axiom.

Chickswithticks' Lyme Story

Healthy to Sick...in Just a Matter of Days
Most people with Lyme disease will describe the subtle creeping of symptoms over months, years, or even decades until they realized something was wrong or until they were finally diagnosed.

My Lyme story is atypical, in that I went from very healthy and active to very sick, almost in a matter of days.

In August of 2013, I decided to clear out an area of my yard that had been untouched for the 7 previous years we lived in our house. I spent about a week pulling weeds and overgrowth from a shady, treed and rocky area, and because I didn't know what poison ivy looked like, I wound up with a very severe rash on both of my arms. A nuisance, but tolerable.

After 2 weeks of scratching, the rash started appearing in other places. I had taken the summer off to be with my children and was scheduled to go back to work the following week. I wasn't too excited to start working again with this ugly and uncomfortable rash, so I got a short course of Prednisone to help clear it up. The doctor told me to take the first dose with food, so I ate a salad with shrimp on it.

About 20 minutes later I went into anaphylaxis. I recognized what was happening and was able to call 911 in time and luckily they were very fast. The paramedics spent 45 minutes saving my life on my front doorstep, and I was given even more steroids at the emergency room to stop the allergic reaction. On top of that I was advised to finish up my taper pack of Prednisone. Note: steroids suppress your immune system.

A blood test revealed I had developed an allergy to shellfish, a food I had eaten all my life. It seemed like an unfortunate turn of events, to have the poison ivy and then the life threatening allergic reaction at the same time. I had no idea how bad things were about to get.

Over that next week I felt unwell but chalked it up to the Prednisone. By then it was Labor Day weekend. My husband was working out of the country during all this so I took my children to the National Zoo and did some more gardening and tried to plow through not feeling right. On Monday of the holiday weekend, also the day before my children were to start the new school year, I became much sicker and thought I was having a heart attack. A friend took me to the ER where I found out my blood pressure was really high (normally it is low) and I was having tachycardia (a high heart rate). The ER doctor told me I was dehydrated, gave me a bag of saline and sent me home. I have not felt right since.

So began my journey. I developed more and more symptoms and felt poorly all of the time. My heart raced and pounded out of my chest even when I was sleeping, I was severely lightheaded, fatigued, shaky, I could not sleep at night and had a feeling of malaise at all times. More symptoms began and kept changing, all over my body. My blood sugar fluctuated with highs and lows despite a careful diet, I started losing weight, lost my appetite, had a constant tummy ache, my skin was flushing and I got hives, I started feeling anxious and sad and over emotional. It was as if my entire body was completely out of whack in every way. Could it be perimenopause? Was it my hormones or my cortisol or my thyroid or my adrenals? I spent all of my time researching my symptoms but they were all over the place.

I went from doctor to doctor trying to find an answer. Cardiologists, Endocrinologists, Neurologists, Allergists, multiple Internists, test after test after test, vials and vials of blood, all coming back "NORMAL!" I even had 2 Western blots, knowing I live in a highly endemic area for Lyme disease. Herds of deer are in my yard daily, I gardened in this same yard and have 2 dogs who at the time slept with us. Not to mention all of the time outdoors with my children for sports and nature walks. Both Western blots were negative and since I had none of the symptoms listed on the CDC page for Lyme disease...no headache, no neck ache, no joint pain, no fever, no known tick bite, no bulls eye rash...I didn't think of it again. I have since learned it is a law in Virginia for doctors to notify patients that a negative does not mean you do not have Lyme, and that it should always be a clinical diagnosis. No doctor gave me this important information.

Multiple friends suggested I had Lyme disease. I tried acupuncture hoping it would set me right and the acupuncturist within 5 minutes of talking to me told me he thought I had Lyme disease. No, I insisted. I was tested, twice. I was negative, and at the time I actually believed the blood test was accurate. Plus, I didn't have the "right" symptoms that mainstream medical websites told me I would have if I was exposed to Lyme disease. One friend had me watch Under Our Skin, *the documentary about Lyme. (Highly recommend this movie if you have not seen it, and there is a follow up to it out now called* Emergence.) *Fascinating, but it further solidified my belief I didn't have Lyme since none of the people in the film had my same collection of symptoms.*

I practically had to be hit with a 2x4 by my friends to consider it was Lyme all along. I learned the Western blot is about as accurate as a coin toss and does not test for 2 very Lyme specific bands. That you need to pass a "pre-requisite" ELISA test before you may even have a Western blot performed and then you have to have 5 positive bands for it to be considered positive for Lyme disease. Most people have no idea they were bitten by a tick. *Many never develop the rash. There are over 300 symptoms of Lyme and it can imitate many other diseases, including but not limited to fibromyalgia, chronic fatigue syndrome, MS, ALS, Alzheimer's, Parkinson's, psychiatric disorders and depression, arthritis, ADHD, autism, lupus, and "the aches and pains of growing older." Most doctors have no training in Lyme and rely on the very outdated CDC and IDSA guidelines, so it is often missed.*

I finally got myself to a local and highly recommended integrative medicine doctor. I didn't know it at the time but she is also an LLMD—meaning a Lyme Literate Medical Doctor. Our first appointment was for one hour. Within that hour she recommended I get tested for Lyme, which she thought I may have, through IGeneX lab in California. They are the gold standard for Lyme testing and most doctors have never heard of them, or if they have, they are suspect of the results. My test came back unquestionably positive, meeting the CDC criteria.

I am still angry and sad and disappointed that I spent over 5 months going to doctors begging for an answer when it took one doctor who is trained to recognize Lyme less than 60 minutes to help me. For many with undiagnosed Lyme, it takes much longer, even years or decades to figure it out. How different my life would have been if I would have been correctly diagnosed at the beginning—possibly when I was first infected—and a short, inexpensive course of antibiotics may have been all I needed. I remember how I was dismissed by the first practitioner I went to. She ran blood work and referred me to a cardiologist. When nothing was revealed by either, she looked at me point blank and said, "I don't know what to do with you." She was done with me.

I was told by all of the other doctors after her I was perfectly healthy and that it was probably stress—even though the only thing in my life that was stressful was the fact I knew I was very sick and nobody was taking it seriously because all of my lab work was always in range.

The thing is with Lyme, if you see the tick, or get the rash, and you get it treated right away with a therapeutic dose of antibiotics, you are probably good. But when ticks are the size of a poppy seed and they hide in your parts or in your hair and they anesthetize you when they bite you so you never feel it and you never get a rash and doctors—even in highly Lyme endemic areas—are not well informed about Lyme, you can get very, very sick. By the time you know something is wrong you have lost that precious window to effectively treat it. The Lyme bacteria leaves the bloodstream (hence why the blood test is often unreliable) and corkscrews itself deep into your body where it can hide from both your immune system and antibiotics. Then it forms a sticky substance over itself called a biofilm, making it even more difficult to ever get rid of it.

Being bit by a tick is like being stuck with a dirty needle that you don't know what's in it, so you don't really know how to treat it. Ticks carry more than just Lyme disease. There are a whole host of different co-infections as well as viruses and who knows what else, that they regurgitate into your bloodstream. As if that isn't tricky enough, there are about 100 strains of Lyme disease in the US and about 300 worldwide. Oh, and by the way, the traditional Western blot tests for...ready...one strain. The Western blot was developed over 25 years ago, for statistical purposes, not diagnostic, yet it has never been updated.

Since my diagnosis on February 1, 2014 I have been in continual treatment with oral antibiotics, months of IV antibiotics that I administered myself through a port in my arm leading to my heart, more natural herbal and homeopathic remedies, a very long list of supplements, Reiki, earthing and essential oils. I wish I could write that I am better, and that I was in remission. Unfortunately, as is the case with tens of thousands of people worldwide (maybe more), I have only become sicker with treatment. Lyme is very hard to eradicate. It can hide, it can form a biofilm over itself to unleash on you at a later time, it can go into cyst form, and when it does die it releases toxins into your body that can make you even sicker than when it was alive (it is called herxing which is slang for a Herxheimer reaction, and is just as bad as the name sounds). If you have any of the many genetic mutations (like I do) that hinders your ability to detox well, it makes everything even harder. Same goes for mold or heavy metals (mercury or amalgam fillings for example), if you have those stored up, that is another issue to address. Add in that you may not know what other co infections you are dealing with, and that Lyme can cause an autoimmune response in your body and reactivate dormant viruses you already had, and you are dealing with a very complex illness.

The first month of treatment some of my initial symptoms went away for good but completely new ones appeared. I started getting the moving arthritis and thought, where were you when I needed you, I might have realized it was Lyme sooner! Some of those have resolved, but now I am dealing with debilitating leg weakness and nerve pains. I have lost my ability to stand or walk for long. I use a cane, and when I am having a really bad day, a walker or a wheelchair. Some days I cannot drive. I have numbness, burning, tingling and back pain, and I hope that this peripheral nervous system damage can be reversed. Right now my Lyme is masquerading like MS (2 different neurologists have cleared me through MRIs and a lumbar puncture as not having MS, both believe it is entirely tick borne for me, and by the way, it is widely believed many with MS actually have Lyme disease at the root). To say Lyme disease has drastically altered my life is an understatement and there doesn't seem to be an end in sight. Some days I am functional and some days I am not, so far I haven't had a day where I have felt as good as I did before becoming ill. I would have preferred to have made this website AFTER I had recovered, because everyone likes to read a happy ending, but treating Lyme is like peeling an onion, with many complicated layers, and I know it will take time before my body recovers from this.

I recently read a great list, written by another "Lyme warrior," as we are called. It was a list of things she learned from late stage Lyme. One really spoke to me. To paraphrase, she said that asking "Why Me?" just proves to the Universe that you haven't learned the answer yet, and nothing goes away until it teaches us what we need to know. I guess I will be struggling with Lyme for a little while longer because I admit I have not learned this yet. I had already had my share of struggle in my young lifetime. I had another very serious illness as a teenager where I slowly (mostly) recovered from waist down paralysis (now my doctors think this may have been Lyme disease at work back when I was 16—tick paralysis—and living in a different highly endemic Lyme area of the country) and then when I was pregnant with my first child, my seemingly very healthy first husband died suddenly of a massive heart attack. So I already knew REALLY well how important health is and what to assign importance to in my life. I didn't think I needed more lessons, but my epic battle with Lyme disease is telling me otherwise. The only good that has come, and the only "reason" I can see, is I had the rest of my family tested and found out 3/4 of us had Lyme. My hope is my suffering from this disease will now have headed off any future suffering for my children, since we were given the opportunity to know they were infected before they fell ill from this disease as well.

The most genuine way I can express my gratitude to my dear friends who helped me toward the right diagnosis is to pay that forward. This site is created with that purpose. I have become a walking and talking Lyme-o-pedia of knowledge and resources which I share freely here (and on my Twitter and Facebook pages!) to raise awareness. What happened to me is not unusual, and keeps happening, so let's all help each other by getting the word out what Lyme really is—a plague that is growing worldwide but that most doctors, insurance companies, and governments refuse to acknowledge.[213]

Nancy's Lyme Story

My Life Is Ticking Away

I am Nancy Wheeler, age 68, and I am infected with Lyme/Bartonella. My story is my own, but I have come to understand that it is similar to others.

I arrived at age 67, basically in perfect health. No medications, no sickness, and still functioning on my own. One day, in April of 2014, I was walking our two dogs in the woods on our land adjacent to our house. Everything went as usual or so I thought. To make a long story short, later on that same day, I discovered what looked like a speck of dust on my left calf. I carefully removed it with a tweezers and realized that it was a tick. I thought the head was out, so I flushed it down the toilet, put some ointment on the post and continued my day.

About three days later, my left ankle was swollen and then four days later, my knee on my left leg was suffering and aching. Seven days after the bite, I was at my family doctor's office. He didn't think it was anything although it was plain to see the bite mark. He said, "No bulls-eye rash, it is not Lyme," and sent me on my way.

The following week I was back and demanded a test for Lyme. He reluctantly did it and gave me a prescription for amoxicillin and sent me on my way. Some time later, my phone rang and I was told the Lyme test was negative. I was told I had rheumatoid arthritis and to come back and get some steroids. He called in a doxy prescription for 10 days and I refused the steroids.

When I returned to his office a month later, I was in even worse shape. The hot potato game began. It was a trip from one doctor to another. None would acknowledge Lyme and things continued to decline. I was basically unable to walk and four Lyme tests were negative.

I had all I could take and looked up a local Lyme support group. They sent me a list of all the LLMDs. Most required large sums of money laid out in advance and I realized that my benefits I had worked hard for for 31 years were no good.

I found an LLMD who was more than 100 miles away who took benefits. He did bloodwork of his own and it was finally confirmed that I had Lyme and Bartonella.

I spent the next six months on a roller coaster of pills, supplements and continued to go ever farther downhill. Almost a month later, I ordered the IGeneX test from California. It arrived the same week that my left foot locked up and refused to move. My husband forced me to the emergency room at the local hospital.

When I arrived, they wanted to know why I was there. I explained that my foot wouldn't move, was extremely painful and my husband said, "She has Lyme disease." Of course, they said, "there's no Lyme Disease in Virginia" and so on...

One of the doctors looked at me and said, "You look like a refugee from a concentration camp." A few months later another said, "Emergency rooms are for sick people."

When they noticed on my record that I lost 75 pounds, they decided to admit me. Three days later, nothing had been done.

That same day an infectious disease doctor came into my room, told me to take some steroids, and see a Rheumatologist. I reluctantly took the steroids and was transferred to a rehab centre. Three weeks later my IGeneX results came back and Lyme was in four of five of my blood factors. I also went to a biologist/nutritionist who took a single drop of blood and you could see the spirochetes flowing through my blood and white cells were embedded with Bartonella.

When I went to the LLMD, they would not venture in IV therapy for fear of being caught. I went back to my family doctor of twenty years and showed him the results of my blood tests. He refused to acknowledge them or treat my Lyme/Bartonella. He said I was self diagnosing and needed to see a Rheumatologist.

I am currently detoxing, taking supplements and going to do bee venom therapy. If I go for IV antibiotics, I'll have to sell my house, rob a bank or beg relatives for the $25,000 I'll need that my 31 years of work benefits won't cover.

Why should any sick person be forced to get treatment underground or go bankrupt trying to get well.

I want someone to help us. We are a very sick group— thousands, millions are desperately looking for help. I am on a cane and hold out hope for remission.

Don't forget me please.

Sophie's Lyme Story

Filled with Nightmares and Rage
At just 14 years of age, Sophie knew exactly what she wanted to do as a career—become a doctor to help others with Lyme Disease.

Sophie is the daughter of Mindy Haber, a psychotherapist in New York and the author of Lyme Rage—*her family's harrowing journey to save Sophie from Lyme Disease. I had the privilege of interviewing Mindy about her story. Here's what she had to say. Please read her book for more. As a mother of a Lyme disease sufferer, her book really struck a chord.*

Sophie's illness began with a bad cough, headaches, a migraine diagnosis, blurry vision, and difficulty walking. The worst symptom of all was her neurological rages, and violent nightmares.

She was eventually in a wheelchair, she couldn't walk. Before we knew what it was, we were running to the emergency room, with Sophie screaming at the top of her lungs, flailing. It was terrifying.

I felt isolated in my own family. My other daughter didn't get it. My husband didn't get it.

When we finally figured it out, we consulted with Dr. Daniel Cameron in New York who is a Lyme-literate medical doctor.

Treatment-wise, we tried everything. From Buhner's herbal support to heal it naturally to all sorts of antibiotics and psychiatric drugs like Abilify and Respirodol to manage her rage. We tried Skull Cap, Japanese Knotweed, Sarsaparilla, and Eleuthra for fatigue. If she got tired, boom, it would bring on the rage quickly and other things that would trigger the autonomic nervous system.

Complex illness requires a sustained effort over a longer period of time than we are used to dealing with. It takes a long time to recuperate from this type of illness. We are in the mindset of immediacy, soundbites, immediate gratification, and are not prepared for the relapses along the way. This illness to wellness is not a linear process.

We looked at everything as a point of progress— everything had an impact.

If something worked, I stuck with it.

I found that people tended to do better who exercised as a form of detox and to strengthen the body. Sophie had to relearn how to walk before she could exercise in any way. It took a long time for her to regain stamina.

She was symptom free for 2.5 years and recently had a pain in her side—was it her kidney, a urinary tract infection, we did not know. Again, trusting doctors, we gave her medication but she still had pain. We hospitalized her and she was placed on IV antibiotics, with no change, no improvement.

A nurse practitioner friend who has Lyme recommended the BioMat—a medical device with far-infrared Rays and negative ions that is designed to relieve pain, improve immune function, and reduce inflammation. For Sophie, it worked well. After three sessions of using it, she was up and walking without pain. We were so tired of using painkillers. And they really didn't help much. After the third treatment she was able to attend school for a full day without any pain.

Sophie is still neurologically affected by Lyme. There's a slight cognitive processing delay—she can't process emotions quick enough and has some emotional dysregulation as a result. That said, she's doing great. She's a year ahead of her peers and is in advanced math and science and she keeps on fighting.

We can't say it's cured. But we can say that she's much, much better. I was always in her corner, believing she would get better. We were never going to stop trying to find an answer.[214]

To get a copy of Mindy's book, visit https://www.amazon.com/Lyme-Rage-Mothers-Struggle-Daughter/dp/1936940914

Penny's Lyme Story

Charting My Own Recovery

I'm a forty-something wife to a wonderful husband, a mom to two great boys, and an elementary school teacher. I live in Canada. I've also been battling Lyme disease since January 2011. At this point in time, I appear to be winning the battle, but it was a long road to get here.

I've always been a rather private person, so baring my soul about my Lyme disease is not easy. But I am compelled to tell you my story in the hope that someone else may be helped by it. If it weren't for information I gathered from the media—the radio, the Internet, magazine articles, blogs—I do not believe I would have any quality of life today. When the Canadian medical system could do nothing for me, I had to find my own solution. And I did.

In December 2010, my family had just gone through a very emotionally draining time relating to a surgery that my husband underwent, which resulted in some serious complications. After Christmas, he was stable and our lives seemed to be on the path to normalcy. That is when my symptoms first began.

When I would fall asleep each night, there was a "flutter" in my head or brain as I drifted off to sleep. That's the only way I can describe it. I thought it was very strange, but just ignored it as it wasn't causing me any sleep problems. I also started to get a vibrating feeling throughout my body during the daytime, especially in my legs. I searched the internet for answers to that, and all I came up with was that it could be a perimenopause symptom.

A few weeks later, about mid-January 2011, that little "flutter" in my head became a very strong "pulsation" one night that actually prevented me from falling asleep. It was horrible. My head or brain started to vibrate whenever I was on the verge of sleep. Sometimes I drifted off to sleep, but I would wake up a short time later. This continued all night long.

After several nights of this insomnia, I became exhausted and took a few sick days from my teaching job. Little did I know that I wouldn't be back to work for more than a year.

I went to my family doctor and she had never heard of anything like this. She set up a referral to a neurologist, and prescribed some sleep medication for me. The medication helped a little, but my sleep was still very broken. I was absolutely exhausted during the day. I had never had sleep problems before, even through the stressful times of my husband's many illnesses.

Frightening thoughts raced through my head: Was this the start of MS? Parkinson's? ALS? CJD? What could be causing these pulsations in my head?

Things got worse by February 2011. I became so fatigued and had a general malaise. I was still off work. My doctor was giving me sick notes, a few weeks at a time. It was becoming harder to think, and a horrible anxiety set in. I recall driving to my kids' school to pick them up at the end of the day, and when I got home, I felt so horrible from fatigue and brain overstimulation (that's the only way I know to describe it!), that I went straight to my bed at 4:00 p.m. and pulled the covers over my head to shut out the light and noise. I couldn't sleep, of course. My brain refused to. I would just lay there until my husband got home from work and could take care of the kids. My body was vibrating. I knew something was terribly wrong, but what could it be?

Over the next month, other symptoms appeared: muscle twitching, head pressure, headaches, a throbbing sensation in my head during the daytime, especially when walking or with exertion, a burning pain in my neck, digestion problems, nausea, the chills, tender glands, sore eye muscles, heart palpitations, tinnitus, a constant low-pitched rumbling sound in my ear, air hunger (i.e., feeling like you can't get a satisfying breath), a low-grade fever, brain fog which felt as though I was drunk and unable to think clearly or focus on a conversation, an agonizing feeling in my body, as though all of my nerves were "irritated," weight loss (13 lbs. in about a 2-month period).

I was so physically weak, unable to sleep, extremely fatigued, in pain, overly emotional, and I could hardly think. I dreaded the days when I had to wash and dry my hair, as this became such an exhausting task. I could hardly manage it. Many days were spent laying on the couch all day, awake but with my eyes closed, unable to listen to the TV because the sound bothered me. The days were so long. I was so sick.

I made many, many trips to my family doctor during this time, telling her that this felt like an "infection." In all honesty, she didn't know what to think, but she did her job—she referred me on. I saw several specialists—2 neurologists, an endocrinologist, a sleep specialist, a psychiatrist, and a chiropractor—but no one came up with any concrete answers. They examined me, checked out my scans (CT, MRI), and told me that they did not know what was causing my symptoms, OR that this *must* be stress-related; after all, I had been through so much with my husband's illnesses the past few years.

I learned quickly that specialists have tunnel vision. If you don't fall within their narrow scope, you are dismissed and sent on your way. I was absolutely shocked that no one took this on and really tried to figure this out! Why wasn't anyone admitting me to the hospital? Isn't that what you do when you can't figure out why someone is sick? (Where was House when I needed him?!) Sadly, our medical system just doesn't work that way.

My best advice here, is to never go to the ER unless

it is absolutely necessary. It is not a fun place to be. I was so ill, though, that I was grasping at anything and anyone who might be able to help me. I made 4 visits in total to the ER. The last visit was by ambulance because I had fainted and my young son phoned 911. When I was brought by ambulance, I had such hope that THIS would be the time when I might be admitted to the hospital to have some in-depth testing done. I had the ambulance attendant grab a file on my desk with my medical records and prayed that someone in the ER would finally listen to me and piece this together. But no. They performed an EKG and said that their job was to simply evaluate my fainting spell. They were not interested in investigating my many other symptoms. Because my EKG was fine, and it appeared that I was being followed by other specialists in the community, they released me.

The first 3 ER visits weren't totally fruitless. Although the ER doctors had no idea what was wrong with me, they were the ones who sped up my appointment with the first neurologist, who made the referral to the endocrinologist, and who arranged for an immediate CT scan.

One visit was particularly frustrating when the ER doctor pulled my husband aside *twice* to ask if I was doing illegal drugs! Clearly he didn't believe my husband the first time. And if he knew anything about my character, he would have known how ridiculous that question was. Furthermore, had he known anything at all about late stage Lyme disease, he might have spared me some of the agony I went through in the ensuing months.

Sometime in March 2011, it dawned on me! Through all my brain fog and anxiety, I somehow remembered listening to the CBC radio on my way home from work the previous year, and hearing an interview with a U.S. doctor who had contracted Lyme disease and who was now treating patients for Lyme. I remembered her talking about how Lyme is not properly diagnosed in Canada. I wondered if THAT was what I might have. I searched the internet for that interview with Dr. Maureen McShane, and listened to it. I then did some internet research for Lyme symptoms, and things were beginning to make sense. (Thank you, Dr. McShane, for going public and trying to inform Canadians. Had I not heard your CBC interview, I would likely still be very ill today.)

Where might I have been bitten? Over the past few years, I had been to several places where ticks are found: a cottage in Muskoka, a cottage in Sauble Beach, and two visits to the Pinery Provincial Park where we had walked through grassy, wooded areas to get to the beach. In actuality, it could even have been in my own backyard. No, I don't recall a bite or bulls-eye rash, but from my reading, 50% of people don't. Furthermore, the baby ticks (nymphs) are the size of a poppyseed, and are easily missed. I've also been informed that this illness can be transmitted by flies and mosquitoes as well. I certainly came into contact with a lot of black flies up north.

Apparently, this infection can lie dormant in a person's body for weeks, months, or years until one's immune system becomes compromised, allowing the bacteria to multiply and cause symptoms. I suspect this is what happened to me. I had been through such a stressful time in November-December of 2010 with my husband seriously ill after his brain surgery. It is no surprise to me that my symptoms began then.

As I dug deeper, a horror fell over me. It became evident, from peoples' stories, that there were numerous roadblocks to getting proper treatment in Canada. If I had Lyme disease, I might be ill forever or deteriorate further and possibly die. Thoughts raced through my mind. Could this really be true in Canada in 2011? The doctors don't really understand this? They don't know how to treat it effectively? I was panicked. How was I going to get help? Where would I find a doctor? I was definitely too weak to travel.

I really thought my life would soon be over.

From my internet research, I determined that I needed to send my blood to a lab in California that specializes in tick-borne illnesses: IGeneX. My family doctor agreed to sign the requisition for IGeneX, but wanted to send my blood to the Ontario Public Health Lab first. My dear sister-in-law drove me to the lab and then to FedEx to package everything up for its trip to California. It was quite the process.

The Lyme test results came back: negative from the Ontario lab, positive from IGeneX. (This is typical from the many stories I've read about. The ELISA test performed by the Ontario lab is highly inaccurate.)

My family doctor didn't know how to interpret the IGeneX test results, as they are complicated to read, so she referred me to a local infectious disease specialist. In the meantime, I got myself on the waiting list with two

Lyme-literate doctors in the US.

Sadly, any mention of Lyme disease to the specialists I had seen was quickly dismissed. I was cautiously hopeful that the local infectious disease specialist would diagnose me correctly, but he told me that he did not suspect that I had Lyme disease because of the low probability. He said that our medical system works on probability, and that it was more probable that my symptoms were due to stress and anxiety. (Low-grade fevers? Tender glands? Ear rumbling? I. don't. think. so. I couldn't believe what I was hearing. Once again, my hopes were dashed. No help here.) He had a negative opinion of the "for-profit" US labs, and would not consider the very detailed test results I had just received, clearly showing antibodies to the Borrelia burgdorferi *bacteria (a.k.a. Lyme). If I wished, he would offer me a 3-week course of the antibiotic doxycycline...if it would make me feel better. I took the script. But I didn't fill it right away.*

I will be ever grateful to our family for taking care of us, 24/7, for about two months in March and April. My husband had had a health setback, and I couldn't do much of anything around the house, and we needed the help so badly. Thank you, from the bottom of our hearts, for keeping us and our kids together during this very difficult time. xoxo

And to our friends and church family who brought meals, provided rides for our kids, and prayed for us, we are so thankful for you.

In June 2011, six months after the onset of my symptoms, I had two separate appointments with Lyme specialists—in two different US states. I really wanted two opinions to be sure of my diagnosis. Both doctors spent about two hours each with me, taking my history, examining me, and looking at my IGeneX lab work. Both doctors diagnosed me with Lyme disease, and possibly the co-infections of babesia and bartonella. Both doctors recommended long-term oral antibiotics, probiotics, and various vitamins and supplements. I had to make a choice between the two doctors, and chose the one who was located closer to me. I continue to make the 3-hour trip to see him regularly.

The past year has felt like an eternity, but my LLMD has restored my health to a great degree and has given me my life back. I started on a course of antibiotics in June 2011 and I continue to take them today, more than a year later. The antibiotics have been switched up from time to time to outsmart those stealthy spirochete bacteria. There have been a few bumps in the road with regard to side-effects, but generally, I have tolerated the meds quite well.

My healing has followed the path that my doctor described to me, and that I have read about extensively. It is a slow process to reduce the bacterial load in your body, as these spirochete bacteria are slow-growing and are only susceptible to the antibiotics when they are in their growth phase. The progress seems slow at first, but many months down the road, you start to realize that you're feeling quite a bit better than you were, and you start to have some hope. Periodically, I have flare-ups of my symptoms from bacterial die-off. These are called Herxheimer reactions. These reactions should not be feared, but welcomed. It means the meds are working. They always say that with Lyme treatment, you will feel worse before feeling better, and that is certainly the case when you first start on antibiotics.

My 13 lb. weight loss didn't last, unfortunately! I've regained 23 lbs., likely from a messed up metabolism caused by the Lyme and various medications I've been on.

I'm happy to say that I'm back to work on a modified schedule, with the hope of returning to my regular teaching job in the fall. I don't know how much longer my treatment will be. LLMDs usually treat until symptoms are gone, plus two months. I'm not quite there yet, but I do see the light at the end of the tunnel. Many of my symptoms have disappeared, and others have lessened substantially. My progress is still "up and down," sort of a "two steps forward, one step back" pattern. I still have fatigue, but I'm sleeping much better, and I've finally been able to stop taking sleep medication. I am so thankful for that!

There continue to be challenges and hills to climb, but despite them, I'm enjoying life again.

Raven's Lyme Story

Wilderness Parks No More

Three long years of suffering and it is time to look back. I had always treated my body as if it was immortal. It was a foolish attitude but probably born of a harsh childhood and my will to survive. So the sudden embrace of disease and disability was quite a shock to me.

It was late spring 2002 and I had just returned from hiking in the desert canyons. Despite the heat, I enjoyed clambering through the palms and stream beds while taking photos. I returned home to an intense work schedule.

I had been working many hours and not eating properly. I was entering menopause and had problems with night sweats and insomnia. I had constant problems with sinus infections and every spring would come down with bronchitis that would take months to resolve.

That weekend, I felt a type of fatigue that I had never experienced before. I remember being at a party and having to lean on a kitchen counter. The next day I was sitting in bed watching television when a small brown spider crawled on my arm and bit me. I killed it instantly and didn't think much about it.

The next morning as I was running water in the bath, the sound of the water hurt my ears. Crumpling a paper bag was excruciatingly painful to hear. The top of my hand felt numb. I never noticed any tick bites but had found ticks on me after hiking in the local California mountains. Later in the week, I had a series of short, sweaty fevers and the numbness crept up my arm into my head and neck until the entire right side of my body was numb.

A few days later, I developed double vision.

The first doctor I saw thought it was a pinched nerve in my neck but later sent me to a neurologist. My first neurologist was an elderly man who seemed serenely out of touch with the times. Although his office staff used computers, there was not one to be seen in his office. He gave me the routine exam and didn't have any answers for me. After my first MRI showed a small spot on the pons area all he could say was that it was some kind of inflammation. He had a visual evoked potential test done that came out slightly abnormal. At this time I was still seeing double.

He told me about spinal taps and said I could wait and see if things resolved. I became impatient and went to a university MS center for another opinion. They did a Lyme ELISA and it was negative. I had a spinal tap done and they could find nothing in the CSF that indicated MS. So I went home and began researching on the Net.

The first thing I changed was my diet. Regular healthy meals became a requirement as well as supplements. Sleep seemed to be the only escape from the pain and sensory distortions. I began to do Yoga and my attitude to work went through a shift. I let go of having to do so many things just right. My stress levels dropped.

I would have good weeks and bad ones. My subsequent MRI revealed that the spot was healing. In the early spring of 2004, I again felt very fatigued. I ignored it and did gardening in the sun—it was a hot day and it felt good to sweat and do some physical labor.

The next day, I thought I had an intestinal flu. After the gastric disturbance I came down with bronchitis. After three days, I felt burning pain in my head with intense buzzing. Then a massive wall of fatigue descended that lasted for months. I went back to the old neurologist for another MRI. This time, it was a spot on the cerebellum— very close to the original area on the pons.

I made an appointment at another university MS center. After looking at my case, the doctor told me she thought it was MS. She suggested I go on Copaxone and gave me a promotional kit for the drug. I went home to consider it. I spent the rest of the day in a fog of despair.

I never called the toll-free number on the package. Something was nagging me.

There had to be something I was overlooking. I sat down at my computer and Googled "MS and Infection" and found Dr. David Wheldon's site.

Reading his clear and direct account of his wife Sarah's illness was so familiar. I had such a strong feeling it was some kind of infection. I asked if he knew a doctor in the US who was knowledgeable about the Vanderbilt protocol for Chlamydia Pneumoniae—*the disease he had her treated for. (I did not find out I had Lyme until years later.)*

He put me in touch with a Dr. Powell in Sacramento. For the first time, I had some hope that I could be well and healthy again.

He put me on the Vanderbilt therapy for C.Pneumoniae after my tests came back very high. He told me it would also treat Lyme if I had it. I began taking antibiotics in August '05 but the full treatment cycle really began in September.

I took different combinations of antibiotics that always included either Flagyl or Tindamax. The herxes were painful and tough to get through but I made it through five years of treatment. Many improvements happened in just the first year.

Much later, I was tested through IGeneX and they found Lyme and Bartonella.

I must have had a load of C. Pneumoniae *that went*

wild when Lyme entered the picture. What complicates our treatment are the many co infections. (Mine included many viruses.) But today, I am grateful to have my life back and will continue to be vigilant.

And I have given up hiking in the wilderness parks forever!

Judy's Lyme Story

My Life Was Forever Changed

I was seventeen when I pulled an engorged tick from my head. We threw it away, I went to bed and that was that.

Little did I know my life would be forever changed.

That was the summer of my senior year of high school. A short time later my legs from my knees down were raw oozing sores. My mother took me to many doctors, all with no diagnosis. They said dry skin or possibly I was allergic to a poodle. That same year my blood sugar would fluctuate with no apparent reason.

Fast-forward ten years; I am married with one child and another on the way. I noticed a lump in my throat, diagnosis a multi-nodular goiter. I was put on thyroid medication. Later that year I had hives the size of silver dollars all over my body. No diagnosis but after visiting the allergist it was determined I had a mold allergy. A few years later I had the goiter removed and half of my thyroid, only to have it grow back with more surgeries to follow.

Gallstones were removed, a total hysterectomy, a frozen shoulder and a visit to a surgeon for a large lypoma that suddenly appeared on my arm. I kept going to my Endocrinologist and telling him I was so tired. He would say that I was a working mother, with a husband and children and it was just the stress.

Now many years had passed. My boys were grown and my husband had a great job, life was good! My job was very stressful at the time and my legs began to ache at the top, like tight rubber bands. Nothing relieved the pain that at times was excruciating. Each of my toenails, one at a time fell off, to have a new one grow on. The doctor was puzzled and couldn't find a cause. The emotional symptoms and pain began to get worse. I felt like I was moving in fast motion and losing control. I went to a rheumatologist who said he thought I had rheumatoid arthritis. He did multiple tests and discovered a spot on my lung. He sent me for a PET Scan, which did not show cancer. I had fallen three times in my own home for no apparent reason that year. I would awaken at times with my hand drawn into a fist. Something was very wrong. I quit my job but God provided for me to continue a portion of the job from home.

In May 2012 the real nightmare began. My husband and I had gone on a wonderful hike and to a craft fair for a great anniversary date. About a week later, as always in the spring, I broke out with poison ivy on my arm. I was determined not to have to go get the annual steroid shot so I treated myself at home. It was beginning to look a little better. A few days later I noticed a really strange cough, kind of a hollow sound. Then I lost my voice and this really strange round spot was on my arm. I was not feeling well at all. Everyone said that looks like you have a bullseye on your arm. I decided to call the doctor for an appointment. *Wow, he said, you really have a bad case of infected poison ivy.* He gave me a big steroid shot and sent me home. A few days passed and I couldn't hold my head up. I was so sick. I couldn't think, I couldn't speak in sentences. The words would not come. My husband practically carried me back to the doctor. Fortunately, the same doctor was not there and by this time I had the bulls-eye rash on my back, legs, chest and thighs. The doctor took one look at me and said *you have Lyme disease.* She put me on Doxycycline for 10 days and ran the usual Lyme tests. She told me to come back and see the doctor at the appointed time. I did not get better and the cough and shortness of breath were terrible. The aches and shooting pains were getting worse. Night sweats so bad my hair was soaked, insomnia to the point of not sleeping for nights on end. To our shock the lab tests came back normal and the doctor who said I had infected poison ivy said I did not have Lyme disease. They actually made me feel like I was making this whole illness up in my head. THE TEST RESULTS WERE NORMAL!

My husband and I began to research everything we could about Lyme disease. I could not focus on anything. I could not read or watch TV, much less work. I was in bed or on the couch all day. I quit talking. My life was a shell of what it had been. My gait was now a shuffle, bouncing off the walls when I walked.

I was fortunate to get an appointment with an LLMD about 3 hours from our home. He taught me so much and the supplements paired with antibiotics were helping a little but really didn't solve the problems.

The next step was IV antibiotics, which I chose not to do. I sought help through an herbalist for a while but got very, very sick and made my first visit to the ER.

One night I was on Facebook a gentleman said he had a way to give you back your life after Lyme disease. He introduced me to the GB4000 Rife Machine. I know God put him in my path because it has totally changed my life. I have faithfully used it every other day for over two years. Along with supplements and a diet of no sugar, no gluten or dairy and a lot of faith in God I am determined to live a full life. Yes, the pain still exists at times and I have had to realize I cannot always do the things I once could, but life is good and I feel very blessed.

Judy Steele

Sue's Lyme Story

Canada Refuses to Acknowledge Lyme

My name is Sue Thomas, and I am 55 years old.

My story begins in May of 2011 with the bite that showed up on my leg. I went to the doctor a few days later as I wasn't feeling well, flu like symptoms. The bite itself was red with a red ring inside. The Dr. gave me 10 days of antibiotics as it appeared I had a skin infection from the bite. We both assumed I have been bit by a spider as neither of us had any education on ticks. I continued to have pain in my leg that didn't go away and continue the flulike symptoms with nothing showing up in blood work.

Weird symptoms start showing up, bottom of feet

hurt, headaches, night sweats, couldn't sleep at night, arthritis showing up in all my joints, pain in gallbladder, spleen, heart, and air hunger. Doctors run more tests, and still nothing showing up. So I started investigating what it could be.

The more research I did, the more I realized it must have been a tick, and that I had Lyme disease. Eventually, my Doctor did the ELISA test, which of course came up negative, as I had been bitten a year and a half earlier. This test only shows up a recent infection. This is the only test my General Practitioner can order if the ELISA test comes up negative. Even though I had all the symptoms, when my general practitioner sent me to the infectious control Doctor in Edmonton, she told me there is no Lyme Disease in Alberta. She wouldn't order the western blot, even though my General Practitioner requested this specific test. She also informed me as I was leaving, that I could pay, and send my blood to IGeneX in California to be tested for Lyme.

I have been on sick leave, as I could hardly walk without a cane, so the Village of Alliance people raised funds to help me get the testing done through IGeneX. In October 2013, I received positive test results for Lyme Disease, which my Doctor has sent to this same infectious control Doctor, and we've yet to hear back from her.

There are no Lyme Literate Doctors in Alberta, so my Doctor and I are researching how to treat it ourselves, as I can't afford to fly to the United States to be treated there. The ILADS (International Lyme and Associated Disease Society) protocol is to treat with IV antibiotics, as oral antibiotics are very hard on your digestive system, but my Doctor can't prescribe me IV antibiotics without the consent of the Infectious Control Doctor. As a result of no response, I am being treated with oral antibiotics off and on, and since October, 2014, at least I have been able to walk without a cane. The residents of Alliance made donations to help pay for tests, and treatments, as I am waiting for government assistance. I started the paperwork in August, 2013 for CPP Disability and AISH, and here it is now August of 2015, and AISH and CPP Disability have denied Lyme Disease, and I am still appealing.

Even though my MD has clinically diagnosed me as having Lyme Disease, Canada refuses to acknowledge this diagnoses. This stress is a crime to put on someone who is ill.

My GP is still pulsing me on antibiotics and Mepron, as it seems to keep it in check, but not in remission. I have been treating since June of 2015 with Cannabis oil, and I feel the brain fog is getting better, but there's still a long road ahead yet.

Through research being done by Lyme Literate Doctors in the United States, Borrelia burgdorferi *spirochetes (Lyme Disease)* have been found in blood, saliva, and tissue samples of patients diagnosed with MS, ALS, and Alzheimer Disease. Lyme Disease is called "The Great Imitator" as it is often misdiagnosed as these other diseases. Canada has the highest rate of MS in the world. This is not a coincidence. Research is proving it is spread through blood, saliva, in vitro, in fact all body fluids. The Red Cross does not screen blood for Borrelia burgdorferi, and the Government of Alberta doesn't recognize

Chronic Lyme. We need to change this, or it will become a pandemic.

I hope your book brings out the truth of how many people are suffering. In my small community of Alliance, I know of 2 other people diagnosed with Lyme Disease, and also know 2 other people that know they have Lyme, but are not bothering to get tested. All of us were bitten in Alberta, but no Lyme here, we are told.

Wish you the best for your son, and keep on educating people.

Janet's Lyme Story

Self-Diagnosed on Facebook
I don't remember a bullseye, but because I had a vegetable garden I got a lot of mosquito bites. Shortly after I got bitten, I woke one morning with a horrific pain in my head and neck. My husband took me to the hospital and the Drs just looked at me and didn't conduct any tests, then gave me an antibiotic and told me it was a virus...hmm.

Abx for a virus??

While on bedrest, I was in so much pain all over all I could do is cry. I had two young children (this was 1981-1982 in Massachusetts), and I had difficulty taking care of them. I felt like I had a fever but when I took it, it was below normal.

So begun my hunt for a diagnosis. Friends would call and tell me to turn on Oprah. That's what you have! So whatever the flavor of the day, I would do as much research as I could. No internet in our house yet.

I went to the chiropractor several times a week for adjustment for my neck (it was so stiff it was impossible to move it) and would come out and be in just as much pain as before the adjustment. The Chiro thought I had TMJD and sent me to a dentist where I got braces and a night guard after.

I went to a rheumatologist and he diagnosed me with Fibromyalgia and soon after the fatigue was debilitating...Chronic Fatigue Syndrome. I applied for SSDI and got it several months later.

I joined a support group and had the internet (1990s), so more research. Someone in the group mentioned a doctor who tested for everything, including Lyme... Negative...but the tests were not like they are now, and the doctor didn't know to look for symptoms as well.

I met people on the internet who mentioned a doctor in New Jersey, and after a week at his clinic, I came home with medications, supplements, etc. No relief after months of course. Then I found a doctor in New York...also spending a week at her clinic, came home with the same and no relief.

There were a lot more doctors but too many to mention. We spent thousands of our own money and we were not getting anything for it.

Then a hysterectomy in 2000 and we moved to Pennsylvania in 2001. I felt better after the surgery, but I was also on a very strict diet—only organic foods.

In the last 6 months I noticed a Facebook friend talking about having Lyme, and I decided to join the Lyme Disease and other Lyme groups. I mentioned my symptoms and a lot of people told me it sounded like Lyme, Babesia and Bartonella. I asked for recommendations and about 6 people mentioned one name of an LLMD who is only a half hour away.

The LLMD agreed that these were present even though test results were negative. I also have Mycoplasma Pneumonia and Chlamydia Pneumonia (not std!).

I've seen the LLMD several times and will see her again soon for more test results. I'm sure this is chronic Lyme and coinfections.

I understand your son is sick. Children being sick is the worst and I am so sorry. My daughter was diagnosed with Lyme and Babesia, and she can't afford treatment. She's applied for SSDI recently. She has a son who is 16 months old.

I hold your son in my prayers. Fondly, Janet

Pam's Lyme Story

My "Chronic Tonic" Protocol

I was first infected at the age of 7 (1970) with Rocky Mountain Spotted Fever and by the age of 8, I was showing signs of chronic Bartonella and by the age of 9, I was showing the symptoms of late stage Lyme disease (Lyme arthritis & other symptoms). I may have had more tick-borne infections at that time, but no one was looking for them or their signs, so I learned to live with the ups and downs.

I had periods of my life where I was plagued with different symptoms (narcolepsy, extreme pain, pseudo-blockages in my intestines, major female troubles and so on) and I was bedridden for periods of time as well, then at the age of about 30 I realized that I could no longer work outside the home. I was given so many misdiagnoses, from MS and Fibro, to psychological diagnoses. In 2002, I had a Neuro tell me that I had Bell's Palsy due to Lyme disease—but I wasn't ready to hear that— even though I had been looking into that possibility since 2000! But, I was in denial.

It wasn't until 2007, when I was 44 years old, that I found a LLMD that agreed to treat me—the late, great Dr. Edwin Masters (RIP). I used antibiotics for a full 12 months and only got worse. I believe there were a number of reasons for this, not simply just because I was using antibiotics. I now know that my body was badly compromised and couldn't detox very well (likely MTHFR mutations).

I stopped all treatments as I was beginning to have seizures, passing out regularly and a ton of serious issues with cognitive function, my intestines shutting down and more. I quite honestly thought I was going home to die. I even called my kids to come up and we had "the talk" of what to do once I was gone.

Fortunately, my husband was not ready to give in just yet and he found a holistic doctor not far from us that agreed to treat me, even though she said she knew nothing of these infections, but she was willing to learn. At first, after doing her intake of me, she said she wanted me to just go straight to the hospital due to my adrenals crashing—but I refused as I knew that I would have a fight on my hands keeping them from giving me steroids since Lyme isn't even recognized as a threat here.

As I said, my practitioner knew nothing of these infections, but since there was no one else in my state willing to treat those who had Lyme and other tick-borne infections, I decided to start treatments with her and help her learn all I could. I kind of felt like it was my one last chance.

The first 6 months all I did was detox and get my organs and systems in my body to balance back out using herbs and acupuncture. My adrenals were crashing, I had Hashimoto's Thyroiditis, serious issues with my digestive system along with all the symptoms of Lyme, Bartonella, Babesia, chronic Rocky Mountain Spotted Fever and more, so we had our work cut out for us.

After the first 6 months, we agreed I would start on the "Chronic Tonic" herbs.

Although my Practitioner had me make the medicinal tea differently than what is instructed from Misty Meadows site, I used all the herbs listed and in the amounts listed. It only took 2 months of using this medicinal tea before I started really feeling some decent improvements in my symptoms. I used this medicinal tea for a total of a full 12 months.

Three months after starting the "Chronic Tonic," we added in Houttuynia—also made into a medicinal tea for my Bartonella infection. I used this medicinal tea for a total of 9 months and finished the same time as I finished my Lyme treatment. At this point I didn't seem to have many symptoms of either infection left, although it was obvious that my nerves hadn't healed yet.

We started treatment for Babesia, which proved to

be quite stubborn for me. We used many herbs—often changing them every 2 weeks, tons of acupuncture and many changes in my diet to help me get through. This is also why it's taking me so long to put together what all I did for Babesia—there were so many herbs that were used to support the different organs I was having issues with, like my spleen, liver, intestines (always), even my kidneys for a while. After treating for a full 12 months, we decided it was time to take that nerve racking "trial run" without any treatments, only life had a way of really testing me.

My father-in-law was doing quite poorly due to Alzheimer's disease. He had been living alone, and although family was just across the driveway, he was good at hiding how he was declining. Once it was discovered how poorly he was really doing, my husband and I set out and remodeled a bedroom and moved him in—to my delight. Three months later, he passed away, so although it was a grueling time physically and emotionally, to my absolute delight and surprise, I did not relapse—although I did spend some time waiting for the "other shoe to drop"!

Then the unthinkable happened in the summer of 2014—I got re-infected with Lyme! I went into denial/ shock, but started my herbs once again at 3 months post bite, and treated for 5 months and haven't had any symptoms since then, although I do still struggle with my health because there was considerable permanent damage that was done to my body from having untreated infections for 40 yrs.

Ruben's Lyme Story

A Veteran Left Sick and Stranded
My name is Ruben Sims and I am a retired analyst with sound credentials and decades of experience. I was selected best in the Air Force in 1978. I was the First Enlisted man to become a "Certified Cost Analyst."

I am also a veteran with Lyme disease and I am now seeking to save lives by sharing critical information, knowledge and skills.

After thirty-three years of being misdiagnosed and mistreated care by United States Air Force and Veterans Administration healthcare systems, I learned I had Lyme disease from a Costco Magazine article. Throughout my service in the Air Force, doctors were incapable of diagnosing and treating Lyme disease. Instead, they got me addicted to opioids and sleep medications for three decades and left me virtually blind, and prepared for death.

In 2016, I was finally diagnosed with Lyme disease by a Lyme specialist hired by the VA; however, the VA refused her diagnosis and treatment recommendations. So I abandoned the VA for private healthcare. Since then my vision is restored and I have begun a whole new life. I have since endured agonizing withdrawals from opioids and sleep medications too. I am no longer addicted. Before treatment, I compared myself to a ninety-year-old man. Death seemed a desirable relief from the agony of undiagnosed and untreated Lyme disease. Today, I compare myself to a fifty-year-old man.

Every day, I learn to relive and appreciate life. My

personal experience with Lyme disease led to being punished under the Uniform Code of Military Justice, facing court martial and confined to psychiatric wards several times. I was told I would be on the psychiatric ward until I got better. However, I was discharged as a hopeless hypochondriac instead. The medical justification was, "no disease accounted for my many symptoms."

After fourteen years of service, I was discharged without an income or health insurance, homeless and with a wife and child I could no longer support. My outstanding fourteen-year military career ended in shame. However, I now understand why veterans are literally dying on the doorsteps of their local VA and commit suicide at the highest rates in history. I now understand there are many veterans with Lyme disease just like me.

My goal is share my story to help save the lives of those veterans too. I hope you will help.

Paula's Lyme Story

A Letter to Myself Before Lyme Disease Rebuilt Me into Something Greater

Dear Paula in 2009,

I know this is going to sound strange, but in just a few short months, something is going to happen to you, something you are not expecting, something you didn't ask for or were even aware that could happen. Your life is going to change in ways you never fathomed.

I am writing this letter in hopes to prepare you and bring you some comfort, for what lies ahead is not pretty or easy. I know that you consider yourself a strong, resil-ient woman. I know what you've been through, what you've survived. I am here to remind you that all that strength will be needed and used. All those coping skills will become an asset in ways you never thought you'd have to use them. I am here to assure you that you will survive it, even though there will be times you will cry out to God to call you home, when the pain is so unbear-able it supersedes any other thought.

*I am writing this letter because I know how you think and how you operate, and I want to tell you that what you think and what you know will be challenged. People you trust will fail you, turn their backs on you and walk away. They will mock you because they won't understand what you are going through. I know how frustrated you will become because you won't under-stand it, either. You'll want compassion and support and I am here to tell you that you will get it—but in the most unconventional forms. Don't worry about the ones who let you down and walk away, because they are just going to make room for all the new peo-ple who will come into your life; people who share this journey with you, who understand you in ways even those closest can not. They will inspire you with their stories, educate you with their experience and encour-age you to fight the good fight, stay the course and one day, they will recruit you to join them as a fellow **Lyme disease*** warrior, educator, advocate and supporter.

I am writing this letter because although your body will break down and you will lose sight of the woman you once knew, you will be rebuilt into something stronger and greater. Now listen, you survived all those things before this, and this path will strengthen you even more. It will grow you in a direction you never thought about but are needed in. And as you grow, you will have all the support you need for every step of the way. I need you to remember this part because you will lose every ounce of strength you have. Even the most mundane daily chores will be taken from you. You will be attacked from all sides—physically, mentally and emotionally.

I am writing this letter to assure you that although there will be some very dark moments filled with some of the worst pain you've ever felt, you won't be alone. Your cries will be heard, your tears collected. All your ashes will be saved and restored one day. I am here as living proof that you will survive this pain, the darkness, the despair and even the heartbreak of everything that you will lose. I am here to tell you that pride won't get you anywhere. You will have to ask for help. It will humble you and from there, you will grow. There are lessons to be learned and whether you want to or not, you will learn them!

Now this next part of the letter may be difficult to read and even harder to grasp.

I am writing this letter to tell you that those doctors you've placed all your trust and faith in will fail you on the first part of your journey. They will challenge you and exasperate you. You're going to face some difficult times and hear some not-so-nice things. You're going to feel alone and desperate. You're going to feel lost and hopeless. But I am here to remind you to stay the course. Don't give up because hope is out there. You just need to keep going and connect the dots. You're going to have to listen to others who have gone down this path and you're going to need to filter things and do your own research (that part I know you will love). The frustration will come from the many walls you hit, but keep hitting them, for one day they will crumble and you will see a path that will take you in a different direction.

Please trust me: You want to take this path.

I am writing this letter because as unconventional as this path may seem, it is going to save your life. You won't understand a lot at first but the people you meet on this path will teach you, and they will do so in ways so you fully understand everything and know what to expect. They will stay close to you and they will check in on you. You will never feel alone again. They will empower you with their unconventional ways, empower you to want to get better, to want to make a difference...for others.

I am writing this letter because I don't want you to give up hope. I can't say how long this bend in the road will be, for I am still here on this journey seven years later but so much better than I ever was. I can say now I never thought this day would come—but it did. I will tell you that you will get better but not before you feel worse. That is just par the course but remember these words—you will feel better and you will see your life going in a new direction. I know when you first become sick, you're going to think that this will pass and I am here to tell you that it will but it will take time. It will get worse before it gets better, that is just how chronic illnesses work.

I am here to tell you this illness will forever change your life. It will break you down physically as it grows you spiritually. It will strengthen core values within you that had been ignored and make them a priority. It will change your outlook on life and set your feet on a new path. You won't know where you are going or when you will get there, but that won't matter because you'll enjoy all the stops and people you meet along the way.

I am writing this letter because I know you will find all of this hard to believe. Doctors turning their backs, insurance wars, outdated guidelines by the Infectious Diseases Society of America and the Centers for Disease Control, misdiagnosis after misdiagnosis and failed treatment. I know you and I know how you think. But trust me, it will be bad. It will be frustrating. It will make you scream at doctors and it will reduce you to tears in public settings. You won't care anymore but I am here to tell you don't give up! There will be many stumbling blocks, but you will advance. You will need to lean on these new friends and borrow some of their strength until you regain yours—just remember to pay it forward!

I am writing this letter to tell you to keep pushing forward, don't take no for an answer, when you hit a wall keep pounding until it crumbles and when you feel lost, cry out, there are people who are there to help you. When you feel alone, lift your head and look at the thousands who stand with you.

You won't know or even remember all their names, but you'll know their stories and it's that connection that will forever link you to each other and strengthen one another even from a distance. It's that connection that will take a debilitating disease that can weaken even the strongest, toughest person and make them #Lymestrong.

Love, Paula in 2016
@paulajacksonjones2014[215]

FINAL THOUGHTS

OUT OF THE RABBIT HOLE
AND INTO THE LIGHT

"Begin at the beginning," the King said, very gravely, "and go on till you come to the end: then stop."

—ALICE'S ADVENTURES IN WONDERLAND

This Lyme journey has brought so much darkness. A heavy cloak of darkness that has been so hard to shed. The rabbit hole has felt endless. So much to learn. So much to know. Years of navigating this winding road with so few clear answers and so many overwhelming obstacles standing in the way.

Like Alice, I often wondered "...if I shall fall right *through* the earth!" So many unfamiliar doors to walk through. So many uncharted passages to take. Never knowing which one of these would lead to a positive outcome. Never knowing if we would find light or continue to feel a sense of foreboding.

Above all, there has been a feeling of chronic outrage.

What is outrage but a powerful, often overwhelming

feeling of resentment and anger triggered by what we experience as an injury, an insult, or an injustice? Those of us in the chronic Lyme world are indeed outraged—chronically outraged—Lyme sufferers, caregivers, and advocates alike.

We are outraged by the lack of medical care and support. We are outraged by the lack of reliable and stable diagnostic testing. We are outraged by the outright negation of this disease and its effects on millions worldwide, for more than four decades now. We are outraged that there is a group of professionals—medical professionals—who seem to be personally benefiting and capitalizing on an extraordinary amount of human suffering, which we can easily conclude by their daily and widespread dismissal and mockery of the ill and infirm.

We are outraged by the personal costs of this disease, a disease that continues to go unsupported by the vast majority of the allopathic medical community, the government, and insurance companies alike, causing many to go without medical care, remain ill for a lifetime, go bankrupt, lose their life's savings, their health, their relationships, and sometimes their lives.

Our outrage does not stop here.

We are outraged by the fact that the director of the Centers for Disease Control and Prevention, on camera, shed a tear for those with Zika, calling it "an extraordinary and unusually urgent crisis" and, at the same time, refused to address chronic Lyme, where there are hundreds of thousands, realistically millions, suffering without care or support. We are further outraged by the fact that, according to the *Huffington Post*, "his 'jaw dropped' when he realized how long it would take Congress to move on the issue. 'Three months in an epidemic is an eternity,' he said."[216]

Three months? Lyme sufferers have been waiting for medical attention for forty years while the number of cases has mounted to a pandemic.

We are outraged because on a recent radio show a doctor with the Association of Medical Microbiology and Infectious Disease of Canada (AMMI) said, "I want to stress again, that as tragic as these stories are, these folks, by and large, do not have Lyme disease, and have never had Lyme disease and so there is this misplaced focus on that label, primarily because of this lab in the United States that results have no meaning, but also this tendency of some so called Lyme-literate physicians to diagnosis this on the basis of clinical grounds."[217]

To all doctors, researchers, politicians, bureaucrats, and insurers who negate and dismiss and even mock the suffering of Lyme patients, we beg of you to STOP.

Stop denying and negating the suffering and illness of so many. Stop marginalizing these patients. Stop using your time and medical expertise to harm and invalidate. Not only are you not helping Lyme patients but you are making their struggle exponentially more challenging as they are left to diagnose, treat, and heal it themselves. And thanks to the widespread denial of this disease, Lyme sufferers are left to deal with an uncontainable amount of deserved outrage and anger as they are forced to become their own microbiologists, immunologists, neurologists, rheumatologists, medical researchers, and more. They have been forced to navigate this long, arduous, frightening medical journey with little access to medical support.

The outrage is hard to contain. Not because Lyme sufferers and advocates are "crazy" or have nothing better to do, as our naysayers and denialists would have the world believe.

We are outraged because millions are sick without answers, because we have been treated unjustly for far too long, and because we have been confronted by one roadblock after another, including the long-term promulgation of falsehoods, political doublespeak, and obfuscations.

So we are left with no choice but to hold strong and fight back. Our voices are rising. Our actions are soaring. Our power is escalating.

We are *not* antiscience.

As CanLyme says, "Lyme researchers are advocating for a more complete, open and transparent examination of the illness, and a continued re-evaluation of guidelines as new evidence comes forward. Evidence is abundant that the status quo is harmful."[218]

Above all, at this critical juncture in the Lyme Wars, as things are slowly shifting and our power is surely mounting, what we hope for is that those who are not *yet* affected by chronic Lyme disease and are listening to our pleas will join us in this outrage. This is a war that affects us all. And when it comes to chronic Lyme, our outrage is more than an appropriate response.

Our outrage fuels our activism, which *will* effect change.

Let There Be Light

Along the way, with all the darkness hanging overhead, there has been light. Light in the form of new friends, other advocates, many supporters, countless smart and courageous people all fighting the same good fight.

I am still a mom on a mission. Until such time as my son gets fully well, and until we get the medical system to turn its attention toward this pandemic, my work is not done.

The two are not interdependent. We are not waiting for

the majority of doctors to understand. Healing will continue to come from our own hard work, research, and perseverance, and not from the likes of the allopathic medical community.

In the meantime, I am going to spend more time in the light. I'm going to place even greater attention on hope and faith, on resilience and connection, on gratitude and appreciation, on courage and meaningful action.

I'm going to hang on to hope, along with our best guess at the moment, not holding my breath for conventional doctors to offer anything more than denial and neglect. The very system that we once thought was there to protect and heal us is no longer the bedrock of society that we believed it to be. Save for a handful of humane and heroic doctors who practice with heart, courage, interest, curiosity, and a true moral compass. I'm well aware that without them, we'd have no hope. Something I shudder to imagine.

In the meantime, I'll do my best to remember that our energy flows where our attention goes. So I'm going to focus on climbing out of this dark, dank rabbit hole, while we press on.

I'm going to continue to search for places where light meets dark. Where suffering meets hope. Where fear meets courage. Where humanity and justice reign.

I intend to be present and awake to new possibilities. While discovering the wonders and joys of life that I'm ready to embrace once again.

RECOMMENDED READING

Anatomy of an Illness As Perceived By the Patient by Norman Cousins

Bite Me: How Lyme Disease Stole My Childhood by Ally Hilfiger

Brave New World by Aldous Huxley

Chronic Illness as an Access to Quantum Healing: Passing through the eye of the needle into self-actualization by Jenny Rush

Confessions of a Medical Heretic by Robert Mendelsohn

Cure Unknown: Inside the Lyme Epidemic by Pamela Weintraub

Eat Dirt: Why Leaky Gut May Be the Root Cause of Your Health Problems and 5 Surprising Steps to Cure It by Josh Axe

Ending Denial: The Lyme Disease Epidemic: A Canadian Public Health Disaster: A Call for Action from Patients, Doctors, Researchers by Helke Ferrie

Energy Medicine: Practical Applications and Scientific Proof by C. Norman Shealy, MD

Energy Medicine: The Scientific Basis by James L. Oschman PhD

Everything You Need to Know About Lyme Disease and Other Tick-Borne Disorders, Second Edition by Karen Vanderhoof-Forschner

Gone in a Heartbeat: A Physician's Search for True Healing by Neil Spector

In the Crucible of Chronic Lyme Disease: Collected Writings & Associated Materials by Kenneth B. Liegner M.D.

Lab 257: The Disturbing Story of the Government's Secret Plum Island Germ Laboratory by Michael C Carroll

Lying by Sam Harris

Lyme Brain: The Impact of Lyme Disease on Your Brain, and How To Reclaim Your Smarts by Nicola McFadzean Ducharme ND and Robert Bransfield MD

Lyme Disease and the SS Elbrus by Rachel Verdon

Lyme Rage: A Mother's Struggle to Save Her Daughter from Lyme Disease by Mindy Haber

Medical Industrial Complex: The $ickness Industry, Big Pharma and Suppressed Cures (The Underground Knowledge Series Book 3) by James Morcan and Lance Morcan

Medical Medium: Secrets Behind Chronic and Mystery Illness and How to Finally Heal by Anthony William

Out of the Woods: Healing from Lyme Disease for Body, Mind, and Spirit by Katina I. Makris and Richard Horowitz

Plague: One Scientist's Intrepid Search for the Truth about Human Retroviruses and Chronic Fatigue Syndrome (ME/CFS), Autism, and Other Diseases by Kent Heckenlively and Judy Mikovits

Power vs. Force by David R. Hawkins

Quantum Healing: Exploring the Frontiers of Mind/Body Medicine by Deepak Chopra

Shifting the Lyme paradigm: The Caretakers Guide on a Hero's Journey by Huib Kraaijeveld

Survival Lessons by Alice Hoffman

The Brain's Way of Healing: Remarkable Discoveries and Recoveries from the Frontiers of Neuroplasticity by Norman Doidge

The Structure of Scientific Revolutions: 50th Anniversary Edition by Thomas S. Kuhn and Ian Hacking

The Quantum Doctor: A Quantum Physicist Explains the Healing Power of Integral Medicine by Amit Goswami PhD and Deepak Chopra

The Widening Circle: A Lyme Disease Pioneer Tells Her Story by Polly Murray

This Idea Must Die: Scientific Theories That Are Blocking Progress by John Brockman

When Your Child Has Lyme Disease: A Parent's Survival Guide by Sandra Berenbaum and Dorothy Kupcha Leland

Why Can't I Get Better? Solving the Mystery of Lyme and Chronic Disease by Richard Horowitz

DVD
Under Our Skin —— Parts 1 and 2 (Emergence)

ENDNOTES

1   https://www.lymedisease.org/lyme-basics/co-infections/ other-co-infections/
2   http://www.lymestats.org
3   http://www.bayarealyme.org/about-lyme/ lyme-disease-facts-statistics/
4   http://www.ilads.org/ilads_news/2015/list-of-700-articles-citing-chronic-infection-associated-with-tick-borne-disease-compiled-by-dr-robert-bransfield/
5   https://en.wikipedia.org/wiki/Gaslighting
6   http://www.nationalacademies.org/hmd/~/media/Files/ Report%20Files/2013/Partnering-with-Patients/pwp_meeting-summary.pdf
7   http://orthomolecular.org
8   http://orthomolecular.org
9   http://jama.jamanetwork.com/article.aspx?articleid=245777
10 http://www.housemd-guide.com/house-med/2007/04/ house-great-diagnostician.html
11 http://discovermagazine.com/2007/medical-mysteries/ the-real-dr-house
12 http://www.providencejournal.com/article/20130809/ NEWS/308099923
13 Pema Chödrön, *The Places That Scare You*, Shambhala (2002) p. 4
14 Mark Prigg published: 22:53 GMT, 29 May 2014 | UPDATED: 06:07 GMT, 30 May 2014 http://www.dailymail.co.uk/sciencetech/article-2643339/The-bacteria-longer-humans-Lyme-disease-discovered-15-million-year-old-amber.html
15 https://www.sciencedaily.com/releases/2008/06/080629142805.htm

16 Kate Lunau, January 7, 2016 Inside the guts of the Iceman—Maclean's magazine http://www.macleans.ca/society/science/inside-the-guts-of-the-iceman/

17 http://www.seranogroup.org/serano_docs/a_very_short_history_of_lyme_disease.pdf

18 http://www.lymeneteurope.org/forum/viewtopic.php?t=5133

19 http://www.ncbi.nlm.nih.gov/pubmed/836338

20 http://extension.entm.purdue.edu/publichealth/insects/tick.html

21 http://canlyme.com/just-diagnosed/

22 https://www.lymedisease.org/lymepolicywonk-the-cdc-the-fda-and-lyme-disease-lab-tests-two-tiered-tests-igenex-the-c6-and-the-new-culture-test-2/

23 http://www.poughkeepsiejournal.com/story/news/health/lyme-disease/2014/03/26/so-called-lyme-wars/6907209/

24 "The Complexities of Lyme Disease, A Microbiology Tutorial: Part 1" by Thomas M. Grier, MS, from The Lyme Disease Survival Manual, 1997

25 *Journal of Neuroinflammation*—Lymestats.org

26 Inquisitr November 8, 2015

27 http://www.cdc.gov/lyme/index.html

28 http://www.idsociety.org/Lyme_Facts/#sthash.47tIMshk.dpuf

29 http://cid.oxfordjournals.org/content/43/9/1089.full

30 Valley View: Lyme is most misunderstood disease since AIDS, Holly Ahern *12:08 a.m. EST November 9, 2014*

31 drjoneskids.org

32 http://www.ncbi.nlm.nih.gov/pmc/articles/PMC266646/pdf/jcm00080-0058.pdf

33 http://www.lymedisease.org.au/transmission/

34 http://www.wholehealthinsider.com/newsletter/lyme-next-aids/

35 https://sites.google.com/site/drjoneskids/transmission-methods

36 http://www.wholehealthinsider.com/newsletter/lyme-next-aids/

37 http://www.nytimes.com/1989/07/18/science/doctor-s-world-lyme-disease-transfusion-it-s-unlikely-but-experts-are-wary.html

38 http://canlyme.com/just-diagnosed/co-infections/specific-co-infections/

39 http://www.scientificamerican.com/article/new-cause-for-lyme-disease-complicates-already-murky-diagnosis1/

40 Lyme disease symptoms fueled by vaccines, Posted by: Abby Campbell, staff writer in Vaccine Dangers August 15, 2015, Natural Health 365

41 http://www.ncbi.nlm.nih.gov/pubmed/3190104
42 https://www.lymedisease.org/372/
43 http://www.huffingtonpost.com/dana-parish/lyme-the-infec-tious-disea_b_9243460.html
44 Under Our Skin, documentary
45 http://www.lymenet.de/lymeals.htm
46 http://www.macleans.ca/society/health/could-canada-cause-multiple-sclerosis/
47 http://www.thespec.com/news-story/3870220-canadians-trapped-in-lyme-disease-limbo/
48 http://www.ncbi.nlm.nih.gov/pubmed/15617845
49 http://www.nationalmssociety.org/Symptoms-Diagnosis/Other-Conditions-to-Rule-Out/Lyme-Disease
50 http://www.samento.com.ec/nutranews/pdfs/nnutranews1003_high.pdf
51 http://www.wpr.org/chronic-lyme-disease-major-healthcare-crisis-doctor-says
52 https://en.wikipedia.org/wiki/Lyme_disease_microbiology
53 http://www.huffingtonpost.com/dana-parish/lyme-the-infec-tious-disea_b_9243460.html
54 http://www.cdc.gov/lyme/stats/humancases.html http://www.ncbi.nlm.nih.gov/pmc/articles/PMC3879353
55 http://www.cdc.gov/media/releases/2013/p0819-lyme-disease.html
56 Lyme researcher and former Lyme physician in Hope, British Columbia, Dr. Ernie Murakami
57 Lyme researcher and former Lyme physician in Hope, British Columbia, Dr. Ernie Murakami
58 *The Nature of Things*, CBC
59 http://www.lymediseaseassociation.org/index.php/about-lyme/cases-stats-maps-a-graphs/940-lyme-in-more-than-80-countries-worldwide
60 http://ilads.org/
61 https://youtu.be/l7MvboE0AGw
62 http://www.cdc.gov/hiv/statistics/basics/ataglance.html
63 http://report.nih.gov/categorical_spending.aspx
64 lymestats.org–created by Alison Childs
65 Polly Murray, *The Widening Circle: A Lyme Disease Pioneer Tells her Story,* St. Martin's Press (1996) p. 101
66 Polly Murray, *The Widening Circle: A Lyme Disease Pioneer Tells her Story,* St. Martin's Press (1996) p. 101

67 http://canlyme.com/lyme-basics/symptoms/
68 http://www.drlwilson.com/articles/brain_fog.htm
69 http://www.telegraph.co.uk/news/celebritynews/11881516/
    Phones4U-billionaire-John-Caudwell-devastated-after-whole-
    family-diagnosed-with-Lyme-disease.html
70 http://www.telegraph.co.uk/news/health/news/12048122/
    Phones4U-billionaire-John-Caudwell-says-11-family-members-
    now-diagnosed-with-Lyme-disease.html
71 http://www.dailytelegraph.com.au/newslocal/
    inner-west/lyme-disease-sufferer-hopes-sen-
    ate-inquiry-will-answer-questions-for-australians/
    news-story/812b3bd58cc801c1d89efb230584f2c2
72 http://willtherebecake.org/2015/11/11/
    success-rates-of-various-lyme-treatment-options-a-personal-study/
73 http://www.etonline.com/news/167014_avril_lavigne_breaks_
    down_tears_over_her_battle_with_lyme_disease/
74 http://underourskin.com/blog/?p=191
75 Michael Schopmann, lawyer, Lake Success at a Lyme rally,
    November 9, 2000
76 http://rel-risk.blogspot.ca/2015/10/i-believe-so-i-dont-have-to-
    know.html?m=1 RELATIVE RISK BLOG—"I Believe So I Don't
    Have to Know" Saturday, October 31, 2015
77 http://rel-risk.blogspot.ca/2016/01/absent-entities-in-ld.
    html?m=1
78 By Harriet Hall—MyMedClinic, All About Care,
    "Does Everybody Have Chronic Lyme Disease? Does
    Anyone?" https://www.sciencebasedmedicine.org/
    does-everybody-have-chronic-lyme-disease-does-anyone/
79 http://montrealgazette.com/health/
    opinion-lyme-disease-is-very-real-but-its-no-epidemic
80 *The Nature of Things*, CBC
81 www.donna-y.com
82 http://www.ilads.org/ilads_news/2015/list-of-700-articles-cit-
    ing-chronic-infection-associated-with-tick-borne-disease-com-
    piled-by-dr-robert-bransfield/
83 http://calgaryherald.com/news/local-news/lyme-disease-patient-
    living-in-her-car-after-being-discharged-from-banff-hospital
84 http://reachwhite.com/blogemilyreachwhite/2013/4/5/
    at-least-it-isnt-cancer

85 https://www.youtube.com/watch?v=f5_Bdj5d0Mo http://www.
    tiredoflyme.com/uploads/9/4/9/4/9494510/lyme_disease.pdf
86 Desmond Tutu, *No Future without
    Forgiveness* http://www.goodreads.com/
    quotes/165597-ubuntu-speaks-of-the-very-essence-of-being-human
87 http://badlymeattitude.com
88 http://www.kevinmd.com/blog/2015/11/the-joy-has-been-
    sucked-out-of-medicine-heres-why.html
89 http://jemsekspecialty.com/ncmb-remarks/
90 David Bornstein, "Medicine's Search for Meaning," New York
    Times September 18, 2013
91 http://vitalitymagazine.com/article/medical-research-fraud/
92 http://www.greenmedinfo.com/blog/has-drug-driven-med-
    icine-become-form-human-sacrifice Posted on: Thursday,
    December 29, 2011 at 11:00 a.m.
93 http://blog.oup.com/2008/02/specialization/#sthash.0lF-
    SimHn.dpuf
94 http://mdmunk.com/2015/01/21/flood-of-information/
95 http://www.ncbi.nlm.nih.gov/pubmed/22579043
96 Herd behavior in medical profession, October 31, 2008 By Dr. S
    Venkatesan
97 "Running for Cover—The Herd Instinct Among Physicians,"
    Issue: Summer 1996, Volume Number: 1, Issue Number: 2,
    Author: Russell L. Blaylock, MD
98 http://journals.plos.org/plosmedicine/article?id=10.1371/jour-
    nal.pmed.0020124
99 http://chriskresser.com/behind-the-veil-conflicts-of-interest-and-
    fraud-in-medical-research/
100 http://kimbertonclinic.com/wp-content/uploads/essays/essay2.pdf
101 The Blacklisted News website
102 Bushman & Baumeister, 1998; Kernis, 2003; Kernis,
    Grannemann, & Barclay, 1989
103 http://www.cbc.ca/beta/news/canada/manitoba/undi-
    agnosed-illnesses-leave-doctors-with-bad-bedside-man-
    ners-health-columnist-1.3322574
104 http://www.webdc.com/pdfs/deathbymedicine.pdf
105 http://www.webmd.com/osteoarthritis/news/20080708/
    fda-warning-cipro-may-rupture-tendons
106 http://articles.mercola.com/sites/articles/archive/2013/09/25/
    fluoroquinolone-antibiotics.aspx

107 http://www.fiercepharma.com/story/levaquin-users-slap-jj-800m-rico-suit-claiming-pharma-giant-hid-serious-sid/2016-01-21

108 http://ahrp.org/former-fda-commissioner-charged-in-federal-racketeering-lawsuit/

109 http://philpapers.org/profile/37495

110 http://www.vaccinationdebate.net/web3.html

111 https://books.google.ca/books?id=EQHPoGs6CvIC&pg=PA27&lpg=PA27&dq=no+batch+of+vaccines+leonard+scheele&source=bl&ots=Zd1BJGOgqn&sig=YMpnSbUNNFIGXdWyzmbfXHE0I3E&hl=en&sa=X&ved=0ahUKEwiql9q20tPOAhVV_mMKHTyIDj8Q6AEIITAB#v=onepage&q=no%20batch%20of%20vaccines%20leonard%20scheele&f=false

112 http://www.ncbi.nlm.nih.gov/pmc/articles/PMC2828219/

113 http://www.publichealth.org/public-awareness/understanding-vaccines/goes-vaccine/

114 https://www.youtube.com/watch?v=cT6An0jA8Vw

115 http://traceamounts.com

116 http://www.nytimes.com/2012/12/17/health/experts-say-thimerosal-ban-would-imperil-global-health-efforts.html?_r=0

117 http://articles.mercola.com/sites/articles/archive/2015/12/01/another-flu-vaccine-flop.aspx

118 http://www.cbc.ca/news/health/flu-vaccine-paradox-adds-to-public-health-debate-1.2912790

119 https://healthimpactnews.com/2015/march-2015-settlements-in-vaccine-court-117-vaccine-injuries-and-deaths/

120 http://www.ncbi.nlm.nih.gov/pmc/articles/PMC1949105/ Stories for life Introduction to narrative medicine Author: Miriam Divinsky, MD CCFP FCFP

121 https://www.functionalmedicine.org/files/library/six-core-principles.pdf

122 http://www.nature.com/nbt/journal/v26/n7/box/nbt0708-743_BX3.html

123 http://www.bibliotecapleyades.net/ciencia/ciencia_vibrational-medicine.htm

124 http://www.oprah.com/health/Energy-Medicine#ixzz3sjenCbiR

125 https://www.washingtonpost.com/news/opinions/wp/2016/02/26/the-robot-doctor-will-see-you-now-if-we-can-ever-get-out-of-the-waiting-room

126 http://www.ncbi.nlm.nih.gov/pubmed/14519082

127 http://journals.plos.org/plospathogens/article?id=10.1371/journal.ppat.1003796

128 http://www.aapsonline.org/liegner/Gibson-Letter.pdf

129 http://www.edwardgoldsmith.org/53/the-medical-industrial-complex/

130 http://www.lymenet.de/literatur/stricker_lautin_burrascano.pdf

131 http://www.thelancet.com/journals/laninf/article/PIIS1473-3099%2811%2970034-2/abstract

132 http://www.ilads.org/ilads_news/wp-content/uploads/2015/09/EvidenceofPersistence-V2.pdf

133 Under Our Skin 2: Emergence

134 Under Our Skin 2: Emergence

135 https://www.linkedin.com/pulse/cdc-lyme-programs-routinely-flout-federal-procedures-luche-thayer?trk=pulse-det-nav_art

136 http://cid.oxfordjournals.org/content/52/3/364.full

137 http://www.forbes.com/sites/judystone/2015/09/04/lyme-deaths-from-heart-inflammation-likely-worse-than-we-thought/

138 http://owndoc.com/lyme/dying-of-lyme-disease-case-fatality-rate-nearly-100/

139 http://www.lymeblog.com/modules.php?name=Blog&file=display&jid=2178

140 http://owndoc.com/lyme/dying-of-lyme-disease-case-fatality-rate-nearly-100/

141 https://www.lymedisease.org/ny-teen-death/

142 http://sci.tech-archive.net/Archive/sci.med.diseases.lyme/2006-04/msg00501.html

143 http://www.nbcnews.com/health/three-die-suddenly-rare-lyme-disease-complication-2D11733669

144 http://ireport.cnn.com/docs/DOC-1037462

145 https://www.psychologytoday.com/articles/200709/munchausen-unusual-suspects

146 http://healthimpactnews.com/2014/boy-removed-from-family-father-jailed-over-lyme-disease-disagreement/

147 http://lymestats.org/

148 https://www.gofundme.com/w3b5nvuc

149 http://www.casewatch.org/board/med/jemsek/charges.shtml

150 Tina J. Garcia is a Lyme patient and founder of Lyme Education Awareness Program, L.E.A.P. Arizona at www.leaparizona.com http://www.publichealthalert.org/joseph-jemsek-md-the-power-of-truth.html

151 http://underourskin.com/news/
feeling-pressure-update-dr-charles-ray-jones

152 https://docs.google.com/document/d/19VQxBXX-
Vp1zshfhwlvfMl1oHP8RW6q9is3H6yawOc14/
edit?copiedFromTrash

153 http://www.ohioactionlyme.org Read the charge sheets: Posted
by blogger, activist, and Lyme sufferer Beaux Reliosis to Michael
Moore (documentary filmmaker) May 24, 2015

154 http://owndoc.com/lyme/
dying-of-lyme-disease-case-fatality-rate-nearly-100/

155 http://spectator.org/articles/64944/
how-medical-industry-profits-broken-patent-system

156 http://www.nytimes.com/2008/09/07/technology/07unbox.
html?pagewanted=print&_r=1

157 http://www.ncbi.nlm.nih.gov/pmc/articles/PMC2870557/

158 http://www.historyofvaccines.org/content/articles/
history-lyme-disease-vaccine

159 http://www.lymediseaseassociation.org/index.php/aboutlyme/
controversy/vaccine/261-lymerix-meeting

160 http://lymeblog.com/modules.
php?name=News&file=article&sid=496

161 http://www.actionlyme.org/LYME_FACTS.htm

162 http://badlymeattitude.com/2016/01/21/petition/ http://bad-
lymeattitude.com/2015/08/26/help-wanted-lyme-aids-2-0/

163 http://www.michaelchristophercarroll.com/work1.htm

164 http://www.amazon.com/Lyme-Disease-Elbrus-Rachel-Verdon/
dp/1470178397

165 https://www.smashwords.com/profile/view/RachelVerdon

166 http://www.thedogpress.com/editorials/Plum-island-
LymeDisease_Andrews1.asp

167 https://sites.newpaltz.edu/ticktalk/social-attitudes/
story-by-smaranda-dumitru/

168 http://www.rense.com/general67/plumislandlyme.htm

169 http://www.history.com/news/ask-history/
what-was-operation-paperclip

170 http://www.theatlantic.com/health/archive/2014/05/
when-viruses-escape-the-lab/371202/

171 http://journal.sjdm.org/15/15923a/jdm15923a.pdf

172 http://tv.greenmedinfo.com/
aldous-huxley-the-ultimate-revolution-1962/

173 The truth about Lyme disease, Anne Kingston, March 24, 2014 http://www.macleans.ca/society/health/the-truth-about-lyme-disease/

174 Lymestats.org

175 http://www.cbc.ca/natureofthings/blog/climate-change-impact-canadians

176 http://www.macleans.ca/society/health/the-truth-about-lyme-disease/

177 Interview with Jim Wilson

178 *MacLean's* magazine, "Health Canada's new Lyme disease plan: You act, we'll watch," Anne Kingston, July 30, 2014

179 Interview with Jim Wilson

180 http://www.gmagnottafoundation.com/about/

181 Facebook post—Lyme sufferer, Toronto. November 28, 2015 (Joan Pifer)

182 Posted on OHOH Canada—a closed Lyme Facebook group—December 2, 2015

183 Lisa S.

184 Dr. Ernie Murakami M.D. Clinical Associate Professor Emeritus, UBC

185 http://canlyme.com/2015/05/12/dr-ben-boucher-discusses-lyme-disease-on-cbc-radio/

186 Lyme Disease: The Real Truth by Lia Grainger—*Reader's Digest Canada*, June 2011 http://www.readersdigest.ca/health/sickness-prevention/lyme-disease-real-truth/

187 http://www.theglobeandmail.com/news/british-columbia/federal-scientists-eager-to-share-their-research-now-that-muzzles-are-off/article27171269/ "Federal scientists eager to share their research now that muzzles are off" Mark Hume, Vancouver, *The Globe and Mail,* published Sunday, November 8, 2015 9:21 p.m. EST Last updated Sunday, November 8, 2015 9:22 p.m. EST

188 http://www.nationalobserver.com/2015/11/30/news/open-letter-canadian-physicians-justin-trudeau

189 http://www.cbc.ca/news/health/lyme-disease-1.3585784

190 Post Lyme Disease Awareness November 18, 2015 (Michelle Thompson)

191 http://badlymeattitude.com/2015/10/26/of-truths-and-lymes/comment-page-1/

192 Tina J. Garcia, Founder, Lyme Education Awareness Program (L.E.A.P.) www.leaparizona.com Posted 18 October 2013 by Dawn Irons, M.A., LPC http://pha-usa.blogspot.ca

193 http://www.rollingstone.com/music/features/
kris-kristofferson-an-outlaw-at-80-20160606

194 http://www.thesundaytimes.co.uk/sto/newsreview/arti-
cle1611767.ece

195 http://www.usmagazine.com/celebrity-news/news/yolan-
da-foster-reveals-bella-anwar-hadid-also-battling-lyme-dis-
ease-2015910#ixzz3sCeD8R7W

196 http://radaronline.com/celebrity-news/yolanda-foster-lyme-dis-
ease-kyle-richards-real-housewives-beverly-hills/

197 http://www.truth-out.org/news/item/24027-irate-lyme-disease-
patients-storm-dinner-party-at-idsa-headquarters

198 http://www.lymedisease.org.au/wp-content/uploads/2015/11/
Lyme-like-illness-inquiry-final-00000002.pdf

199 https://www.facebook.com/notes/heather-rolfe-reid/new-ca-
nadian-lyme-organization-takes-lyme-horrors-to-the-pub-
lic/10153580126291020

200 https://www.facebook.com/groups/657758067709230/

201 http://www.prnewswire.com/news-releases/the-steven--alexan-
dra-cohen-foundation-grants-65-million-to-bay-area-lyme-founda-
tion-300194081.html

202 https://www.sciencedaily.com/releases/2016/05/160519101035.htm

203 https://www.guideline.gov/content.aspx?id=49320

204 https://www.change.org/p/the-us-senate-calling-for-a-congres-
sional-investigation-of-the-cdc-idsa-and-aldf

205 http://www.truth-out.org/speakout/item/33256-why-is-the-cdc-al-
lowing-a-private-group-to-determine-federal-policy-on-lyme-disease

206 https://www.linkedin.com/pulse/we-may-need-whistleblow-
er-address-lyme-epidemic-jenna-luche-thayer?trk=prof-post

207 https://www.linkedin.com/pulse/we-may-need-whistleblow-
er-address-lyme-epidemic-jenna-luche-thayer?trk=prof-post

208 Anthony William, *Medical Medium: Secrets Behind Chronic and
Mystery Illness and How to Finally Heal,* Hay House (2015) p. 213

209 Anthony William, *Medical Medium: Secrets Behind Chronic and
Mystery Illness and How to Finally Heal,* Hay House (2015) p. 213

210 http://www.mayoclinic.org/diseases-conditions/infec-
tious-diseases/expert-answers/infectious-disease/
faq-20058098

211 http://healthimpactnews.com/2015/vaccines-and-retrovirus-
es-a-whistleblower-reveals-what-the-government-is-hiding/

212 http://healthimpactnews.com/2015/vaccines-and-retroviruses-a-whistleblower-reveals-what-the-government-is-hiding/

213 http://chickswithticks.weebly.com

214 Interview with Mindy

215 http://themighty.com/2016/04/lyme-disease-letter-to-my-self-before-my-diagnosis/ Paula Jackson Jones, President and Cofounder, Midcoast Lyme Disease Support & Education, a nonprofit 501(c)(3) organization in Midcoast Maine Email: paula@mldse.org Website: www.mldse.org

216 http://www.huffingtonpost.com/entry/tom-frieden-cdc-zika_us_5747574ae4b03ede4414498c

217 http://canlyme.com/2016/05/25/cbc-radio-show-bc-almanac-interviews-doctors-with-opposing-opinions-on-lyme-treatment-lyme-testing/

218 http://canlyme.com/lyme-basics/lyme-myths/©

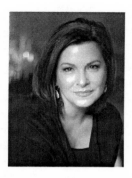

ABOUT THE AUTHOR

Lori Dennis is a mom on a mission. She is also a Registered Psychotherapist who works in private practice in Toronto, Canada.

Ever since her adult son fell ill in the fall of 2012, her only focus has been to help him get well. Little did she know at the start of this medical odyssey just how deep and unending this rabbit hole would be.

While helping her son navigate his medical journey from "no answers" to continued recovery, she was determined to write this book to help others navigate this long and arduous path from illness to wellness—the overwhelming and complicated trek that comes with having chronic Lyme disease. She was also determined to provide a platform for other Lyme sufferers to have their voices heard in an effort to end the madness. A madness where millions are suffering around the globe while mainstream medicine continues to turn its back on the sick and infirm.

Lyme Madness can also be found on:
Facebook: https://www.facebook.com/lymemadness/
Twitter: https://twitter.com/LymeMadness
LinkedIn: https://www.linkedin.com/in/loridennis

CPSIA information can be obtained
at www.ICGtesting.com
Printed in the USA
LVOW11s1958170117
521258LV00003BA/350/P